Macrobiotics For Dummies®

P9-DGC-102

Universal Macrobiotic Life Principles

These macrobiotic principles are the map by which we discover guidance that leads to truth — our personal compass to self-revelation.

- ✔ The Principle of Opposites: Everything exists in opposition.
- ✔ The Principle of Change: Everything changes!
- ✔ The Principle of Cycles: All beginnings have endings.
- ✔ The Principle of Non-Identity: Nothing is identical.
- ✔ The Principle of Front and Back: Every front has a back.

Macrobiotic Principles of Awareness

These principles help you establish a personal philosophy for the purpose of designing a more creative and meaningful life.

- ✔ Develop a generous spirit: The Principle of Abundance.
- ✔ Embrace responsibility and admit faults.
- ✔ Discover life via personal experience.
- ✔ Develop your intuition.
- ✔ Cultivate active appreciation.
- ✔ Make friends everywhere.
- ✔ Respect your elders.
- ✔ Be mindful of ecology.
- ✔ Practice economy of life: Vivero parvo.
- ✔ Discover humor.
- ✔ Practice self-reflection.
- ✔ Perfect the art of living.

Macrobiotic Food Principles

Think of the seven macrobiotic food principles as the foundation from which you build new health and sensitivity. Each is covered in much more detail in Chapter 3.

- ✔ Enjoy principle, secondary, and pleasure foods.
- ✔ Emphasize seasonal and local foods.
- ✔ Be mindful of quantity and quality.
- ✔ Avoid dietary extremes.
- ✔ Chew your food thoroughly.
- ✔ Take the minimum required.
- ✔ Use the *Power of Five* in food preparation: The five food groups, flavors, textures, cooking styles, and colors.

Macrobiotics For Dummies®

Cheat Sheet

The New Multicultural Macrobiotic Dietary Template

Here's my basic template for a macrobiotic diet. Variations for specific dietary needs are presented in Chapter 6.

Principle foods:

- **Whole grains:** Approximately 25 to 30 percent by volume for the amount of food consumed for one day

- **Grain products:** Approximately 5 percent per day (as in 1 to 2 slices of bread or 1 to 2 servings of pasta)

- **Vegetables:** Approximately 35 percent of the day's total percentage of food from greens, roots, and ground varieties

- **Beans:** Approximately 5 to 10 percent beans or bean products (tempeh, tofu, and so on), either canned or dried

Secondary foods:

- **Fruits:** Approximately 5 to 10 percent as fruits, according to sweet cravings

- **Beverages:** Grain-based teas, herbal teas, vegetable juices, and so on

- **Oils, nuts, seeds, and limited dairy products:** Approximately 5 to 10 percent natural vegetable oils, nuts, seeds, or limited dairy products

- **Reduced animal protein:** Approximately 5 to 10 percent of fish (preferable) or meat (optional)

- **Swing percentage:** Additional percentage of whole grains or more vegetables, according to your needs

- **New foods:** Devote a small percentage of your dietary template to exploring new foods, such as sea plants or fermented foods (sauerkraut, pickles, miso, and so on)

Pleasure foods:

- **WYW:** *Whatever You Want* means exactly that. Enjoy a small amount of your favorite foods.

"Foods" to Be Avoided

In attempting to change the way you eat and obtain the most positive result, you need to limit foods that contribute to inflammation, cause blood sugar swings, and increase cravings. Here's my list of "no-no" foods:

- Any food containing white, brown, or any other refined sugar

- Maple syrup, barley malt, rice syrup, and agave syrup

- Fruit juice

- Milk, cheese, cream, butter, ghee, yogurt, and ice cream

- Refined oils

- Caffeine

- Alcohol

- Recreational drugs

- Medications (with some exceptions for current prescriptions)

- Heavy use of spices

- White rice and white flour

- Foods containing chemicals, preservatives, dyes, and insecticides

For Dummies: Bestselling Book Series for Beginners

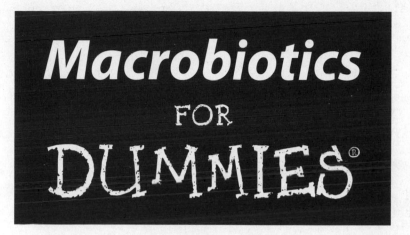

Macrobiotics FOR DUMMIES®

WITHDRAWN
LIFE UNIVERSITY
LIBRARY

by Verne Varona

WILEY

Wiley Publishing, Inc.

Macrobiotics For Dummies®

Published by
Wiley Publishing, Inc.
111 River St.
Hoboken, NJ 07030-5774
www.wiley.com

Copyright © 2009 by Wiley Publishing, Inc., Indianapolis, Indiana

Published by Wiley Publishing, Inc., Indianapolis, Indiana

Published simultaneously in Canada

For general information on our other products and services, please contact our Customer Care Department within the U.S. at 877-762-2974, outside the U.S. at 317-572-3993, or fax 317-572-4002.

For technical support, please visit www.wiley.com/techsupport.

Wiley also publishes its books in a variety of electronic formats. Some content that appears in print may not be available in electronic books.

Library of Congress Control Number: 2009925032

ISBN: 978-0-470-40138-5

Manufactured in the United States of America

10 9 8 7 6 5 4 3 2 1

WILEY

About the Author

Verne Varona has become known as one of the most energetic and dynamic health educators in the country. During the past thirty-five years, his lectures, workshops and media appearances have motivated thousands of people to take better and more conscious care of their health.

A nationally sought-after speaker, Verne is a frequent speaker at health expos, public institutions, educational foundations and in public seminars. Verne studied Oriental Medicine and Macrobiotics at Michio Kushi's East West Foundation of Boston, Massachusetts (1970-1974) and with Herman Aihara at Vega Institute.

He is a frequent guest on a variety of media where his research expertise, humor, and entertaining teaching style make him a welcome and often repeat visitor. For five years, Verne was the nutritional consultant and cofounder of a popular Los Angeles medical group with a clientele that featured well known entertainment and athletic professionals.

Verne's first book, *Nature's Cancer-Fighting Foods,* was published in June 2001 by Prentice Hall Press (now Penguin Books). It is currently in its twelfth printing and is used as a textbook in a number of academic health and wellness institutions.

In 2006 he created a production company, Exceptional Films, to make feature-length films on topics relating to health and wellness.

Verne divides his time between New York City and Miami. Please visit his Web site at www.vernevarona.com.

Author's Acknowledgments

The reward of counseling comes from the open feedback clients give about what seems to work and what doesn't. This validates the work, helping to make it personalized and more effective. Thank you for your faith and feedback.

I thank the following friends for seminar sponsoring and bringing me before their audiences. This teaching and counseling opportunity helped me shape the content of this book.

Sandy Aquila, Nebraska (Omaha Healing Arts Center)

Zlatko & Jadrenka Pejic, Croatia (Makronova Institute.)

Joao & Maria Borges, United Kingdom (One World Family)

Alvin Pettle, MD, Toronto, Canada

Diane Bradshaw, Salt Lake City, UT

Carol & Jim McElroy, Invermere, Canada

Ray & Marie Butler, Scotland

Ruska Porter, Los Angeles, CA (Tuesday Night Group)

Terry Rex Cady, Seattle

John Belleme & Sandy Pukel, Florida (Taste of Health Holiday Cruises)

Larry Cooper, Santa Barbara, CA (Health Classic)

Julie & David Greenhalgh, Abu Dhabi, UAE

Mark Scholtz, MD, Los Angeles, CA (Prostate Cancer Research Institute Conferences)

Carl Ferre, Chico, CA (GOMF Summer Camps)

Judy Grill, Washington, DC

Peter Temars, Amsterdam, Holland

Joel Huckins, San Francisco, CA

Glenda Twinning, Dallas, TX

Eduardo Longoria, Austin, TX (Casa Luz)

Francisco Varatojo (Instituto Macrobiotico de Portugal)

Gerard Lum (Peninsula Macrobiotic Community)

Vesna Vulksa, Toronto, Canada

To my literary agent, Bob Silverstein, for his perseverance, his attentive ear, always sage advice and unflappable faith. Yo Bob, you de best!

To Diane Steel, Publisher, and the folks at Wiley, for believing this was the right time, the right book, and the right author.

To Tracey Boggier at Wiley who diligently went to bat for this book and helped me to learn Dummies-speak.

To Tim Gallan, Senior Project Editor at Wiley, whose crack editorial skills and friendly suggestions always turned out to be smart choices for making this material more personalized and readable. You're the best, Tim!

To Vicki Adang, Wiley copy editor, for her detailed notes and editorial diligence.

To Melisa Dufty from Marketing at Wiley for her can-do attitude and aid in handling the cover.

To Terry Shintani, MD, JD, MPH, for his exemplary work in disease reversal, professional dedication, and loyal brotherhood. Mahalo nui loa!

To Edna Johnson, for the extended generosity of her Florida home and writerís guesthouse sanctuary.

To David Kerr, macrobiotic scholar and samurai surfer, who generously helped me with all things related to Hufeland and the Ohsawa–Gurdjieff connection.

To friend and ace cook, Melanie Waxman, for her positive spirit and prompt recipe support. Big yum!

To Jamie & Kasia Travena and *The Macrobiotic Guide* (www.macrobiotics.co.uk), for featuring my writing, their constant support and promotion of my UK counseling.

To Wonder Cook Christina Pierello, who also came to my recipe rescue offering tasty wisdom.

To Bill Tara, Michael Rossoff, Phil Chen, Matt Chait, and Jimmy Israel, fellow teachers, friends, and travelers, for their wisdom and presence.

To Ron Kotzsch, author of *Macrobiotics, Yesterday & Today,* for the inspiration of his detailed research and gentle, candid clarity.

To Patrick Verre, French Macro Chef and food stylist extraordinaire, who on a moment's notice prepared beautiful food that I could photograph for this book's cover. Merci bien de votre aide, mon ami!

To my good friend and noble English gentleman, David Saunderson, for his visionary enthusiasm, wit and confidence in my work.

To Jack Bone, man of many talents for introducing me to all of this once upon a time in 1969. Cheers 2U.

To the memory of Ruska Porter, who laughed at all my jokes and encouraged me to expand my teaching.

To my daughters, Sara, Desire, and Haley. Their love helps me keep an essential perspective.

To my wife, and unsung super woman, Dawn Southgate-Varona, for some extraordinary help with the kitchen chapters, rewrites, suggestions, editing, and general brilliance. Your support, dedication, and love is nothing less than heroic. Now, finish *your* book!

Dedication

This book is thankfully dedicated to the inspirational teachers and exceptional clients I've had the good fortune to counsel, both of whom contributed to the academic and experiential nature of this work. The wisdom of my teachers has given me a magnificent framework that helps to unify things when all seems fragmented; seeing them with greater trust, clarity and confidence.

Over the years, generous feedback from many clients has helped me to shape and refine this work; making it more adaptable, cohesive and of critical importance, FUN!

My deepest gratitude to influential teachers: Herman and Cornelia Aihara; Jacque Yvette Delangre; George and Lima Ohsawa; Michio and Aveline Kushi; and Duncan Sim, for their insight, dedication and commitment to elevating human health and happiness.

Publisher's Acknowledgments

We're proud of this book; please send us your comments through our Dummies online registration form located at www.dummies.com/register/.

Some of the people who helped bring this book to market include the following:

Acquisitions, Editorial, and Media Development

Senior Project Editor: Tim Gallan

Acquisitions Editors: Tracy Boggier, Erin Calligan Mooney

Senior Copy Editor: Vicki Adang

Copy Editor: Megan Knoll

Technical Editors: Emily Nolan, Patti Santelli

Editorial Manager: Michelle Hacker

Editorial Assistants: Joe Niesen, Jennette ElNaggar, David Lutton

Cartoons: Rich Tennant
(www.the5thwave.com)

Composition Services

Project Coordinator: Katie Key

Layout and Graphics: Claudia Bell, Reuben W. Davis, Melissa K. Jester, Melissa K. Smith, Christin Swinford, Christine Williams

Proofreaders: Melissa Cossell, Jessica Kramer, Christopher M. Jones

Indexer: Potomac Indexing, LLC

Publishing and Editorial for Consumer Dummies

Diane Graves Steele, Vice President and Publisher, Consumer Dummies

Joyce Pepple, Acquisitions Director, Consumer Dummies

Kristin Ferguson-Wagstaffe, Product Development Director, Consumer Dummies

Ensley Eikenburg, Associate Publisher, Travel

Kelly Regan, Editorial Director, Travel

Publishing for Technology Dummies

Andy Cummings, Vice President and Publisher, Dummies Technology/General User

Composition Services

Gerry Fahey, Vice President of Production Services

Debbie Stailey, Director of Composition Services

Contents at a Glance

Table of Contents

Introduction

· ·

During some challenging times many years ago, I owned a car that was in dire need of repair. To fix what it needed would have exceeded its actual worth, so I made a practical decision to do minimal maintenance and get as much out of the car as I could until it completely failed me.

After spending nine months driving this wreck, I was able to finally purchase a new car and realize the extent of what I had been tolerating. I got so caught up in the challenge of adapting, of coping, and finding temporary short-cut solutions that the stress just became familiar. I had no marker to compare it with until I drove that new car.

Then my perspective immediately changed. My drive was lush and quiet; those familiar engine fumes from my junker were suddenly not assaulting my sinuses. It rode like it floated on air, held me comfortable in a seat with no jutting spring surprising me at inconvenient times. I had a car with decent power and good handling — and it wasn't going to explode at any moment and leave me stranded. What a difference! Why did I put up with that piece of junk for so long?

I realized, in a similar vein, there were other things in my life, similar to my puke-green junker, that were also in need of changing but that I had neglected because they had simply become tolerable: a relationship that had run its course, an unfulfilling job I loathed, and an immediate need for more planning and discipline in the way I was caring for my health.

Currently, you may be tolerating circumstances in your daily life that deep down you feel undeserving of. And maybe you suspect something more positively challenging and rewarding is possible. Sometimes difficult situations can seem normal because they've become so familiar and we become comfortably distracted in the struggle of bandaging symptoms and coping.

Our health and how we temporarily relieve problems can be a good example of this mindset: Some of us are used to seasonal sickness for which we may get flu shots or take other medications. Because waking up is difficult and we feel sluggish and cranky, we run for our morning coffee to avert those symptoms. For monthly menstrual cramps, women purchase over-the-counter medicines and hope for the best. The same goes for headaches. For problems of stomach acidity, we take something alkaline such as Tums, Alka-Seltzer, or even Prilosec and wait for the heartburn to go away. We want to be in control, and these efforts are about that goal. But they're only short-term solutions. At some point, we need to wake up and realize that we've visibly aged beyond our years. And then, we wonder if this is normal?

This method of dealing with our health is *not* normal. And I assure you, a new opportunity to prove otherwise exists. It exists in the form of taking a daring road trip. Test driving a new body for a little while to check out its performance — a test drive that begins with a change of nourishment, a renewed perspective, and a healthier lifestyle as expressed in the pages you're about to read.

The keys to that ride are in your hands. I wish you an exciting trip full of adventure, recovery and discovery.

About This Book

Health is truly universal. It is a natural condition that should be available and affordable to all, not just the privileged few that have the discretionary income to purchase expensive supplements, "alternative" treatments, imported foods, or exotic remedies from remote corners of the globe. Good health is our birthright and the goal of *Macrobiotics For Dummies*.

This book offers a refreshing take on macrobiotics, emphasizing a body, mind and spirit approach. Instead of relying on Asian traditions, this book offers a multicultural perspective and outlines the little-known principles of macrobiotics in detail, along with practical examples of how they apply to daily life. Additionally, a number of different templates for beginning dietary change offer more flexibility so that readers can choose an approach that works for them, customizing it at a later time, after they've experienced positive changes in their health.

Macrobiotics (a compound Greek word meaning *large* or *great life*) is a philosophy of dynamic living. It provides practical and inspirational tools for enhancing and balancing health, elevating judgment, stabilizing moods, improving mental clarity, increasing intuitive sensitivity and fortifying your internal flow of energy.

- ✔ **Physically**, macrobiotic dietary philosophy is based on solid nutrition and the traditions of self-healing from numerous long-lived cultures. The foods recommended have fed the world's traditional cultures for thousands of years and are based on our human design, our relationship to the environment, seasonal growth and our individual health condition.

- ✔ **Mentally**, macrobiotic thought embraces ancient and time-tested principles that offer universal perspectives for harmonizing our mental and emotional lives. These principles offer unique perspectives that can enable you to transform fear into faith and judgment into love.

- ✔ **Intuitively**, macrobiotics helps us to relax more internally, which helps to develop a greater awareness of the present moment. That awareness allows us to recognize, and eventually trust, our intuitive voice.

✔ **Spiritually**, macrobiotic philosophy also embraces the "energetic" world. It can be seen as the vehicle that moves us to developing higher judgment or an elevated consciousness; a path that is based more on the recognition and development of intuition, not just intellect or analysis. Numerous spiritual practices are encouraged to create a stronger energetic communion. The result of a macrobiotic lifestyle is the achievement of a physiology that's more sensitized to energy and allows us to play in both worlds of matter and spirit.

Ultimately, the task of living a macrobiotic life requires that we cultivate all of the various realms that influence our health, freedom and happiness; from dietary, physical and emotional, to intellectual, creative and spiritual. The goal of a macrobiotic lifestyle is to transform the mundane into the magnificent and discover that we always have the choice to live a truly great life.

Conventions Used in This Book

You're occasionally going to see technical terms in this book. I italicize them and provide definitions. The recipes in Part IV of the book use English units rather than metric. (So temperatures are in Fahrenheit, measurements are in cups and ounces, and so forth.)

What You're Not to Read

This book is full of helpful information, which can save you time having to hunt cover-to-cover for inspiration, techniques, suggestions, or helpful sidebars. The sidebars are the grey text boxes that contain information or anecdotes that supplement the chapter text. The arrangement of the book allows you to skip around and read selectively. Information that might seem a bit technical is marked by a Technical Stuff icon. That text is relevant but not completely necessary.

Foolish Assumptions

Of course, this book is not for everyone! *Macrobiotics For Dummies* is for

✔ Anyone who's healthy and wants to remain that way

✔ Anyone who's afraid of becoming sick

✔ Anyone who is sick and committed to healing

✔ Anyone who cares for a loved one

✔ Anyone who wants government out of his or her food and healing choices

✔ Anyone concerned about the welfare of today's children

✔ Anyone concerned about the care of the elderly

✔ Anyone concerned about the environment and planetary health

✔ Anyone tired of paying premium prices for junk food

✔ Anyone wanting to make changes in the health care system

All others don't need this book.

How This Book Is Organized

Macrobiotics For Dummies is organized into six parts. Each part addresses a body, mind or spirit aspect of the adventure we call macrobiotics. This layout makes it easy to find the topic of your choice. Here's a brief overview of what you'll discover in each part:

Part I: Getting Started with Macrobiotics

The chapters in this part are your road map to a macrobiotic path of healthy living. In this section, I discuss macrobiotic philosophy, principles and dietary information. In addition, I also present the body, mind and spirit aspects of macrobiotics, the sound nutrition behind the dietary suggestions, and practical ways to handle and eliminate cravings for food that doesn't support our health.

Part II: Healing the Macrobiotic Way

Healing ourselves from degenerative disease or acting as our own advocate to prevent sickness requires that we understand all the factors that influence good health. The chapters in this part address the broad concept of healing in practical and doable terms, including suggestions for healing common diseases. I explain what to avoid in order to sustain good health, and I reveal the factors behind extraordinary healings and show how we can marshal body, mind, and spirit to achieve health renewal.

Part III: Planning and Preparing Your Macrobiotic Adventure

Planning and preparing is half the work, and when you can do it in an organized and efficient way, it makes everything easier and more inspirational. This part explains how you can make healthier lifestyle changes to support a new way of eating and great tips on creating a macro-friendly kitchen.

Part IV: Morning to Evening Recipes: Your Dietary Path to Wellness

Of course you have to eat, and having a guide to creating delicious meals makes it less of an effort and more exciting as an adventure. This part offers delicious and easy-to-follow recipes that will have you leaping around your kitchen like the galloping gourmet you really are — or want to be. It's just a matter of practice! Some helpful advice for handling social situations and making healthy restaurant choices makes this adventure one that you can share without feeling like you're restricted from socializing.

Part V: The Part of Tens

This part presents helpful information in lists of ten items each. You can read about the ten sure-fire ways to handle sweet cravings, as well as the ten tips for prompt and permanent weight-loss, tailoring your macrobiotic journey more to your personal needs.

Part VI: Appendixes

Appendix A gives you a sample menu for a whole week of macrobiotic meals. Appendix B provides some historical information on the founders of macrobiotics.

Icons Used in This Book

This book uses icons—small graphics or images in the margins—to mark certain paragraphs of information that you may find useful. Here's an explanation of the helpful icons I've used in this book.

When you see this icon, you'll find a helpful nutritional tip, lifestyle suggestion or some information that can be of practical use.

This icon reveals critical information worth remembering and often summarizes a point.

The Warning icon cautions you against something potentially harmful. Be sure to read and heed the information with these icons.

Here and there, I delve into nutritional detail or physiology about how the body works. This icon tips you off to a road sign that says "Brain Work Ahead." If you're not technically oriented, or find yourself getting a headache over your right eye as you attempt to read such detail, simply skip it, because it exists only to enhance your understanding and tends to be more a more detailed explanation.

Where to Go from Here

Like most *For Dummies* books, this one is set up so you can read any chapter in any order (except backwards) and still come out ahead. You really don't need to read every word from cover to cover (although I will be flattered and your friend forever), but only what interests you. You may find an interesting-sounding sidebar that prompts you to read something you may have passed, so an open mind is a good thing.

This book is based on what I was exposed to by macrobiotic teachers many years ago and the personal refinement that I have added and found to be very successful among thousands of clients. It chronicles the subjects that I have studied with passion to learn more about why people do or don't heal. The body, mind, spirit aspect has always been a part of macrobiotic teaching; however, it has really not been emphasized. This book is an attempt to include all aspects of healing and the emphasis of macrobiotic principles, which are usually worded in complex terms with archaic references to physics. Considering them over the years and finding ways to explain how we can use them in daily life makes them more real and more accessible as another tool for personal growth.

Don't forget, the proof is in the pudding, as the cliché goes. You need not appreciate theory, but do experiment with the practical application. Macrobiotics can be appreciated for its complexities and references, but in the end, the day-to-day experience of transforming your health is what makes all the difference and allows you better insight to the true meaning of "a great life." Happy adventuring!

Part I
Getting Started with Macrobiotics

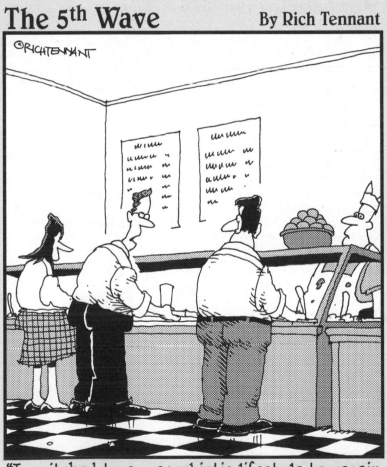

The 5th Wave   By Rich Tennant

©RICHTENNANT

"I switched to a macrobiotic lifestyle to regain a more harmonious balance of mind, body, and buffet line."

In this part . . .

The chapters in this part are your road map to a macrobiotic path of healthy living. In this section, I discuss macrobiotic philosophy, principles and dietary information. Additionally, the body, mind and spirit aspects of macrobiotics, the sound nutrition behind the dietary suggestions and practical ways to handle and eliminate cravings for food that doesn't support our health, are all comprehensively detailed.

Chapter 1

Choosing the Macrobiotic Path to Healthy Living

In This Chapter

▶ Explaining what macrobiotics is all about

▶ Connecting the body-mind-spirit dots

▶ Looking at the basics of macrobiotic eating

Your life revolves around the many choices you make on a daily basis. This word, *choice,* is familiar, but many people misunderstand the role of choice in healing. Choice determines the quality of your life and presents the opportunity to empower or enslave, create safety, offer challenge, and invite love or keep it distant. Because you are always making choices, recognizing the possibilities of choice is the first step toward creating a happier and healthier life. Through the risk of choice and the surrender to its trials and tribulations, you can uncover a primary and powerful tool for self-healing.

There are many paths to self-realization. Some paths seem to be direct routes; others follow more variation. However, like a vehicle you depend on to get you from place to place, your health carries you through life, fortifying you for challenges and providing you with resiliency to adapt to difficulties in order to pursue, undaunted, your journey.

Choosing the macrobiotic path requires more attention — that is, *presence* — and accountability for the many ways you need to nourish yourself. This chapter walks you through the basic tenants of macrobiotics. May you find resonance and revelation in the adventurous journey that lies ahead.

Defining Macrobiotics

Macrobiotics is a compound word adapted from Greek that means "large" or "great" *(macro)* and "life" *(bios).* Hippocrates used the first recorded term of *makrobios* to describe a particular group of individuals who followed a natural way of life and were known for their good health and longevity. In early Western literature, macrobiotics was described as a more fundamental and natural way of life with dietary principles centered on grains, beans, and vegetables.

Macrobiotics defines itself as a comprehensive way of life, offering invigorating principles that guide and educate with practical tools to strengthen the body, mind, and spirit. Recognizing that we are composed of many bodies — physical, intellectual, emotional, creative, and spiritual — macrobiotics offers unique nourishment to sustain growth and elevate judgment. The ultimate goal of macrobiotics is to create freedom from fear, from sickness, and from living lives of indifference. Creating a "great life" is the goal of macrobiotics.

I heard a quote that has remained with me because it contains a truth that resonates deeply. It comes from German philosopher Arthur Schopenhauer (1788–1860): "The two foes of human happiness are pain and boredom." The reality of this quote can be confirmed by the millions of individuals throughout the world who are suffering from pain and witnessing firsthand how this state negatively influences every aspect of their lives. The ability to live happy, passionate, and vital lives of inspiration, depth, and meaning can be compromised by indifference or pain, be it physical, emotional, or spiritual.

To truly live a *great life,* you must feel at home in your own body. This means existing with a certain level of comfort about your health, sensitivity, and fears.

A little macrobiotic history

Classical authors, including Aristotle, Galen, Herodotus, and Lucian, used similar forms of the word *macrobiotic* in regard to health and longevity. In François Rabelais's *Gargantua and Pantagruel,* a famous Renaissance satire about the foibles and follies of the newly emerging modern civilization, the French avant-garde, writer, doctor, and humanist has a chapter on macrobiotics. In 1797, Christopher Hufeland wrote a popular book on healing titled *Makrobiotik, or The Art of Prolonging Life.*

In 1958, macrobiotic philosopher and teacher George Ohsawa met a distant relative of Hufeland and by 1959 began using the term *macrobiotic* to promote his teachings. During a New York visit, he took note of Zen's popularity

in America and, in what seemed like a savvy marketing decision at the time, added it to macrobiotics. Ohsawa's book *Zen Macrobiotics* attempted to capitalize on the popularity of Zen as taught by popular teachers, Alan Watts, and the works of Dr. Daisetz Teitaro Suzuki. Interest in Zen was high among the '50s "Beatnik" movement, which evolved into what we now know as the hippie generation.

Michio Kushi, a student of macrobiotic innovator, George Ohsawa, had come to America to teach macrobiotics, eventually, Kushi dropped the Zen compound and created a diet that was less strict and confining from the original one Ohsawa had proposed in translated works.

The Heart of Macrobiotics: Nourishing Body, Mind, and Spirit

Our health and happiness depend on the way we nurture each realm of our life. We can discover a more balanced and unified health when we nurture body, mind, and spirit. Too much emphasis in one area can potentially weaken other areas.

I've had clients who were all brain and didn't seem to live in their body, and I've had clients whose focus was exclusively on the physical at the risk of ignoring other realms. The way we eat can influence our mental and emotional state. Conversely, our thinking, the way we perceive situations and react to them, can influence our body functions. Emotional states are known to influence our hormonal levels, digestive secretions, and even immune health.

I'm not saying that all areas need equal attention; however, we do need to cultivate deeper relationships with areas we've ignored. Each area requires some nourishment and self-challenge for growth.

Nourishing the body means

- Taking nourishment from balanced whole food sources
- Challenging your physical endurance
- Exercising regularly for better circulation and oxygenation
- Performing deep breathing exercises to help release respiratory acids
- Getting quality sleep and rest

Nourishing the mind means

- Developing your intellect and judgment
- Identifying and articulating your feelings
- Challenging and changing behavioral patterns that don't serve you
- Establishing a personal philosophy, a moral code, and personal rules of conduct
- Setting goals regarding your health, finances, education, body, creativity, relationships, and so on

Nourishing the spirit means

- Discovering a more meaningful life or purpose (see Chapter 10 for more on this)
- Making time for regular worship, prayer, or visualization

✔ Developing more sensitivity to the "energy world" ("sending" prayer, yoga, T'ai Chi, acupressure are some examples of "energy therapies")

✔ Practicing meditation, if not as a spiritual practice, then as a destressing technique

✔ Cultivating and trusting intuitive impulses

Many people fall somewhere between being at home in their bodies and feeling out of place in their bodies. We've lost the understanding of what foods truly nourish and sustain us.

How eating well can bring balance

We've become estranged from the normal functioning of our body. We need "outside" help; now, we need caffeine and nicotine to get going each day; suppositories to move our bowels; alkaline tablets to neutralize excess dietary acidity in our stomachs; sleeping pills to fall asleep; statin drugs to normalize blood pressure; analgesics for pain; and insulin to regulate blood sugar.

Originally, our body functions were designed to work naturally, without the "benefit" of medications. Treating symptoms has become so ingrained as an immediate therapy that we think nothing of popping a pill to soothe our complaints, ignoring the side-effect consequence of many medications. Our refined food diets with excessive amounts of sugar, salt, chemicals and animal products are prime reasons for such dysfunction and must prominently figure in any attempt to foundationally change these conditions.

While exercise can be a helpful therapy, it is still limiting because a lack of dietary balance can undo the benefits of what you've earned from exercise.

Not knowing how to reverse these conditions puts us at a gloomy disadvantage because we end up feeling out of control and victimized by poor health. Most of us falsely assume that many of these conditions are the natural consequence of aging and therefore irreversible.

The very simple act of eating nourishes and sustains your physical well-being and is one of the most basic functions that ensure your daily survival. It's a simple black-and-white premise: If you don't eat, you cease to exist. So, eating properly is the key to restoring your health.

Eventually, beyond securing quality food, you must address the larger concerns of balancing food groups, eating for your needs, and becoming sensitive enough to interpret the messages your body continually broadcasts.

Eating a "macrobiotic diet" isn't simply a matter of choosing between *good* and *bad* foods, but more about knowing what foods create health and what foods are compatible with the way you are designed and the lifestyle you've

chosen. Thinking about foods in moralistic terms of good and bad only encourages rebellious behavior and is often cited as a cause of eating disorders. Ultimately, it's not just about how _long_ you live, but more about how _well_ you live.

How the mind and spirit contribute to good health

Spiritual questions help you to find meaning in your life. They may include some of these: How did I help others? How much of my heart do I share? How much distress have I caused others? How forgiving am I? How well do I love? These questions reflect your happiness and tell you about the life you're living better than questions such as, How much status have I achieved? How much am I earning? What material possessions have I acquired? A healthier question to focus on is, How well am I living?

It's easy to get lost in the information vacuum of nutrition: diets, nutrient evaluations, supplements, herbs, food combinations, assorted theories, and recipes. Then the mental and spiritual aspects of health take a backseat to the latest health fads.

Since mental and spiritual aspects of daily living directly influence our health, they are inseparable from the physical and not to be ignored. Our emotional patterns need to be examined and ways of thinking or narrow perspectives need to be redefined. No one ever said that this stuff is easy. You can make some dietary changes in a heartbeat, but feeling bitter or resentful, emotionally isolated or overly critical of others needs to change because such attitudes do not support good health or peace of mind. A mind and spirit overhaul often requires much self-reflection, outside support, and an enduring will to change.

Experiencing nature can offer a healthy contrast to a frenetic fast-paced city life that seems insulated from natural elements. Exposure to nature can help you feel a deeper and more calming communion with a larger aspect of life. Such experiences give you a measurable sense of scale, allowing you to shift in perspective and invite change that inspires.

Demystifying Macrobiotics: Updating Macrobiotics for Modern Times

From chopsticks to futons, three-piece suits to seaweed consumption, archaic yin-yang principles to Japanese martial arts, the introduction of macrobiotics to the West by Japanese teachers presented many aspects of their culture as a part of the macrobiotic package.

As young adults in the tightly knit Boston community of 1970, many students (myself included) of well-known Japanese macrobiotic teacher Michio Kushi (esteemed student of George Ohsawa) went out of their way to emulate Kushi; some even spoke in broken English accents, despite having English as their primary language and not being able to speak a word of Japanese. Others wore three-piece black suits (as did Kushi), bowed as a greeting, acted very formal, and even took up smoking (at the time, there didn't seem to be a Japanese teacher of macrobiotics who didn't smoke). We mixed Japanese words into our conversations with a sense of exclusivity: A condiment made with sesame seeds and salt was not called "sesame salt," but by its Japanese name, *gomashio;* white radish was called *daikon;* sitting on your calves with knees bent was called *seiza*. We were young, impressionable, and engrossed in demonstrating the oldest known form of flattery: imitation.

Some of us grew out of this emulation act, while some are still doing it. In the last 15 years, macrobiotics has undergone a quiet revolution of cultural reorientation. With the deaths of many community members and even teachers, the bedrock of the belief system — that food exclusively changes all — has eroded into a practical reality now realized by many (save for the macrobiotic myopic). Today's practitioners understand that there are many paths to healing where each individual can best serve himself by discovering his own balance point. For some individuals, the need to explore psychological aspects of healing may be the perfect complement to a whole foods diet. Some may find greater balance with spiritual disciplines, while others focus on physical work, like aerobic activities, that goes along with a balanced eating plan.

No one-size-fits-all paradigm exists. While a whole foods way of eating is foundational, it is by no means the solitary path to healing.

Setting the record straight on macrobiotic falsehoods

Over the years, I've met many people who told me that they had stopped eating macrobiotically. I debunk the more common reasons people quit the macrobiotic lifestyle in the following list:

- ✔ **"It was too strict — I couldn't eat that way."** There is really no "macrobiotic diet." Macrobiotics is a dynamic philosophy of principles, and some of these principles focus on what foods best suit the way our bodies were designed. The length of our intestines, digestion secretions, and tooth structure reveal that we should minimize how much animal protein we eat. Highly concentrated and artificial foods, such as refined sugar, weaken our immunity and mess with our blood sugar, promoting wide swings that result in moodiness and fatigue.

The so-called macrobiotic diet suggests a template of principle foods of grain, bean, and vegetable, with smaller quantities of secondary foods that include sea vegetables, fruit, and (optional) animal proteins (see Chapter 3). If you can't eat a certain way, find elements of whole food eating that feel better. This book offers a number of different starting points, making transitions easier and more appealing.

✔ **"I'm not Japanese. Everything macrobiotic seems to be Japanese."** Your foods and lifestyle don't have to conform to anything Japanese. The people who originally promoted macrobiotics in this country were Japanese, so this misunderstanding is understandable. However, if you research your own culture, you're sure to find identical practices from its ancient traditions. Most early cultures that had developed agricultural practices ate the same whole foods.

In search of culture

It's common to seek a cultural identity if you don't have one. Having a sense of belonging, of commonality, and of ritual helps us mark time with familiar ceremony. Because America is somewhat of a melting-pot culture, we may share a lack of cultural history and ritual tradition. Many turn to religion to fulfill that void in their lives. For those not religiously motivated, a movement with a strong ideology can often become the substitute, allowing us to adopt another culture and new codes of behavior or belief systems. This was a common theme among many of the early Boston macrobiotic community members.

After several years of life in the Boston macrobiotic community, I developed a better understanding about the essence of macrobiotics. Then I began to question things that were supposedly "macrobiotic." I donated my floor futon and bought a familiar (and natural fiber) mattress; I found a table that had chairs, instead of sitting in Japanese *seiza* position before a low table. Although I still ate with chopsticks, I found some quality wooden spoons and forks to use as well. I began to call vegetables by their American names and research other cultural cuisines with a focus on adaptive macrobiotic principles. I had trained myself to think in terms of opposites (yin and yang), but realized that this wasn't a linear concept of opposites but a very complex philosophy with many layers that required much more thought than just extreme labeling. I went from thinking in black and white to realizing that there were many shades of gray.

Immersing myself in Japanese culture was a powerful and broadening experience, and I grew to appreciate its uniqueness as a traditional culture practically opposite from Western culture. However, it also gave me an appreciation for things Western.

At some point in our quest for what feels authentic, we have to admit what feels natural and what feels contrived. I still appreciate Japanese culture, but having studied other cultures and the roots of my own, adopting some rituals and creating my own, I now have a greater sense of identity from this journey.

✔ **"I just crave all the bad foods you shouldn't eat."** Many cravings are rooted in a physical or psychological basis. Cravings are how your body talks to you, so you need to understand this language and find effective and natural ways to handle your cravings. See Chapter 5 for some practical strategies to overcome cravings and make eating less stressful and more pleasurable.

✔ **"There's too much salt in the diet."** In the early days of macrobiotics, many Japanese teachers recommended far more salt than was necessary. Although you need quality sea salt, the amounts needed are minimal.

✔ **"There's nothing fresh in the diet — everything's cooked."** This revision of macrobiotics that you hold in your hands heartily suggests eating fresh foods, such as salad or vegetable juices. The only exclusions are for people who have intestinal inflammation or those with nutritional deficiencies where raw food can often be an irritant. With raw food, many nutrients remain locked in the cellulose layer. The heat from cooking softens these plant cell walls, making nutrients more available.

✔ **"I couldn't get the whole yin/yang thing — it was too heady for me."** There's enormous value in understanding the concept of opposites and how they influence all phenomena. But this has been overconceptualized and is overwhelming to many. In this book, Taoist terminology of *yin* and *yang* is replaced by the more easily understood *expansion* and *contraction*.

✔ **"I don't have time to do all that cooking."** You mean you don't want to spend the rest of your life in the kitchen? I can't blame you! I offer many shortcuts for reducing cooking and preparation times. See Chapter 13 for some advice.

Examining our dietary fall from grace

Since the Industrial Revolution ("Ah, yes, I remember it well . . ."), dietary patterns and habits throughout the world have undergone a gradual yet dramatic shift in quality, production, and availability. Although we have a multitude of foods, in terms of healthy quality, it's been a downhill ride.

Technological developments, mechanized methods of farming, chemical preservatives, food coloring, and artificial flavorings have become staples for nearly 90 percent of commercial foods. In our hurried pace of life, we have made the poor choice of opting for mass production, added sugar, and fat over quality and balanced food groups.

A macrobiotic approach uses whole foods that contain nothing artificial, encourages local farming, has proved to be far more sustainable and ecological while economically, in the long run, lowers food bills.

What follows are my top ten detrimental food-related changes that have occurred in the past 150 years.

Whole grains have gone A.W.O.L.

Somewhere along the line we began *polishing* whole grains, thus stripping away valuable vitamins, minerals, and fiber. Today we have wheat bran, wheat flakes, wheat germ, and so on. What happened to *whole* wheat? White rice was originally brown rice with seven layers of bran that were milled off.

Whole grain has been a staple food of many cultures for thousands of years. The most common forms of whole grain, which are really grain products, are bread, pasta, crackers, muffins, and pancakes. Real whole grains are cereals that still have their original form intact: brown rice, millet, unhulled barley, quinoa, buckwheat (technically a seed), and others. Giving whole grain as feed to animals and then eating them makes them into our personal grain processor. Go direct! Eat whole!

We're steak-and-potatoes people

As we've reduced complex carbohydrates (from whole grains) and increased refined foods and various sugars in our diets, we crave the dense and salty quality that meat gives us.

We can't seem to get enough: We start some mornings with bacon, eggs, and sausage, have a meatball sandwich or chicken or tuna salad for lunch, and complete this animal feast with steak, lamb, or veal for dinner. Reducing or eliminating the amount of meat we eat isn't just about chemicals, hormones, and other synthetics added to animals' feed, but the fat and protein content and the toxic substances produced when our bodies break down the meat.

Excessive animal protein has been linked to colon cancer and a host of other diseases. (There's an ethical argument as well, but not everyone is sympathetic to that.) What I am sure about is that if everyone were required to kill, butcher, and prepare the meats they favored, animal protein as a dietary staple would plummet. It's so convenient to buy a neatly packaged chicken breast from the market and go home and pop it in the oven that we rarely reflect on the steps we didn't have to endure that make this possible.

"Just a spoonful of sugar . . ."

Shakespeare wasn't thinking about sugar when he gave Romeo the words, "What's in a name? That which we call a rose by any other name would smell as sweet." But when you think about white sugar, honey, molasses, brown sugar, maple syrup, barley malt, and agave syrup, and all their different properties, they still share the same acidity and inflammatory effect in our bodies. True, some may have a little bit of minerals, but they're all predominantly sugar, no matter how you slice it.

Once upon a time, we enjoyed the naturally sweet taste of fruits, which we ate fresh, or dried, cooked, or canned in winter. A little honey or maple syrup also proved memorable on special occasions. Today it's a sad and tragic story. The average North American consumes nearly 140 pounds of refined sugar each year, not including corn syrups, honey products, and miscellaneous edible syrups like sorghum. This figure also does not include an additional 24 pounds of artificial sweeteners! It's estimated that the average teenage boy drinks more than 800 cans of soda yearly! The most assaulting thing we do is wash down a good meal with soda, milkshakes, fruit juice, alcohol, or milk. This isn't digestive friendly; it's an act of intestinal war!

Long ago sugar was considered a luxury food and most frequently enjoyed by royalty. The mind-boggling increase of simple sugars in the modern diet parallels the increase of disease, debilitation and premature death.

"Isn't ketchup a vegetable?"

The main vegetables in the fast-food world are tomatoes, potatoes, lettuce, and a sprig of throwaway parsley. Save for these, many people wouldn't know a vegetable if it hit them in the head.

Additionally, the adoption of pesticide and herbicide farming, freezing, canning, and using artificial preservatives to facilitate long durations of storage and transport have contributed to the deterioration of vegetables' quality.

"But it looks like a fruit . . ."

Hybrid species of uniform fruits sprayed with toxic chemicals have replaced wild and naturally cultivated fruits. In many examples, modern fruit has lost some of its naturally sweet taste and tends to be larger. This has also given way to the juice industry, where artificially flavored, colored, and sweetened concentrates seem to be everywhere and are consumed daily by many.

Did you say "vegetable protein?"

Say the word protein and most people immediately think of some kind of meat. In the Western world, the word meat has become synonymous with the word *protein*. But for the majority of the rest of the world, concentrated sources of protein come from beans and bean products. Today much of these protein sources are fed to livestock instead of people.

Depending predominantly on bean protein, as opposed to animal protein, makes good ecological sense. The foods that we eat greatly affect our environment. Raising animals for food in large "factory farming" operations ends up using tremendous amounts of natural resources such as land, water, and grain. At the same time, these operations are responsible for water pollution, erosion of soil, and greenhouse gases. A plant-centered, whole-foods diet uses fewer resources and does not impair our environment to any degree similar to a diet that emphasizes animal products.

Don't believe that gas is a given when you eat beans. You can do many things to avoid this problem (see Chapter 6 for additional tips). I recommend avoiding certain food combinations and using sea salt when cooking beans or not combining the complex sugars of beans with simple sugars of fruit. When these two different sugars are combined, the simple sugar ferments the more slowly digesting complex sugar, and the result is a fermentation that is gaseous.

Junk food is everywhere!

Almost daily we are faced with an onslaught of vending machines, fast-food restaurants, food courts, and street vendors selling anything that's fast-food related. Ready-made foods, sodas, ice cream, candy, flavored coffee, and other sugary, salty, or spicy foods and beverages are the featured players. Nutritionally, there's nothing wholesome about these foods, yet they've flourished.

"Autopilot" agriculture and a perilous environment

Because of massive demand, most large-scale farming is dependent on mechanized agriculture, relentless pesticide and herbicide spraying, and soil additives for the crop yields that are necessary to make substantial profits. Chemicals and hormones have altered the quality of livestock feed, causing growth hormones and chemical residues to be passed on in meats and animal byproducts, such as milk, cheese, and butter. Currently, nearly 100 percent of cattle are fed five or six sex hormones to accelerate weight gain.

"Don't mess with my salt"

Mine salt, with much of its trace mineral compounds removed and artificial ingredients added (to prevent discoloring, to bleach color, to help pour more freely, to help with potential iodine deficiency, and so on), is but a shadow of its former self.

Real salt from the sea, with its mineral matrix intact and none of the artificial ingredients added, can be found in natural food markets as "solar evaporated sea salt."

Welcome to "Artificial Land"

Not only have we infiltrated our foods with chemicals, hormones, and synthetics over the last 100 years, but those substances have found their way into our water, air, building materials, housewares, clothing — pick a random category and it's guaranteed to contain some chemical toxins. It's estimated that more than 25,000 chemicals can be found in cosmetics alone.

In some way, all of these chemicals pose a direct threat to our health. The body, in its wisdom, attempts to store chemicals and toxins in fat cells to keep them from accumulating in the bloodstream. Still, they affect us, in terms of liver function, brain tissue, nervous system health, and blood chemistry.

The benefits of macrobiotic eating

The preceding sections tell you how tough it can be to eat healthy in today's world. But after decades of observing the effects of balanced whole foods on thousands of clients, friends, and family members, as well as drawing on my personal experience, I've seen a sensible macrobiotic diet result in the following:

- Greater energy, endurance, and vitality
- Regular and effortless bowel function
- More stable moods as a result of a regulated blood sugar profile
- A reduction in systemic acidity, which means less inflammation, more muscular flexibility, and better absorption
- Better digestion simply by reducing dietary extremes
- Deeper and more restful sleep with a reduction in the previous amounts required
- More mental clarity, better memory, and more coordinated physical responses
- Reduced physical stress
- Prompt and permanent weight-loss
- Better circulation of blood and lymph fluids
- Greater tendency toward optimism and less negativity
- Less emotional rigidity, more vulnerability, and more openness

The rest of this book shows you how you can achieve these benefits.

Chapter 2

Applying Macrobiotic Principles to Your Daily Life

In This Chapter

▶ Considering universal principles

▶ Becoming more self-aware

The foundation of macrobiotics is based on a number of universal principles that are simply natural laws of life and change common to many religious movements and ancient spiritual teachings. Many of these principles have become New Age sound bites, philosophical colloquialisms, and glib adages that roll off the lips of many but seem to be understood by few.

I've never felt comfortable identifying myself with a movement, especially one fraught with a bit of notoriety because of the perception that it may be a "fanatical" Japanese food movement, which it's not. Instead of focusing on one spoke of the macrobiotic wheel, I'd rather say that I try to live by macrobiotic principles.

The principles outlined in this chapter can provide greater life meaning, adventure, and amusement after you understand them. They are ancient, time-tested principles from cultures and ideologies that demand reverence and expression. Some of them can be found in the New Testament, in Talmudic works, throughout Greek literature, in the sacred texts of India's Charak-Samita, and in the Chinese medical book *The Yellow Emperor's Classic of Internal Medicine.* You many also identify the voice of Asian sages, as well as Western scholars.

These principles can exert a powerful influence on our mental, spiritual, and physical health. Collectively, they each contribute toward unifying body, mind, and spirit for healing or general well-being.

What makes these principles universal is both their age and commonality among different groups around the globe. Their core teaching is a timeless wisdom that always leads to the same conclusion: God, the universe, nature, and all expressions of creation are undeniably one.

This chapter illustrates some core universal principles that offer an enhanced way to expand your perspective for a more dynamic way of living.

Understanding Universal Macrobiotic Life Principles

Although principles tend to apply predictably within certain parameters of life and creation, they're not absolutes, nor are they "rules." To survive and thrive in this life, principles offer practical insight and a conscious awareness that make the game more meaningful to play.

In modern life, principles are omnipresent. They are at the foundation of systems like math and geometry and help develop ideas into concrete realities, as in government, finance, and even battle. Principles are woven into scientific revelation and theoretical physics, just as they are the basis of various astrological and numerological systems; and they are inherently connected to psychological behavior, spiritual thought, language, and the traditional medicine of developed cultures.

Principles are time-tested, logically deduced, and confirmed. They frequently appear as inexplicable patterns that become apparent only when everything seems to fall into place. They are natural wisdom you can trust when you're unsure of everything else.

Principles exist independently of any opinion or belief you may have about them. It's a bit like gravity — believing or not believing in gravity doesn't change the daily action of gravity in our lives. It just exists. It is, ultimately, not your agreement and identification with these principles that changes your life. It is your experience of them that transforms you.

The following macrobiotic principles are the map by which we discover guidance that leads to truth — our personal compass to self-revelation.

The Principle of Opposites: Everything exists in opposition

An unprejudiced view of all phenomena around us reveals the presence of constant *polarity* — the motion between opposite poles, which is life's essential mechanism of movement. Polarities govern the cycle of birth, growth, and decay of everything, be it of the material, mental, or spiritual realm. They are nature's paradoxical reality.

The pairing of extremes and all degrees in between permeates our lives; light and dark; hot and cold; masculine and feminine; dry and wet; vegetable and animal — the list is endless.

These laws of polarity have been called the *heritage of humanity*. They are always at work, influencing our lives and personal interactions.

Principle of Opposites, Sub-Law 1: All polarities are complementary yet antagonistic

Clichés can be viewed in a larger context when seen through the eyes of the Principle of Opposites. Here are a couple of well-known examples:

- After a storm comes the calm.
- As soon as man is born he begins to die.
- Failure teaches success.
- Absence makes the heart grow fonder.
- Familiarity breeds contempt.
- You always hurt the one you love.
- Truth is the mother of deceit.
- United we stand, divided we fall.

Polarities are, essentially, extremes. Yet, as much as they may be in opposition, they also have a complementary nature. That's the paradox of this principle. You can get a better understanding of balance by being able to identify extremes.

We've all seen the black and white Tao symbol (also referred to as the yin yang symbol). In it, you can clearly see both polarities in black and white. However, within the large white area, you see a dot of black; within the large black area, a dot of white. Polarities always contain a bit of each other; therefore nothing is solely black or white. Within the dark of night is the subtle light of stars, and within the bright hot sun of midday, there is cool shadow.

It's like saying someone is strong. Of course, no one is *all* strength; he has to have some weakness. Therefore, using the symbolism of the Tao sign we can translate this statement as, the amount of strength this person has exceeds his weakness.

The Principle of Opposites is easy to misunderstand because referring to things in terms of fixed classifications often leads to rigid thinking. You have to remember that this principle has many layers of depth. If you limit yourself to thinking in pure black and white terms, you omit an important spectrum of gray.

Principle of Opposites, Sub-Law 2: Opposites attract, like repels like

The principle sub-law of "opposites attract and like repels like" can be illustrated with an analogy of magnets. I remember being taught about magnetic north pole and south pole when I was a kid in science class. Placing one magnet's north to another's south created immediate attraction — they'd lock together. But when you attempt to put the south end of one magnet with the south of another, they repel (and you look a bit feeble trying to make them stick). There are always degrees of opposition, but the greater the degree, the greater the attraction. There are many examples of this law in chemistry, food preparation, and even relationships.

Opposites represent extremes. As applied to health, understanding how to identify extremes and recognizing the natural laws between them allows you to find a more balanced state. For example, on the acid-alkaline scale, beans, which are protein rich, contain more acids. You can neutralize some of these acids by soaking them, applying longer cooking times, adding sea salt, and eating small portions of fermented foods with bean dishes. These acid-reducing practices can eliminate, or at least minimize, some of the gas-producing acids, making the beans more digestible and their nutrients easier to absorb. In this case, using alkaline elements to neutralize excess acid creates a better balance.

Principle of Opposites, Sub-Law 3: Everything in the extreme changes to its opposite

In classical Chinese philosophy, it is said that all opposites you experience in life are better understood in reference to the perpetual authority of one principle over the other. Considering that all conditions are subject to change into their opposite, no one principle can always prevail. All phenomena are cyclical and move in a repetitive rhythm of reversal that results in all phenomena eventually transforming into their opposite.

Some of these transformations include

- Light changes into dark
- Health transforms into sickness
- Poverty develops into wealth
- Concealment becomes revelation
- Submission grows into power

Because opposites are the extremes of one principle, it is said that all phenomena have within them the seeds of their opposite; so sickness has the seeds of health, just as health holds the seeds of sickness; poverty contains the seeds of wealth, just as wealth holds the seeds of poverty. In universal reality, no phenomena is completely without some degree of its opposite.

Opposites in everyday life

The natural laws that govern opposites are numerous and can be applied to every aspect of life, including health management, the way you look at the world, and living a life of greater significance. These universally applicable laws are based on common sense, the invisible energy world, and native human intuition, rather than a pragmatic mindset that examines things more analytically.

Using the terms *contraction* and *expansion,* here is a practical example of how opposites in regard to food affect our health balance: Overeating, which fills and expands us, produces acidity, for which we are commonly advised to take some form of alkalinity as a remedy. An alkaline substance can neutralize excess acidity because the two are opposites. Fasting, the opposite of overeating, can also work, but it may make you overeat later or result in cravings for something distinctly acid, such as sugar.

The Principle of Change: Everything changes!

> *"Nothing endures but change."*
>
> — Heraclitus (540–480 BC)

That change is so pervasive in daily life makes it almost futile to describe and analyze.

In the face of everything being temporary, nothing really remains stable. You can see examples all around you; in nature, things are either growing or in a state of decay; virtually everything, from work to passions, moods, fashion, success or failure, and even friendships, is subject to the principle of change.

Two of the most common illustrations of this principle are the Life Cycle and the Moisture Cycle.

- ✔ In the **Life Cycle,** a small seed sprouts and continues its growth cycle, developing roots, stem, branches, blossoms, fruit, and seeds, and then drops to the ground to repeat the cycle.
- ✔ In the **Moisture Cycle,** water evaporates from exposure to the heat of the sun and ascends until it condenses and returns to the earth as rain.

Everything in life goes through change cycles. Emotionally, this can be very destabilizing, because people naturally seek security and comfort by attempting to exert more control in daily life. Yet, change is deceptive. It's a reoccurring instability that's beyond human control. For any measure of peace, accepting change requires surrender, trust, and acceptance of this cycle.

In a larger context, the Principle of Change offers insight into many domains. Even atoms, which modern science once considered the unchanging building blocks of matter, change. Modern physics has increasing evidence that matter is actually a form of energy that is the same thing, but in different states. The stars and the sun, which seem to have remained the same forever, also change or inevitably disappear.

Therefore, *everything* changes — particularly the attention you'll give to the principles in this chapter. Some will resonate with you; some will not. At a later time, based on your evolving perspective, others may take greater importance.

When you understand the law of change, you gain patience and faith. Recognize that only one thing can truly resist change, and that is simply change in itself. For what is known about the nature of phenomena, it's the only absolute.

The Principle of Cycles: All beginnings have endings

Nothing in this universe is exempt from beginnings and endings. All beginnings have endings. All endings have beginnings. It's part of the birth and life cycle. Surely you know this; however, how can this principle be of value?

In the rhythm and repetition of nature, we constantly observe change. This reminder of change makes life more dynamic and more meaningful. For the ever-changing world around us, our most secure moments are those that we find ourselves present in. Not the future, not the past, but the present, where life unfolds before our eyes.

For me, this understanding has always been a consolation because during periods of stress and difficulty, I was able, in knowing that all beginnings have endings, to understand that change was inevitable. It bolstered my patience and reinforced my faith. You may be at the beginning, or you may be at the end. Be present with it, because it shall soon transform before your very eyes.

The Principle of Non-Identity: Nothing is identical

An ancient Greek philosopher once said, "You cannot step in the same river twice." All phenomena around us has its unequaled singularity; whether it be fingerprints, mountain terrain, the structure of rivers, the biology of twins, snowflakes, or even each side of the human face, there will always be some degree of distinction. Even in a physical object made up of molecules and atoms, differences exist because the sum total and combination that each contains is unique.

Presuming that two things are precisely "identical," the mere reality that they are two isolates them because they inhabit two locations in time or space. Considering that everything is in an eternal process of change, nothing can be wholly identical. There is always difference, however subtle.

The Principle of Front and Back: Every front has a back

The idea that every front has a back unites opposites, antagonisms, and even enemies. It reveals that all things exist in this world by their opposites, through relativity. If you have opposites and antagonisms, it means you also have identity in relation to them. Modern industry has created great comfort in our living conditions, but has also brought numerous disadvantages: pollution in our air and land, poisons in our food supply, and degenerative disease. This is simply an example of front and back.

Categorizing extremes provides a window of contrast to measure the relationship between front and back: truth and lies, integrity and deceit, work and leisure, convenience and complication. Each extreme creates more value for the opposite. To some degree, they always co-exist. In what appears overwhelmingly wonderful, there is bound to be a bit of the opposite that remains hidden.

The bigger the front, the bigger the back

In almost everything we examine, front and back are apparent; however, this sub-law refers to the "depth factor." The more magnificent, beneficial, comforting, or whatever the front seems, the more potential it may have of containing an equalized backside.

Modern medical drugs, such as morphine, can help alleviate deep pain, but their backside is twofold: They can be addictive and potentially fatal. Money can bring us great comfort, power, and joy, but it also may become a source of discomfort, instigate suspicion of others, and inspire alienation and depression. Beauty, a quality desired by many, can also become a cause of jealousy, resentment, and conflict.

Understanding front and back and the growth factor of big front, big back gives you the ability to examine things in scale. You can see both sides and are more likely to make healthier choices that contribute to your health and psychological growth.

It's human intuition to suspect that a gift of gigantic proportion may obligate you to a greater payback; that a super-nutrient, one single pill advertised to be the "mother of all nutrients — for only $39.95" may also be a bit of snake oil; or that the most convenient of technology, the cellphone, which allows us to communicate in ways previously impossible, may also eventually fry our brains with concentrated radiation held barely ½ inch from our brain cortex. Our innate understanding of front and back arouses our suspicions.

Chemotherapy, heralded as a cancer treatment, is another example of front and back. The treatment may dissolve a primary tumor, but in many cases, the chemo renders the immune system so weak that it's unable to contain stray cancer cells, which continue to divide and soon manifest another tumor in a different location. *Front and back.*

Macrobiotic Principles of Awareness

What is the secret to a happy, healthy life? How do you acquire stable physical health, mental health, and a sense of peace? The secret lies not only in how you nourish yourself, but in the perspective you maintain that creates your attitudes and values that help you cope with daily life.

Awareness can be considered the first step in your creation process. As you grow in self-awareness, you better understand why you feel what you feel and why you behave as you do. With this understanding, you are given the opportunity to change the things you'd like to change about yourself to create a life that is more meaningful. Your life can become significantly different when you're the one directing your mind, as opposed to allowing *it* to direct *you.* In this regard, becoming more self-aware is the key to lasting happiness. To become more self-aware, you must sharpen your perceptions and observational skills. This isn't something they teach in school.

Your attitude toward life is strongly influenced by your personal philosophy, which plays an integral part in the healing process. Self-knowledge, core values, and deeply held convictions define the personal philosophy of your character. How you experience things, including triumph, loss, happiness, grief, love, death, success, devotion to a cause, friendship, and risk taking, as well as physical, emotional, intellectual, and spiritual growth, depends on the personal philosophy you create to guide you on this earthly journey.

The work of creating a personal philosophy that defines your daily behavior is the work of living a *conscious life* — a life where value is demonstrated by the example you set with an honest acceptance of your limitations and a self-challenging spirit determined to overcome those limitations.

A personal philosophy can enhance your self-esteem and in the process grace your life with abundant meaning. The consistent practice of self-reflection and self-examination — owning your personal opinions and not just those you have mechanically adopted from parents, peers, or educators — allows you to resonate in a higher level of consciousness, one that has a higher value and self-respect for self and self-care.

The macrobiotic self-awareness principles, listed in the following sections, can become your blueprint toward establishing a personal philosophy for the purpose of designing a more creative and meaningful life.

The Principle of Abundance: From one grain come ten thousand

The symbolism of using grain to exemplify the Principle of Abundance is based on the natural growth cycle of one grain. From one grain, thousands may germinate. Nature, in her generous, diverse spirit, gives unconditionally and abundantly.

This principle means to develop a generous spirit that allows you to share yourself with others, without conditions of receiving back. In the end, it is in the giving where we are rewarded.

You can also apply this principle to the economy of cooking. Because of one grain's potential, we try to not waste a single grain; we use the outer leaves of the cabbage; we chop the end of a radish that looks like a rat's tail and use it in our cooking as part of our "no-waste" commitment. Our spirit in food preparation then embodies a sense of gratitude.

It has become a recent theme to "pay it forward," recognizing that selfless acts of random kindness can inspire others to do the same. Thus each act becomes an emissary of love and gratitude, making the world a more harmonious place in the process.

Mea culpa: My fault

Mea culpa is derived from a Latin phrase that translates as "my fault." In Shakespeare's play *Julius Caesar,* Cassius echoes this sentiment in another way: "The fault, dear Brutus, is not in our stars, but in ourselves." This statement summarizes the origin of human failure and pain. It is about seeking an excuse, or "justified reason," on which to blame our personal choices. Sadly, this has become a habitual practice in modern society.

In modern vernacular, "passing the buck" is a common expression for people who blame others. Essentially, this reveals that you are absolving yourself from responsibility. If you maintain the attitude that any situation you find yourself in must have personal meaning — a reason, divine or otherwise, for occurring — then it is best for our individual growth to share responsibility for that situation before you begin pointing fingers. The old saw that says, "When you point your finger, notice that three fingers (of the same hand) point back at you," captures this point of view.

Yet, our modern emotional climate is steeped in blame; we blame our boss, our partners, the school system, government, the weather, our economy, food conglomerates, industry polluters, viruses, fungi, and so on. Although each of these factions has its part, when you point fingers, you avoid some degree of personal accountability.

On one hand, this tendency is reinforced from childhood when you connected self-blame with being in trouble, shame, getting caught, or being on the receiving end of punishment. Most of us were subject to black-and-white thinking on the nature of blame.

When faced with conflicting circumstances, you must ask yourself, what is my part? Did you not check the facts? Or were you swayed by fact, when intuition was silently screaming a warning to avoid the situation? Did you make choices out of fear? Was there a greed factor in what you did or believed? Or was it just a desire for acceptance?

A more embracive perspective suggests that you create or allow everything that happens in your life. If you adopt the perspective that recognizes and admits some fault in a particular situation, you can change your situation! But if you see it as the fault of another, you can only remain a victim of the circumstance. The result of such thinking is pain, suffering, and often a sense of hopelessness.

Mea culpa is a call to personal surrender and spiritual coping strategy. It requires a sense of optimistic faith that by seeing your individual part, you'll grow and benefit from the situation at hand.

"Non credo": Do not believe

Non credo is another derivative of a Latin phrase that means "do not believe." In its pure intention, *non credo* means to discover for yourself by personal experience. This supports the process of self-inquiry, exploration, and discovery, as well as allowing the faculty of intuition its contribution.

The distinction between belief and experience is emphasized by this principle. Belief is identified with thinking and memory and often is built on what you feel to be the truth based on what you've been taught. Experience is the result of what you gained from personal knowledge.

You can theorize about climbing Mount Everest. From previous testimony of experienced climbers and detailed terrain maps, you can understand its difficulty, the challenge of extracting oxygen from thin air, the requirement for a superior level of fitness, knowing what foods to take, the necessity for many clothing layers, and so on.

However, to actually trudge up the mountain, go through the symphony of emotions, experience the anxiety of danger, bond with fellow climbers, submit yourself to severe weather, and achieve the final triumph of reaching the summit offers an unequalled experience that conceptualizing about it can never match. In this example, belief is intellect's emissary.

Ultimately, *non credo* means to question, challenge, and attempt to experience everything from a more comprehensive viewpoint. It's the difference between someone describing the taste of an exotic sweet fruit and actually tasting it. Personally, I'll take the fruit.

Develop your intuition

Intuition is one of the most common characteristics of humanity. It is not merely an extra sensory response. It's an essential and universal response that many of us hear yet ignore or don't know how to cultivate.

The resonance of our instinctive responses connect us to a larger sense of the mysterious world we call the energetic or spiritual world. Intuition is not logic or analysis. It's an instinctive perception that we are all born with and use every day, usually somewhat unconsciously.

There's an indescribable feeling of connectedness when you hear a random voice in your head offer a suggestion that you impulsively obey and later discover to be a wise choice or, in some cases, a life-saving choice. You must be able to identify and trust that voice if you want to develop this powerful ability.

Naturally, there are many "voices" in our head that at any time may be giving us commands, making judgments, or instilling fears; you have the voice your parents, your anxieties, and societal norms. However, the voice of intuition is a clear and distinctive voice that is suggestive yet not pushy. The work is in recognizing it — and then trusting it.

You can cultivate your intuition by playing risk-free games, such as guessing who may be calling when you hear the telephone ring; who sent the letter that you're taking out of the mailbox; or what direction is the shortest way to your destination without using a map.

All of these circumstances require listening to your inner voice and some degree of self-questioning. If the doorbell rings and you ask yourself, will it be man or woman, one or two people, and what color shirt or dress will they be wearing, don't attempt to guess. Intuit. That means, immediately after you ask yourself the question, see, with your mind's eye, how many people are there, or what color are their clothes, whatever, but intuit. *Guessing* deals with the mind and reasoning. *Intuiting* is about seizing your first primary response from that inner voice.

When you become accustomed to that voice and can clearly recognize it, you can begin to develop your intuition further by asking yourself questions and seizing your first intuitive response. The more you develop your ability to recognize this voice, the more confident you grow that you always have a secret resource to guide and sustain you.

Food can also enhance your intuitive abilities. When your body is more relaxed, your intuitive faculty becomes sharpened. Foods that heat us up, like sugar and alcohol, contribute to inflammation or make blood sugar irregular, making us less sensitive to our intuitive voice. It becomes more difficult to delineate the fine line between the voice of fear and the voice of intuition or our inner critic. Intuition requires mental clarity.

Cultivate active appreciation

Studies have shown that cultivating a sense of appreciation can help you maintain a more positive mood, enhancing emotional well-being as well as resulting in social benefits. But appreciation is not just the expression to another of how much they mean to you. Appreciation is a deeply personal attitude of genuine gratitude for life's challenges and for life itself. With a bit of patience, you can cultivate a deeper sense of appreciation that is both heartfelt and demonstrative.

In a larger context, you can place gratitude into two categories:

- **Present picture:** This gratitude level reflects appreciation for your possessions and immediate conditions: your material possessions, your health, home, family, relationships, job, skills, car, someone who has gifted you with something, and so on.

- **Larger picture:** This is gratitude for life itself, your challenges, your ability to think and feel, your level of consciousness, the planet, people making a difference in the world, and so on.

This larger picture level of gratitude is beyond the circumstantial, beyond the temporary state of remembering what you have to be grateful for. In the larger picture, you marvel at everyday existence of life — whatever its circumstances. It's a form of gratitude that emulates unconditional love without expectation. This expression is about living with a mindset of gratitude and forging it to become a part of our identity.

A profound spiritual law is "like attracts like." When you are truly grateful for the blessings in your life and take the time to reflect on them, you begin to attract more blessings to yourself. Why is this? It must be because you create what you focus on.

True appreciation isn't simply the act of mechanically listing the blessings in your life every night just before retiring. *Appreciation is an attitude.* It's a positive and consistent mindset of thankfulness and joy for everything in your life that nurtures you, challenges you, and makes you who you are. If you're willing to work at it, you can develop your mind's ability to effortlessly embody a spirit of appreciation.

One of the best ways to cultivate gratitude is to keep an *appreciation journal.* Not only will you combine the benefits of journaling with the active adoption of a more positive mindset, but you'll also create a nice record of happy memories and a long list of things in your life for which you feel gratitude. For more difficult or emotionally challenging times, this can be highly inspiring to read.

Make friends everywhere

Amigo, acquaintance, associate, boyfriend, brother, buddy, chum, cohort, colleague, confidant, comrade, crony, girlfriend, homeboy, mate, mentor, pal, partner, sidekick, sister — all indicate different degrees of friendship and the fact that we are all touchstones to the evolving reality of a need to connect.

Evening gratitude meditation

Every evening before I retire to sleep, I try to recall experiences throughout the day that I am grateful for: my neighbor's beautiful blooming hibiscus that hangs over his fence and into my backyard; the old man who came into a restaurant during a business lunch I was having and asked the manager to locate the car owner (me!) who had left his lights on; a friend who called to tell me that his lab work confirmed his sickness is in remission; my pregnant daughter who called to tell me that she felt her baby moving inside of her; or the support and encouragement of a friend who read an early draft of an article I wrote and found something inspiring to contribute. So many things happen to you in the course of a day that you can give thanks for. Recall the events of your day and reflect on the many things for which you feel gratitude.

In doing this kind of recall, you remind yourself about life's daily gifts and thereby close your day positively. This positive attitude usually carries over from one day to the next. As you make this a habit, you'll eventually notice that you feel happier, less depressed, and far more optimistic.

Friendships are essential for us to feel more and share more; be a part of community where we enjoy a sense of belonging; seek support and encouragement; and see ourselves in the mirror of human character.

People naturally seek out friendships. Even couples need the support of other couples. During our school years, associations with people are built into our lives. College students usually study and live together. Throughout our lives, involvement in hobbies or sports provides additional outlets to form new associations and friendships. But as we mature, we become more self-conscious about our need to make and cultivate relationships. Unfortunately, as we age and take on more responsibility (family, mortgage debt, job demands, and so on), we discover a lack of time (as well as energy) to cultivate new friendships.

Consider these ideas for cultivating more friends in your life:

- ✔ Join a club with people who have common interests.
- ✔ Join a sports team.
- ✔ Volunteer for a cause you feel passionate about.
- ✔ Make eye contact and smile in public. Introduce yourself.
- ✔ Be bold and risk taking the first step: Start a conversation!

Naturally, you need to be around people to meet people. Then you need to interact with them in ways that are warm, inviting, and nonthreatening. To transform an acquaintance into a friend, *you* need to take the initiative.

Finally, realize that human needs are pretty much the same across the board: We all want someone whom we can trust and depend on; someone who will listen to our feelings and outlook; someone who'll lovingly level with us when they see us deeper than we imagine; someone who's forgiving; and someone to share love and time with. It's really not difficult to make friends; however, cultivating deeper relationships is another story, one that takes time, patience, self-disclosure, vulnerability, intention, creativity, courage, and compassion.

There's a mirror in everyone you meet — family, friends, associates, strangers. Your work is to see them clearly. We all need friends, and we all need to play. Learn to connect with others.

Respect your elders

I consider this principle to be a sub-principle of make friends everywhere (see the preceding section). We should stand in reverence of those who are our elders.

More than 52 million people in the United States provide care for a loved one. These family caregivers typically don't identify themselves as *caregivers*. In many instances, family caregivers don't differentiate their role as one separate from any other of their daily activities. Care giving is simply a part of their life.

In many cultures, from Latin to Chinese, care giving is a natural and expected part of the culture, wherein many societies, the parents move in with their children after the children get married. The parents dutifully help raise their children's children, and when the parents themselves need care, their children are prepared to care for them until the end of their life. Care giving isn't seen as a chore or another role they must play. It's simply an accepted step in the long, continuous life of traditional families.

Honoring these traditions is one of the foundations of a deeply bonded family. When we become caregivers, regardless of what culture we're from, we include many of these traditional beliefs of honor and value for our elders. Even more than respect, we should offer elders our time, our listening, our interaction, and our gratitude.

We owe deep gratitude to our elders; they are our teachers. Every elder should be a respected part of the human community. We must protect them, show them courtesy, and help them live satisfying lives.

Be mindful of ecology

Ecological principles positively influence the health and happiness of society. The way that we manage our environment, maintain our home, our land, the country, and the resources of our planet reflects our gratitude and social consciousness. Being attentive to plant life benefits us because many plants nourish and sustain us. In these times of quantity, we compromise our health by the thousands of chemicals, solvents, and petroleum products used to increase production yields. This results in poorer quality soil and more toxic residues held within the plants that our livers and kidneys have to handle.

Currently, Americans use more than 4.5 billion pounds of pesticides, including nearly 1 billion pounds of "conventional" pesticides used in agriculture, industry, home, and garden. On a daily basis, we are unknowingly exposing ourselves to a toxic assortment of pesticides in our homes, schools, offices, food, and drinking water. Eventually these chemicals make their way into different parts of our bodies, finding refuge in fat tissues.

Developing an ecological conscience means becoming more mindful about what we buy, using cloth bags instead of plastic, recycling, choosing commercial products and packaging from sustainable or recycled sources, buying organic foods when possible, and wearing clothing, particularly undergarments, from natural cotton sources.

Being mindful of ecology is the responsibility of everyone concerned with their individual health, the health of loved ones, and the health of our city, state, country, and planet.

Practice economy of life: Vivero parvo

Economy of life is applied in our diet as a *no-waste* practice. The less food we waste, the more we have for others. For example, this means

- ✔ Lightly scrubbing vegetables before cooking, but not peeling them as a means of cleaning

- ✔ Chopping only the very ends of the vegetable and being mindful of how much you waste

- ✔ Cleaning the outer leaves of the cabbage and using them, rather than automatically throwing them away

- ✔ Eating what is a respectable volume

When you really think about it, the amount of food that we waste or throw away in stores, restaurants, and homes throughout America is staggering.

One application of a no-waste practice can be to simply adopt a more whole foods dietary approach. Consuming only a part of food eventually contributes to malnourishment. The daily eating of refined sugar and synthetic chemicals detracts from a healthy body and life. Eating whole foods give us the entire array of vitamin and mineral matrixes, allowing better digestion and absorption of trace nutrients.

Vivero parvo is a Latin phrase that means "take the minimum." Applied to food, this means to eat for our needs and not to completely satisfy our appetites. Of course, there's nothing wrong with having a big appetite; in fact, it's a sign of good health. However, if you always completely satisfy your appetite, you lose your will and energy for other appetites. If you have strong passions for things you want to do in life, not eating to excess comes naturally because you're feeding other appetites. "Eat less, do more" is an ancient proverb that may apply to you.

In a lecture, I once heard Michio Kushi remark that "Economy is the practice of gratitude." Hearing that quote moved me profoundly because it helped me understand a more meaningful way of expressing gratitude in a social context.

Discover humor

Having the capacity for humor is a characteristic of good health. We are born with a sense of humor and either develop or suppress it. Babies smile very early in life, and young children have been observed to laugh naturally more than 300 times a day, whereas adults express laughter merely 15 times a day. Somewhere along the lines of evolving maturity, we lose this natural gift. It may be discouraged by social norms as we grow or based on our upbringing and family environment. Although kids tend to laugh unconditionally, adults usually laugh when they have a justifiable "reason" or when a group situation offers a more permissible atmosphere.

Restoring your sense of humor gives you permission to be authentically human and unmask the humor in everyday life. Allowing yourself to enjoy something humorous and respond without controlling your feelings is a unique way to experience being in the moment. In that humorous instance, you think neither of the past nor future, but only the present. In that momentary place, you are face to face with joy.

Recovering a sense of humor demands that we let go of a need to control and surrender to what we naturally find humorous, without worrying about who's watching, how we look, or what others will think. The advantage of humor is the opportunity to be fully engaged in the moment. Laughter has a novel way of putting you there with full attention, joyful and present.

Developing a humorous outlook also allows you to discover new and healthy ways to minimize stressful situations. Part of humor's therapy is not only in laughing with others but in giving yourself permission to laugh at yourself. It can help you to navigate life's disappointments and upsets, making your circumstances temporarily more tolerable as you develop new ways to reframe challenging issues. The best part of all is that humor, the "Vitamin H" of holistic medicine, is free, can be shared with anyone, and tends to be contagious.

Practice self-reflection

The practice of self-reflection is centuries old and rooted in some of the world's great spiritual traditions. Past advocates of this practice ranged from the Christian desert hermits to the Japanese samurai. Contemporary followers include Albert Schweitzer, Benjamin Franklin, and Bishop Fulton J. Sheen. However, one of the Founding Fathers of the United States, Benjamin Franklin, had a fairly comprehensive and systematic approach to the art of self-reflection. Franklin developed a list of "13 Virtues of Conduct" that he followed faithfully to his dying day. The list helped Franklin evaluate his conduct relative to a specific virtue, making self-reflection a cornerstone of his daily life.

Self-reflection is when we take time to look back on our lives, our actions, and our surroundings, or to align ourselves through meditation to bring us calm, clarity, and into the present moment. This introspection becomes a conscious effort to know more about our nature, evolving character, and purpose.

If you think about it, you never really multitask. You do several things in succession or alternatively, but rarely can you actually do several things *at the same time*. This new concept of time-saving multitasking robs quality, focus, and engagement from our tasks at hand. Focusing on whatever task you're doing is a form of daily meditation. Such a single-minded focus allows you to produce work that is of your own vision, reduces stress, and often improves work-related skills because of the intentional concentration that you apply. The opposite of this kind of focus would be to drive your car while you chat on a cellphone, apply makeup while peering in your visor mirror, pet the dog, sip a cold beverage, adjust the radio, and check out the scenery.

The many forms of self-reflection can open up new areas of character and self-awareness to explore. Its effect is healing and transformative.

The following sections present four styles that provoke a deeper awareness, sensitivity, and strength for the challenges we face.

Self-monitoring meditation

Self-monitoring is the awareness that you maintain of yourself in all that you do. This reflection takes the form of a daily, sometimes even momentary, accounting of your thoughts, behavior, and interactions with and to others. You put aside your self-absorption long enough to do a quick assessment of your behavior. Are you fair in your dealings with others? Sensitive to circumstances of the moment? Compassionate? Mechanically performing an activity with your mind in a distant place? Are you working toward your highest vision and not allowing your fears or self-limiting beliefs to hold you back?

Deep relaxation meditation

A deep relaxation meditation is a daily meditation that grounds your energy, produces a sustained calm, and gives you clarity and insight for the day ahead or the one just passing.

Can you sit in silence and quiet your inner noise, focusing on your breath, allowing all thoughts to drift by like clouds that you watch when laying on the grass during a sunny afternoon? In this state, you have no attachment to any thought. They float by, more follow, and they continue to pass, but all the while you focus on your breath, inhaling and exhaling.

By this focus, you liberate yourself from the grind of thinking. It's not easy, but with consistent practice, it becomes easier. The effects can be positively and profoundly sustaining, on physical, mental, and energetic levels. Essentially, it's a brief vacation to the world of renewal.

Meditation in action

Meditation in action may be one of the most difficult forms of meditation you do in daily life. It requires a mindset in which you remain focused on the present moment in all that you do. It requires immense concentration and total immersion into whatever you're doing. You become so absorbed in the moment that it feels timeless, and you find strength in your tasks because you're 100 percent present.

Meditation in nature

Try a nature meditation — whether it's beneath stormy clouds, before a dramatic sunset, within the sounds of crashing beach waves, within a forest environment, or beneath a brilliant full moon.

Say you've chosen a forest thicket to do your brief meditation. You sit comfortably on a tree stump, take some deep breaths, close your eyes, and go inside yourself. Immediately, you realize you are immersed in noise — the noise inside your head reminding you to finish a work task your associate asked you to complete; the noise nagging that your front automobile brakes need to be checked; the noise telling you not to forget to stop at the market to pick up some onions and salad greens; and countless other noises. As you sit in mediation, your body has slowed down, but your mind is still flying, thinking, worrying, and planning.

After some breathing and re-focusing, your mind begins to quiet down, and then you suddenly hear another kind of noise — the sounds of nature that you completely missed before: birds singing, the hum of crickets, the distant chirping of stream frogs, the wind rattling tree leaves, the whoosh of small birds darting by, the wind breezing by your ear. These are the sounds of nature that become pleasurably audible when your mind finally quiets. This type of meditation allows you to feel the bigger self and helps you become more attentive to things outside yourself.

Perfect the art of living: "Welcome to the picnic"

I had a Japanese philosophy teacher who taught macrobiotic theory and had a unique way of explaining the art of living. He explained his philosophy of life in a mesmerizing baritone with his thick accent articulating every word:

We have made a long journey from infinity to earth with a brief "stop-over." Maybe lasts 75 to 90 years. For you, I hope more. But soon, the visit is over. Then we go back infinity. Compare 3.2 billion years of human evolution to 80-year visit; it makes this visit very short — like the blink of eye. Just a short rest. Or maybe like an afternoon picnic, happy time. Time for friendship, time for sharing, time for play. Therefore, my opinion is, make life like a picnic. Happy time. Welcome to the picnic!

When I first heard this many years ago, I dismissed it as an amusing but simplistic philosophy. His accent and concept were entertaining but seemingly naive in scope. Years later, I read a quote by psychologist Eric Fromm: "Man is the only animal for whom his own existence is a problem he has to solve." Suddenly the words of my Japanese teacher echoed a renewed meaning. Maybe life *should* be like a picnic, I thought.

Over the years I've learned that one way to make this picnic more pleasurable and rewarding is by creating health that you have a measure of control over. Good health is the foundation for a joyful life. You benefit physically, emotionally, and spiritually when this foundation is strong.

Understanding the power of food and how it influences your quality of life is a good place to begin. The next step is discovering other ways to nourish your health — what works, what doesn't, and why. As you become strong in body and mind, you begin to enjoy an increasing measure of control over your life and body. Things work right. You develop the energy, endurance, and mental clarity to discover more effective solutions to personal challenges.

This is the beginning of true freedom — freedom from sickness, fear of sickness, and patterns of pessimism.

Welcome to the picnic! Make it memorable. Make it fun.

Chapter 3

Applying Macrobiotic Food Principles to Your Daily Diet

. . . .

. . . .

*W*e have the ability to condition our bodies and control our health so much more than we imagine. But most people don't take advantage of that capability, and their only dietary control is the use of stimulants or depressants: They drink coffee to get a jolt from the caffeine, or they have a cigarette for the stimulus of nicotine. By the end of the day, they're all keyed up, so having an alcoholic drink becomes more appealing as a way to come down. Beyond these extremes, few people really know how to influence their health, mood, and energy level with food.

Macrobiotic food principles offer a practical dietary structure to ensure you receive better nutritional balance and absorption. The seven common-sense principles presented in this chapter offer helpful ways to balance your nutrition, reduce cravings for foods that don't support your health, and make what you eat more satisfying and digestible.

The common-sense and time-tested food principles in this chapter complete the body-mind-spirit approach and act as an evolving foundation for good, sustaining health. This chapter also introduces the concept of *food energetics,* the unseen influence of foods' energetic structures.

Although the concept of eating fermented foods at first may seem a bit strange, it's really not when you look at some of the fermented foods we normally eat and the habits of culinary traditions. Have you heard about the "beneficial bacteria" that live in our gut? They help us break down and better absorb our food. This is one of the reasons why yogurt or *probiotic* (beneficial bacteria) supplements have been recommended. People who have been on antibiotics for a while tend to be more susceptible to colds, yeast infections, and immune weakness for a time after the round of their medication is finished. The reason? The antibiotics weaken our gut bacteria. The solution? Replace it every day with whole food fermentation. Sources include fermented Asian soy products (miso, tamari, umeboshi) or various pickles of some type made with a salt brine over a period of days, weeks, or months. Fermentation allows us to recover quicker, digest our food more effectively and absorb the strength from the pickling process.

Seven Macrobiotic Food Principles

Think of the seven macrobiotic food principles as the foundation from which you build new health and sensitivity. These principles, which come from rich cultural origins, are universal, sensible, and powerfully effective.

1. View your food choices in terms of principle foods, secondary foods, and pleasure foods.
2. Learn to emphasize seasonal and local foods.
3. Become mindful of quantity and quality.
4. Learn to avoid dietary extremes.
5. Become a *chewsy* eater — eat less, chew more.
6. Take the minimum required (the concept is called *vivre parvo*).
7. Use the *Power of Five* in food preparation: The five food groups, flavors, textures, cooking styles, and colors.

Principle, secondary, and pleasure foods

Western cultures have, for the most part, lost the idea of a principle food, where a meal is not a meal without one or two particular foods. A principle food acts as a central food or group of foods that the rest of the meal revolves around.

> ✔ **Principle foods** are basic sustenance foods, such as whole grains, vegetables, and beans. These foods provide a stabilizing order to daily meals.

✔ **Secondary foods** are supplemental foods that you add to principle foods. They can include grain products, sea vegetables, fruits, animal protein, and condiments. Secondary foods add balance to your diet.

✔ **Pleasure foods** are for those in good health and comprise small amounts of whatever you want (WYW).

Here's the breakdown of how much of these foods you should be eating:

✔ Principle Foods (70 to 75 percent of your diet)

    35 percent vegetables

    30 percent whole grain

    5 to 10 percent beans

✔ Secondary Foods (25 to 30 percent of your diet)

    5 percent grain products

    5 to 10 percent animal protein

    15 to 20 percent other secondary foods (sea vegetables, oils, meats, fruit, beverages) and pleasure foods (WYW)

I explain more about these food categories in the following sections.

Principle foods

A principle food, also known as a *staple food,* forms the basis of most traditional dietary templates. The most common principle foods throughout the agricultural world are whole grain cereals such as rice, barley, wheat, spelt, rye, maize, quinoa, millet, buckwheat, teff, amaranth, and wild rice (technically, a seed). In climates close to the equator, yams, taro, poi (made from cooked, mashed taro), potatoes, breadfruit, sago, plantains, and cassava also have been consumed as principle foods.

Whole cereal grains and beans, as principle foods, contain abundant vitamins, minerals, micronutrients, and long chain fibers. Considering the daily need for vegetables, particularly for Westerners, I also include vegetables on the principle category.

Almost every culture with a developed agriculture throughout the world eats principle foods with at least half their meals. Sit down for a meal in Japan, Korea, India, Ethiopia, Mexico, or Tibet and you can wager that cereals, beans or bean products, and various vegetable dishes will be central to the meal. In these places, a meal is deficient if it's without some sort of whole fiber, such as whole grain. In fact, the word *meal* means grain! Therefore, meal time, ideally, is a time for consuming whole grain.

Somehow, this idea of a principle food has been lost in many parts of the world. Here are some characteristics of principle foods:

- **Availability:** They should be available locally.

- **Economics:** They should be affordable. This is a social consideration, because foods that produce real health should be affordable by all.

- **Sustainability:** Principle foods should be able to support survival if eaten exclusively, at least for a short time.

- **Nutritious:** They should be able to enhance your health nutritionally as well as help regulate blood sugar.

- **Storage:** Principle foods should be able to withstand long periods of time in storage. Dried grains and beans can last years, if necessary, in cool storage.

- **Versatile:** Principle foods should have great versatility in preparation.

- **Taste:** The complex sugars in principle foods break down slowly, offering a natural and mild sweet taste that's as nourishing as it is satisfying.

For what is estimated to be a time span of 10,000 years, humanity's diet has revolved around principle foods. They were revered as the sacred source of life. I like to joke in seminars that the Bible doesn't say, "Give us this day our daily chocolate chip cookies," but rather it makes reference to whole grain as "our daily bread," the "staff of life."

Secondary foods

Secondary foods are nutritionally supportive to principle foods. They contain essential nutrients but are not foods that should be eaten in large proportions.

The following types of foods are considered secondary:

- **Animal protein:** Animal meats, such a red meat, poultry, eggs or fish, can sometimes enhance a meal or satisfy a nutritional craving, but their dietary necessity is questionable. If you want to include animal protein in your diet, the percentage should be very small. This is one of the reasons that I usually indicate "optional" after animal protein inclusions. Dairy food is not a recommended food or food group. If you want to have some dairy food, add it occasionally under the WYW category.

  Although very few vegetarian cultures existed historically, one thing that most cultures had in common was consuming a very low amount of animal protein. Typically, these foods were used sparingly, as a small side dish or even as a condiment, which is a major contrast from the modern boast of considering yourself a "steak and potatoes man." Animal protein, for nutritional, ecological, economic, health, and compassionate reasoning, isn't designed to be a principle food.

✔ **Fruit:** Even though it contains valuable vitamins and some fiber, fruit still contains simple sugar and, for recovering health, is often best taken in moderation, according to craving or social circumstance.

✔ **Sea vegetables:** Typically eaten fresh by many coastal cultures and dried, as storage, or for inland travel, sea vegetables are packed with important minerals that good health requires. Due to sodium content and mineral quality, these are not foods to eat abundantly, every day. This is not a rule, but more of a tendency.

✔ **Condiments:** Nut and seed condiments (*example*: almond, pumpkin, sunflower, or sesame seeds) make tasty condiments as do sea vegetable flakes (you can buy "nori" condiment or Dulse flakes at natural food stores), herbs, and spices.

Pleasure foods

This category can be very misleading. The basic philosophy behind pleasure foods is that, in good health, you should be free to enjoy everything. However, if you're attempting to recover from illness, it is best to eat from this category infrequently.

Eating *whatever you want* (WYW) means taking the smallest amount of the best quality of something you truly desire and allowing yourself to enjoy it fully without fear or worry about dropping dead within five minutes (okay, five minutes may be an exaggeration, but you get my point). If there's a food you feel you must have, seek out the best-quality version of it, and enjoy a small amount. No guilt or remorse is allowed. Sometimes those little pleasures can be medicinal, providing a soothing, even homeopathic effect (the principle of "like cures like") and often stopping the craving instantly.

If you're on a healing path, including a pleasure food category in your diet may be somewhat premature. I encourage you to reframe how you think about eating and your favorite goodies. When you're eating as a part of healing, you're not simply eating; instead, you're taking tasty daily medicine in the form of food for a brief period of time in order to assess its value in your healing process.

Sometimes I work with clients on a healing regime who are having cravings for unhealthy foods. I ask if they feel deprived, and if they answer yes, I ask, "What's the bigger deprival: not satisfying your sweet tooth for seven minutes, or life itself? Mentally, accepting life as the bigger deprival requires a shift in perspective. However, with craving strategies that can help reduce certain cravings for unhealthy treats while regulating blood sugar levels through more frequent eating, the likelihood of defeating a craving becomes easier.

Emphasize seasonal and local foods

In the days before refrigeration, air travel, agricultural chemicals, and mass production made it easy (or at least, easier) to import foods, people could consume only foods that grew within their locality and season, similar to animals in the wild. A large percentage of the foods imported today actually aren't suitable for everyday fare everywhere, because they grow in climates most compatible with their chemical make-up.

Eating local foods is beneficial because it

✔ Keeps you in tune with the energetic subtleties of nature.

✔ Tends to mean that fruits and vegetables taste better because they're allowed to ripen in nature because growers don't have to meet early packing and shipping demands for exportation.

✔ Tends to mean that produce is of healthier quality because it's handled less before it gets to you.

✔ Supports local agriculture and the local economy.

✔ Encourages responsible land development by giving local farmers and pasture owners economic reasons to allow their land to remain open and undeveloped.

✔ Supports efforts to protect against global warming by eliminating transportation pollution.

In warmer climates people tend to eat foods that are higher in simple sugar content (such as tropical fruits), large leafy greens, more raw vegetables, less whole grain, and less animal protein. However, as you look farther north into harsher weather extremes, you discover the need for increased cooking, dietary salt, reduced sweet foods, more grain, hearty dishes such as vegetable stews, and in some cases small amounts of animal protein. These foods inspire warmth and offer more concentrated energy as opposed to the more cooling effect of raw foods, fruits, and spices of warmer climates. It's not a matter of good and bad but of climatic utility.

Sometimes it's not possible to select locally grown food (you live in Indiana but the market sells kale from Arizona, rice from northern California and beans from Mexico). In that case, foods grown in the same latitude can suffice (don't be such an idealist — you may starve!) Make imported foods for the occasional specialty dish and enjoy their variety.

When I lived in a macrobiotic study house in Boston during the early '70s, we used to have several house members that would constantly complain of the cold. While the rooms were indeed cool, the degree of "cold" was relative to each individual. Eventually, it came to light that the complainers were the ones slipping out late at night and stuffing their faces with cheesecake and other kinds of sweet treats. Then they'd return home and raise the heat. Imagine that! Sneaky people, they were. Eventually, our household head put a sign on the wall above the thermostat: "Change your blood, not the thermostat!" That showed them! However, considering I was one of the complainers, it was an embarrassing but memorable lesson.

Be mindful of quantity and quality

Quantity changes quality. *Quantity* isn't just related to overconsumption. Quantity also refers to nutrient excess, such as too much fat, protein, or simple carbohydrates in your diet. The quantity of food, nutrients, and toxic elements from food and the environment can be excessive. Consuming excessive amounts of so-called good food can turn it into bad food during digestion, because overconsumption fosters acidity. Acidity in excess diminishes mineral status and, among other conditions, can be a cause of poor digestion, faulty absorption, and chronic fatigue.

Of all the longevity studies conducted in the last 25 years, the most notable have demonstrated that consuming smaller volumes of food produces better nutrient absorption, increased energy levels, and increased life span. Chronic overeating has been linked to depression, heart disease, cancer, acid reflux (also known as GERD), fatigue, stroke, and bulimia.

Frequently, people place excessive importance on quality of foods. Often, in telling me about their current health, a client will say, "Basically, I eat really *good* food" or "I eat very *well*!" These comments usually refer to the quality of their food, meaning that it's organic, imported, or purchased in health food stores. But that's not the real concern. The concentration of nutrients — simple carbohydrates, fat, or protein — in the food is key to how you assimilate and make full use of these nutrients. This is really the concept of balance. Eating good-quality food doesn't make it a balanced meal. Recognizing that you need to meet a daily quota of complex carbohydrates, protein, and fat is the first step toward creating a more balanced approach to your nutrition.

Avoid dietary extremes

The hallmark of good health is a balanced diet. Unfortunately, there's a lot of misconception as to what constitutes a balanced diet. A balanced diet is not a cookie in each hand. It's a varied diet of principle foods (whole grains, beans, vegetables, sea vegetables) and small amounts of secondary foods. These are traditional foundational foods of balance.

- **High alkaline** foods include sea salt, miso, and soy sauce.
- **Low alkaline** foods include vegetables and sea vegetables.
- **Low acid foods** include grains, breads, beans, and fish.
- **High acid** foods include fruit, sugar, vinegar, and alcohol.

If we place foods in a general scale of acid and alkaline extremes, you can see that principle and secondary foods exist more toward the middle — the safe area. Safe, in this context, means that they don't have excessive acid or alkaline properties, they don't elevate blood sugar, and they're packed with nutrients that can sustain us.

Your principle and secondary foods should come from the low alkaline and low acid groups. Eat high alkaline foods in small amounts, and save high acid foods for special occasions.

Eating excessive acidic foods can foster inflammation, fatigue, mineral loss, and immune weakness. Excessive alkaline foods also create some of the same symptoms. The key is balance and to be slightly more alkaline, as this is what our blood chemistry reveals.

Acidifying dietary factors in your diet come from the excessive consumption of foods containing various degrees of acidity, such as grain products, proteins, fruits, sugar, and vinegar. (Although whole grains are actually a mild acid, the acid content can be somewhat neutralized with the soaking of grain for several hours.) Thorough cooking, the use of sea salt, and ample chewing (saliva has alkaline enzymes) are ways to neutralize acid content of food. Non-food acid sources are principally stress, chemicals in the environment, and pollution. More than $3 billion is spent yearly on antacids — a direct result of poor food combinations, emotional eating, overeating, and acid-based foods.

Excessive acid can produce mild inflammation, causing tissues to swell and, in turn, aggravate joint health, possibly promote cyst or tumor growth, and eventually diminish the body's mineral reserves.

Alkalizing (or neutralizing) dietary factors come from the use of sea salt, reduced food volume, increased vegetable amounts, the inclusion of sea vegetables, and good chewing. Non-food alkaline influences include physical activity (excess acidity produces more muscle acids), breathing exercises with emphasis on exhalation, high altitudes, and calm, meditative states.

Too much alkalinity in the body can weaken you mineral status because minerals have to keep acids in check. Minerals neutralize excessive acids and in doing so, we lose part of these alkaline elements from our bones and digestive fluids. Excessive acid also promotes inflammation. As a matter of fact, any "–itis" condition (gastritis, arthritis, colitis, sinusitis, and so on) will be aggravated by the excess of acids. Because the blood controls its acid levels very carefully and because an excess can be fatal, our tissue fluids and cellular fluids get the brunt of acids.

Your bed is not a kitchen table!

Here's a great acid-generating experiment you can do: Eat a lot of food right before you go to bed! In fact, eat in bed if you can, and then go right to sleep. For one thing, you'll probably end up dreaming more. But although your sleep may be cerebrally entertaining, you'll wake up feeling as if a truck ran you over — that is, if you can manage to haul yourself out of bed at all. You'll feel sluggish and mentally dull, and you'll only want to return to sleep.

In Chinese medicine, it's said that the liver is the guardian of sleep. Deep, sound sleep allows you to enjoy wide-awake, energetic days. That's a good thing. Eating before bed invariably makes you awaken craving a stimulant, like coffee or sugar, just to get through your day. That's *not* a good thing.

But sometimes it's just hard to avoid eating close to bedtime. You've been busy with no time to eat dinner, and you finally arrive home late, famished, and dead tired. So, what do you do? In this case, eat a very small amount and sleep slightly reclined with several pillows. The reason why it's best to wait three hours before going to bed after eating is because this is usually the amount of time it takes for the stomach to empty. For maximum clarity of mind and physical energy for the coming day, not eating for three hours before you hit the sack is best.

Following a dietary path of whole grains, vegetables, beans, and sea vegetables with limited animal proteins (optional) and fruits offers a wide balance that can prove its merit fairly quickly. You'll have better nutrient absorption, greater vitality, increased endurance, and deeper sleep. You'll have a stronger immune system, and in general, your body will function with less of an effort.

Become a chewsy eater

The function of chewing, of grinding food into smaller pieces, exposes more surface area of the food to saliva, which pre-digests foods with its alkaline enzymes. This is the first stage of digestion. Therefore, it's essential to chew your food well for easier digestion and absorption.

The ancient Chinese written language character that describes chewing is composed of the ideograms for *God* and *work*. Perhaps this meant that by chewing, you can digest more thoroughly, eat less, absorb more nutrients, maintain low acidity, develop a deeper calm, feel more present, and as a result feel closer to the spirit because you're not hindered or controlled by a body burdened with toxins or blood sugar swings. In such a calm state, you feel more sensitized and receptive.

I've attended lectures by numerous macrobiotic teachers who echo the party line of chewing each mouthful 50 or 100 times. To me, that seems borderline compulsive, and my impulse is to suggest they get a life!

Instead of counting chews every time you eat, my suggestion is to do this for only one meal per week, and concentrate on taste at your other meals. Allow that sensory experience to encourage continued chewing instead of strict self-imposed rulings that make meals somber and mechanical. That one meal each week in which you chew diligently will make you more conscious of chewing for the rest of your meals. Just chew, taste your food, and enjoy.

Vivre parvo: Take the minimum required

Vivre parvo is a Latin phrase that describes the ideal way for achieving maximum health: taking only what your body requires for nourishment and in terms of how you live. At the root of the gross consumptive mentality for super-sized food portions and the accumulation of material stuff is a loss of gratitude for what's been given, fear that there won't be enough, and an insensitivity to know just how much is really needed.

For most human organisms, excessive fat, animal protein, and concentrated sweeteners — all modern staple foods — may be temporarily satisfying, but in excess they're potentially deadly.

If you have strong passions and things that you want to do in life, eating the minimum, keeping slightly hungry, and being active come naturally because you're feeding a bigger appetite. But if you're bored by your current life, there's no incentive to suddenly discipline yourself.

Consider the volume of food you consume. Cup your hands together as if scooping water from a stream. This hand-shaped bowl is equal to the size of your stomach (minus the top cover). Visualize the amount of food you had in your last meal. Is it bigger than the little bowl your palms create? You're likely to be surprised at how much you eat — and how little of it that your body actually absorbs — when you think of it this way.

Use the "power of five"

An old concept from Chinese medicine, the *power of five* offers your daily food preparation an enhanced sense of variety, helps sustain balance, and adds taste satisfaction to your eating. In macrobiotics, food has five elements, each of which has five variations; here's a breakdown:

- **Food group:** Grains, beans, vegetables, fruits, and animal protein
- **Flavor:** Salty, sweet, sour, bitter, and pungent

> ✔ **Texture:** Watery (like soup), firm (like veggies), crunchy (think crackers), creamy (pudding), and chewy (like grains)
>
> ✔ **Cooking styles:** Steamed, sautéed, water-fried, raw, and grilled or baked
>
> ✔ **Color:** Green, yellow-brown, orange, red, and white

The Western diet is so full of tastes and textures that you can hardly blame someone sitting down to their first grain and vegetable meal for complaining, "It's so bland!"

Different tastes, colors, and textures add a refreshing sense of variety, making the food more palatable and appealing. Eventually, you may prefer simpler tastes and won't need to doctor everything you eat with spices or accents, but for certain occasions, medicinal dishes, introductory meals, and so on, the list of five elements can prove invaluable.

Make sure your meal contains different textures, varied colors, numerous tastes, and a mixture of cooking styles. Typically, the taste people miss most when switching to a grain and vegetable-based diet is the crunchy taste. Be crouton savvy! Small bits of crust (essentially, croutons) in a soup offer a contrast of textures, just like popular boxed crunchy breakfast cereal and the addition of milk. Extremes in texture can be very satisfying.

Think about this: What really makes fish and chips appealing for most people? It's what they put on it! Additions can include salt (for its obvious flavor), ketchup (sweet), vinegar (sour), maybe a spicy dip (pungency), and cole slaw (cooling taste to balance pungent flavors).

The proven virtues of frequent small meals

People who consume smaller and more frequent meals tend to have lower cholesterol, lower blood pressure, and more regulated blood sugar than those who eat fewer, larger meals, according to a study conducted by researchers from the United States Agricultural Research Service's Beltsville Human Nutrition Research Center and the National Institute on Aging's Intramural Research Program.

In the study, a small group of volunteers ate either one meal per day or an average three square meals per day for eight weeks. After that time, they switched to the other diet for another eight weeks. The total calories consumed each day were the same in both groups.

When participants ate one high-calorie meal per day, they lost small amounts of weight and body mass. However, they experienced noticeable increases in both total and LDL (bad) cholesterol levels and blood pressure. They had higher morning fasting and all-day blood sugar levels; longer-lasting increased blood sugar following meals; and a delayed response to insulin, a sugar-regulating hormone. Each of these blood sugar disruptions is a precursor to diabetes.

How about the combination of soup and oatmeal? Yeah, bad choice. It's not an appealing combination, because their textures are similar. However, soup and bread is the yin and yang of texture: something dry, something liquid. A perfect partnership. After eating pot-cooked brown rice with steamed vegetables for a number of days, you'll kill for a piece of bread if you're new to whole-food eating. It's not the bread you're craving but rather the broader range of textures that we are so accustomed to eating.

Table 3-1 lists some examples of the unique tastes that can be added to different foods. Though most foods have components of each taste, we classify a food by its *predominant flavor*.

The more tastes you have within a meal, the more satisfying. For example, you can see kale, tamari, and lemon in the table. You can steam kale easily enough. What can make it especially tasty and more appealing is to combine one or two more tastes with it. You can mix equal parts natural soy sauce (tamari) with fresh lemon juice and use this as a light dressing mixed into the steamed kale. It creates a satisfying citrus and light salt taste mixture that ends up being a combination of three tastes.

Table 3-1		The Five Tastes		
Bitter	*Salty*	*Sweet*	*Sour*	*Pungent*
Kale	Sea Salt	Corn	Lemon	Ginger
Collards	Sea Vegetables Tamari	Carrots	Lime	Garlic
Arugula	Miso	Squash	Sauerkraut	Raw Onions
Parsley	Sesame Salt	Yams	Umeboshi Plum	White Radish
Endive	Umeboshi Plum	Parsnips	Fermented Dishes	Red Radish
Celery	Pickles (Salt)	Fruits	Tamarind	Pickles (Tart)
Mustard Greens		Cooked Onions		Wasabi
Grain Beverage		Cooked Grain		Spices
Bay Leaves		Cooked Cabbage		Allspice
		Cinnamon		

Colors cater to our psychological appetite. If it looks pleasing on a plate, your appetite is likely to be stimulated. But from a visual perspective, a plain brown bowl of simple brown lentils really isn't very attractive. But, there's hope! Switch to a contrasting colored bowl, add a garnish of parsley and maybe some carrot gratings . . . and voilà! You've dressed it up and made it look more appetizing. This sort of change can make a big difference to someone who's first attempting to eat grain and vegetables. Think visual.

The Fermented Food Advantage

It is a fact that fruits ferment naturally. You can also assume because of this fact that fermentation has preceded human history. Fermentation used in the winemaking process dates back more than 8,000 years from evidence found in the Caucasus area of Georgia, USSR. Most research cites the Chinese as the first culture to develop vegetable fermentation.

The benefit of fermentation is from the conversion of sugars and other carbohydrates from grains into beer, juice into wine, carbohydrates into carbon dioxide to leaven bread, and the natural complex carbohydrates in vegetables into preservative organic acids.

Fermentation technology has five substantial reasons that make it unique:

- ✔ It adds different flavors, aromas, and textures to your daily diet.
- ✔ As a result of lactic acid, alcohol acetic acid and alkaline (salt) fermentation, foods can be preserved for longer periods of time.
- ✔ Fermentation adds a rich enhancement of essential amino acids, essential fatty acids, protein, vitamins, and necessary gut micro-organisms.
- ✔ Fermentation detoxes the foods involved over its period of pickling.
- ✔ Fermentation requires less cooking, making it more economical in fuel economy.

At first, the idea of fermented foods may be a bit repulsive, typically conjuring images of a meal plate resembling rotting garden compost. However, that's not the case. Fermented foods have occupied a definitive place in many cultural diets for thousands of years, and they can add remarkable flavor, zest, and variety to most dishes.

In a macrobiotic eating plan, fermented foods help the digestion of fats, complex carbohydrates, and proteins, rendering the digesting food easier to absorb.

Historically, one of the most important reasons for fermenting vegetables, sea vegetables, grains, and beans was to preserve nourishment through harsh weather conditions when fresh foods weren't available. In many Western countries, before refrigeration, foods were dried, pickled, salted, and fermented and then stored in a pantry. Common fermented foods included sourdough bread, sauerkraut (fermented cabbage), aromatic cheese, meat, wine, beer, vegetable pickles (preserved in both vinegar and salt), salted fish, cured ham, and more.

Because fermentation doesn't involve cooking (unlike canning), it preserves some nutrients. Properly fermented foods have the superior health advantage of being nutrient rich and full of fiber, containing plentiful amounts of beneficial bacteria that strengthen intestinal flora. Fermentation makes some minerals more available for absorption in the body, as well as B12 production, while increasing levels of other vitamins, trace minerals, and enzymes. The predominant benefit of adding a small amount of fermented foods to your daily diet comes from its contribution of positive gut bacteria that it provides.

Throughout this book, I present macrobiotics in a multicultural light, but some of the Asian varieties of fermented food technology are just too beneficial to pass up introducing — particularly in regard to healing. Of the many varieties of alkaline fermented foods using sea salt (as opposed to foods fermented with vinegar, such as summer pickles), the ones I've chosen to cover in the following sections tend to have more taste appeal.

Miso

The Japanese word *miso* literally translates as "source of taste." Miso is a savory, high-protein, fermented soybean paste used in many ways but most frequently as a seasoning or soup base. Typically fermented for one to three years, it's made from soy beans, rice (or barley), sea salt, water, and a vegetable culture that contains living enzymes that aid digestion. Miso offers a hearty blend of carbohydrates, vitamins, minerals, vegetarian protein, and essential oils. The older and darker the miso, the more medicinal it is.

Miso's delicious and fragrant aroma is reminiscent of beef broth. In fact, I often refer to it as "vegetarian beef broth bouillon paste." It's estimated that over 65 percent of the Japanese population begins the day with a warm cup of miso soup. Miso's alkaline properties provide a gentle wake-up call that endures throughout the morning.

Miso happens to be a powerhouse of nutrition — a concentrated source of protein that contains 17 amino acids and trace nutrients. It also contains linoleic acid and lecithin, which dissolve cholesterol and make the arteries softer and more elastic, helping to prevent arteriosclerosis and high blood pressure.

The top five worst-tasting fermented foods

If the idea of consuming a food that punches you in the nose like a stinky fist is appealing, you may want to try the following five foods, which were voted in a recent survey as "The Worst-Tasting Fermented Foods." Keep in mind the adages "to each his own" and "one person's delight is another's disgust." Opinions are always subjective. Still, here are some prejudiced verdicts:

✔ Fermented squid guts, or Japanese *shiokara: "Nothing more revolting."*

✔ Pickled pork rinds (American): *"Akin to gnawing on grandmother's thigh."*

✔ Fermented fish sauce, or Vietnamese *nouc mam: "Stench of rotting fish."*

✔ Fermented shark, or Icelandic *hákarl:* "An *ammonia taste you'll gag on."*

✔ Fermented soybeans, or Japanese *natto:* "Smells like ripe feet."

One of the easiest ways to use miso paste is to dilute it in any hot soup, particularly vegetable or bean soup, in a measurement of approximately 1 round teaspoon per serving.

Natural soy sauce

When most people think of soy sauce, they think of those little packets tossed in with Chinese takeout that contain an almost black, salty, thin liquid that's liberally poured over most dishes. Think again. Real soy sauce is light-years from its artificially made commercial cousins. Traditional natural soy sauce is carefully brewed from one to three years and usually contains only grain, bean, sea salt, water, and a grain mold used to initiate fermentation. Most commercial soy sauce sold is aged for several weeks to a month and loaded with sugar, yeast, MSG (monosodium glutamate), assorted chemicals, coloring, and preservatives.

The two common varieties of soy sauce, *tamari* (without wheat) and *shoyu* (containing wheat), have a deep robust flavor and fragrant earthy bouquet as the result of long, slow fermentation. The word tamari is derived from the Japanese verb *tamaru,* meaning "to accumulate." This refers to tamari being a liquid by-product of miso fermentation.

Tamari is a good source of vitamin B3 and a healthy source of vitamins, minerals, and protein. Tamari stimulates the secretion of digestive fluids in the stomach while having a preservative effect on food. It also helps stimulate the growth of healthy bacterial flora within the intestines. It's preferably used toward the end of cooking, as opposed to being added afterward as a condiment.

Tofu

Tofu, which literally means *bean curd,* has been an economical food and a central part of Asian cuisine for over 2,000 years. Well known for its exceptional nutritional benefits as well as versatility in preparation, tofu is made by curdling soya milk, or the liquid from boiled soybeans, with a coagulant in order to produce a food with the consistency of soft cheese. To many, it's pretty bland, but fortunately, tofu easily absorbs the flavors of whatever it's cooked with. You can slice it, dice it, press it, cube it, mash it, or boil it in soups, or you can include it in fried dishes, dips, sauces, dressings, or desserts.

Considering the tofu-making process, it's not exactly a whole food and as such was traditionally used sparingly. However, in recent years, tofu has become a ubiquitous presence on the natural foods scene. You can find tofu in many natural food restaurants and delis, as a dish fried or scrambled, in spiced or herbed baked blocks, and in numerous desserts, such as ice creams, puddings, and shakes. Recently, there has been an anti-tofu backlash screaming to consumers that tofu is an *unhealthy* food.

Eating as little as 35 grams a day (just 10 grams over the FDA recommended amount) is thought, according to medical research, to cause thyroid function suppression within three months in healthy adult men and women. However, this has become an argument of volume. While soy has been consumed throughout Asia for thousands of years, their overall consumption is very small compared to North Americans, who use it in a multitude of soy products, ice creams, milks, cheeses, and so forth. That old adage "quantity changes quality" clearly applies here.

A small amount of tofu on occasion can enhance health while adding delicious variety to meals. Go to any Japanese restaurant and order a miso soup. Unfortunately, it's usually a packaged miso powder with MSG and a mix of unhealthy additives; however, note how much tofu is in the soup; you'll see a couple of cubes floating around. That's it! Yet, in most natural food restaurants, you can see large slabs of tofu being served as side dishes. We are clearly eating too much and rather than take the typical "all or nothing" position, minimum servings of tofu can be a healthy vegetable quality protein addition to your diet.

Tempeh

A controlled fermentation process that binds hulled, cooked soybeans into a cake form makes *tempeh,* which originated in Indonesia and is still a staple there. The beans are mixed with a mold spore starter (a culture of *Rhizopus oligosporusor*) and incubated for two days. The white mycelium of the *Rhizopus* vegetable mold keeps the soybean packed together to form a sliceable cake. As a result of the fermentation process, the soy protein in tempeh becomes more digestible.

Now sold not only in health food stores but also throughout mainstream supermarkets, tempeh is fiber-rich and a healthy source of vegetable protein, minerals, and soy isoflavones and saponins — a class of phytochemical compounds found abundantly in plant sources.

Containing only 157 calories per 100-gram serving, tempeh is low in saturated fat and contains a generous source of B vitamins, iron, calcium, and lecithin, plus essential polyunsaturates such as linoleic acids. These acids are important because they help emulsify, disperse, and eliminate cholesterol deposits and other fatty acids that frequently accumulate in and around vital organs and throughout the bloodstream.

Tempeh is always cooked before eating; you can steam, boil, bake, or sauté it. You can enjoy it with a wide variety of grains, vegetables, or noodles, or use it in soups, salads, and sandwiches. You also can serve tempeh as a delicious main course in place of meat. For many, tempeh has become a protein backbone of vegetarian diets.

In 2008, a new form of tempeh based on barley and oats in place of soybeans was developed by scientists at the Swedish Department of Food Sciences. The benefit of this tempeh version is that it can be produced in regions where it's not possible to cultivate soybeans.

Umeboshi plums

Believed to have originated in China over 2,000 years ago, *umeboshi* (oo-mi-bow-shi) plums, commonly called the "King of Alkaline Foods," are actually a species of apricot called *prumnus mume*. In Japanese, *ume* identifies the plum and *boshi* means "dried."

The plums' abundant citric acid bonds with minerals to help the intestines absorb their alkaline minerals, such as magnesium, calcium, and iron, from ingested foods with ease. Citric acid also neutralizes the lactic acid in your tissues and blood.

In experiments during the 1950s, researchers extracted antibiotic substances from umeboshis. This extract was successful in destroying dysentery and staphylococcus germs. In 1968, an extract isolated from the ume was found to have a germicidal effect on the tuberculosis bacteria.

The plums are mostly valued as an alkalizing digestive aid and an appetite stimulant. It's said that taking 10 grams of umeboshi can neutralize the acidity created by consuming 100 grams of sugar. Small amounts of umeboshi eaten with complex carbohydrates or beans help digestion and absorption. The standard Japanese folk remedy for colds is soft whole rice cooked overnight (called *okayu*) with umeboshi. The plums offer a delicious tangy, salty taste to salad dressings, sauces, vegetable dishes, and dips.

Sauerkraut

Sauerkraut is a decidedly German word (meaning "sour cabbage") for a fermented food that may have originated in China before spreading throughout the European continent thanks to Mongol warriors. It's finely shredded, white cabbage fermented by lactic acid bacteria that ends up with a distinctive tangy, sour flavor. Often confused with cole slaw (a raw cabbage and carrot mixture that gets its sour, acidic taste from vinegar), sauerkraut is commonly used as a garnish with or in sandwiches, with meats and cheeses, and in soups and warm salads.

Researchers have found that the process of fermenting cabbage produces *isothiocyanates,* which are known to prevent cancer growth — particularly in the colon, liver, lung, and breast. Sauerkraut also has strong detoxifying properties. Containing plentiful amounts of probiotic bacteria, which create lactic acid, sauerkraut aids digestion by restoring a healthy balance of beneficial bacteria throughout the intestinal tract.

Not all sauerkraut provides bacterial benefit. Most of the sauerkraut sold in mainstream supermarkets is pasteurized. The pasteurization process destroys all beneficial bacteria, so be sure to read labels carefully and select unpasteurized sauerkraut from health-oriented natural food companies. It's helpful for grain and bean digestion and makes overall nutrient assimilation more effective. Make sure to check expiration dates on all fermented food products.

Vegetable pickles

Vegetable pickles are easy to make and usually only require a salt brine from a salted fermented product (miso or tamari) or plain sea salt. The benefit of vegetables pickles is that they provide a form of alkalinity that you take in very small quantities with your main meals (lunch and dinner, ideally). While this may be novel to a fast-food culture, it has been a part of multi-cultural diets for thousands of years. You can see remnants of this in some food combinations: When you order corned beef in delis, you get a pickle, which helps the digestion of the beef; hot dogs traditionally get sauerkraut; and the dill pickle has been an American culinary staple for over a hundred years. But pickles are not a side dish — they are a small compliment to the meal. Eat too much and the salt will make you thirsty or stimulate sweet cravings.

The soy controversy

The growing popularity of soy products has led to much controversy about their health and safety. Suddenly, soy products are being vilified and branded as toxic. This may be a gross exaggeration, but there's some truth to the idea of the lowly soybean as not all that people-friendly. Soybeans are high in non-nutritive phytic acid, or phytates. *Phytates* are organic acids that exist in the bran, or hull, of all seeds and that can block the uptake of some essential minerals, such as calcium, magnesium, zinc, and iron within the intestinal tract. One of the best ways to significantly reduce phytates from soybean products is through fermentation. Fermented soy foods such as miso and tempeh supply excellent nourishment and are easily assimilated.

The real soy controversy is related to non-fermented soy products such as soymilk, soy nuts, fresh green soybeans, soy sprouts, and soy flour. These products are typically recommended because they contain *isoflavones;* until recently, isoflavones were the nutritional darlings in cancer research. Because the chemical structure of isoflavones is similar in structure to the human hormone estrogen, they effectively combat the action of estrogen and therefore have been touted as offering protection against breast cancer, prostate cancer, symptoms of menopause, osteoporosis, and heart disease. However, some critics warn that isoflavones can increase hyperthyroidism and formation of goiters.

Fermenting soy halts the effect of phytic acid and increases the availability of isoflavones. The fermentation process also creates the probiotic bacteria (the "good" bacteria) that your gut requires, such as lactobacilli, which has been shown to increase the availability, quantity, digestibility, and absorption of nutrients in the body. Fermented soy products include miso, natural soy sauce, natto, and tempeh. What nutritional researchers agree on is that, rather than specific nutrient content, the cultured soy medium is what's responsible for fermented soy's health benefits.

There are many types of pickles that you can simply make at home. Many recipes use a pickle press. Typically made of hard plastic, the Japanese pickle press allows you to make delicious, quick pickles by placing chopped and lightly salted vegetables in the plastic bucket, locking the lid, and adjusting the press. The pressure and salt cause the juices to seep from the vegetables, forming a mild brine. You can make pickles in this way from three hours to three days. Simply drain of the brine (makes a hearty soup stock addition) and add small amounts to your meal.

Another favorite is the miso pickle. Miso pickles are probably the simplest pickle you can make. Known as miso-suke (miso pickles!) in Japan, this is one of the oldest known varieties of pickle making. Requiring a minimum of 1 to 3 months to make, some can be pickled for years! Simply obtain a large amount of miso, slice up some carrots, onions, radishes, turnips, or any other vegetable, and embed them within the miso. That's it! Here are some examples:

One way to do this is with a large glass baking dish where you place a thin bottom layer of miso, layer sliced carrots, and then apply another layer on top. On top of that second layer, place additional vegetables (onions or leeks, for example) and then another layer of miso. Typically, you can get about three to five layers in most baking dishes. Cover and place in an extremely cool pantry or a section of your refrigerator for 1 to 3 months. When you are ready to sample, take several varieties from the miso, and place them in an empty jar from which you can use some for various meals.

Chapter 4

Macro Boot Camp: Basic Training

. . . .

In This Chapter

▶ Exploring your eating habits in terms of the Seven Levels of Judgment

▶ Using the 12 Barometers of Good Health to gauge your overall health level

▶ Tracing the digestive process

▶ Explaining the acid/alkaline connection and busting common misconceptions

. . . .

*B*asic training usually begins with introductory stuff — essentials that you need to know before you're actually let loose in the field. But this chapter isn't your average basic training; I don't yell in your face or make you do push-ups and dig foxholes. I just give you some information to read, reflect on, and see how it may apply to you.

In this chapter, I go over some essential information that explains how you can become better acquainted with your current state of health and how food has the power to heal and transform.

I also explore the Seven Levels of Judgment that offer progressive guidelines for self-challenge, and I explain the concept of acid and alkaline and reveal some time-tested secrets for balancing food groups, strengthening health, and promoting longevity.

The Seven Levels of Judgment

In the 1940s, George Ohsawa designed *the Seven Levels of Judgment* (oddly similar to a system created years earlier by George Gurdjieff) as a way of categorizing a person's judgment growth. These stages of judgment simply relate to stages of human awareness and evolving judgment in our maturing process:

- ✔ Sensory judgment
- ✔ Emotional judgment
- ✔ Intellectual judgment

✔ Social judgment

✔ Philosophical judgment

✔ All-embracing judgment

The lengths of the various levels differ widely. Physical and sensory responses can change in seconds or minutes. Emotional feelings last considerably longer (often days), and the influence of intellectual beliefs can endure for years. Social ideas and movements can last hundreds of years, whereas philosophical schools of thought, such as religions and other ideological systems, can last thousands. In an all-embracing judgment, no time limits prevail — its influence is universal and unending.

One of the noble goals of macrobiotic practice is to elevate your judgment. Making your body healthy and your mind clear is the first foundational step in that process. Using daily life macrobiotic principles and discovering peaceful ways to unify opposites and seek balance is the work of higher judgment.

When we are healthy, have established a reliable sensitivity, and understand how to manage our health, we should be free to eat anything, adapting to different circumstances and eating in a conscious way with pleasure that satisfies each level of eating. Based on our education, environment, personality, upbringing, impulse, and momentary needs, we use many judgment levels in the course of a day. The following sections delve into those judgment levels.

Physical judgment

Physical judgment involves eating mechanically or impulsively. The physical approach to eating is demonstrated by eating without consciousness; rushing to the refrigerator as soon as you enter your home and eating whatever you can to calm your appetite or eating at established mealtimes (even if you aren't hungry) because "it's time to eat" are examples of physical eating. This level of impulsive judgment begins at birth. Babies respond automatically to external stimuli, such as hunger, cold, heat, and so on. Even adults sometimes respond impulsively, such as eating whatever you can get your hands on when hungry and no food has been prepared.

Sensory judgment

Sensory judgment involves the recognition of color, smell, taste, touch, and sound; it begins to develop within a week of birth. The sensory aspect of eating is about stimulating your psychological appetite by varying the tastes of different foods in your meal (salty, sour, sweet, bitter, pungent); utilizing different colors on a plate to represent a full range of phytonutrients; being conscious of the main textures (watery, firm, crunchy, creamy, chewy); and carefully placing foods visually on the plate to stimulate psychological appetite.

Emotional judgment

Emotional judgment stems from emotional attachments to certain foods, habits, and so on. Approximately one month after birth, emotional judgment begins to take root as a baby's personality begins to unfold and she responds to feelings, distinguishes like from dislike, and so on. The emotional aspect of eating is about the feelings you associate with cooking for others, creating new tastes, and finding comfort in using healthier ingredients to recreate old favorites.

Intellectual judgment

Intellectual judgment is driven by nutritional concepts and theories, as well as scientific validation. For people in my lecturing audience that may be prone to a character that thinks predominantly on this level, I would emphasize the *intellectual* theory behind this way of eating; how we could reduce our excessive dietary acid and improve digestion, our assimilation and intake of different vitamin and mineral matrixes; and the value of adding a small amount of fermentation to our daily diet for good intestinal bacterial health and better nutrition. These are all intellectual concepts — "pertaining to intellect."

Around the age of four years, children's personalities become formed, and the reasoning function of the brain begins developing: They become more inquisitive, ask questions, and respond to ideas and concepts and judge them as true or untrue. This progress is the beginning of assumption, conceptualization, analysis, and more-developed mental activities.

Social judgment

Social judgment stems from the social aspects of eating: economics, moral codes, family, politics, and so on. The social impact of eating foods is to be aware of ecological factors and reduce waste in food cultivation; look for foods grown in your area, support local farmers, and don't have pesticides or herbicides that end up polluting the environment; and consider how grain, beans, and vegetables can substantially lower food bills.

By the age of 6, children begin to respond to examples of social behavior; they like conforming to friends and seek to follow social behavior patterns. At this level they become aware of right and wrong, proper and improper, and flexible and rigid.

Philosophical judgment

Philosophical judgment is driven by ideological traits such as doctrines or established religious customs and traditions. These traditions were originally part of the foundations of these teachings; although many of them have fallen by the wayside, some (such as kosher eating or making specific dishes for established celebrations or holidays) still remain.

Also known as *ideological judgment,* this level is based on the experiences and challenges of our growth, successes, and failures. Here, our consciousness develops toward a more philosophical perspective. We begin to question life and seek deeper and more personally significant meaning. All traditional religions and spiritual schools of thought begin at this level. However, this level still contains a dualistic (opposing) perspective such as the division of good and bad: justice and injustice, positive and negative, friends and foes, capitalism and communism, and so on.

All-embracing judgment

All-embracing judgment (which Ohsawa called *supreme judgment*) is the level of universal love and absolute freedom where we are free to embrace all. Here, we are free to play among each level of judgment, according to need. We can eat anything with great joy and appreciation and without fear.

Evaluating Your Health: 12 Barometers

A great way to evaluate your general health and longevity potential is to compare your health with the 12 barometers discussed in the following sections. Each barometer represents an important health quality; in fact, some of these conditions are actually questions that most physicians are trained to ask their patients during a general check-up. Collectively, these barometers reveal the overall quality of your health. Use them as a checklist to determine what areas of your health need attention.

Energy

By far, energy is a main barometer of good health. All human activities — healing, self-expression, self-care, relationships, work life, and so on — require energy. One of the main problems people face today is the "energy crisis" happening in their own bodies. They have become dependent on stimulants (such as sugar, caffeine, and salt) to boost tired, deficient bodies, as well as depressants (alcohol, medication, and so on) to calm down frenetic ones, with no middle ground.

And from triple-caffeinated soft drinks to double espressos and herbal concoctions, they've become addicted to the temporary rush of stimulants. But what happens when you take away the stimulants? Suddenly, you feel like a walking coma. Your body has become so used to stimulants that your natural state of energy is woefully deficient. A flexible whole foods macrobiotic dietary approach can help eventually restore your energy to optimum levels and in the process give you a larger perspective of what it's like to have energy to spare without the need for stimulants or the down swings that come along with them!

Appetite

This general category encompasses the many appetites we have for food, curiosity, sex, intellectual exploration, meaning, and so on. "How's your appetite?" is one of the first questions a competent physician asks a patient. A hearty appetite is a positive sign of sound health, so if you find that your appetite has become consistently low, that may be a cause for concern.

Bowel regularity

On a varied eating plan with whole grains, vegetables, and beans as *principle foods* (the main foods of grain, vegetables, and beans that you eat as staple foods), you're likely to have a very healthy movement once daily. Here's where the discussion get a bit graphic, but stay with me. I'm not talking about a token bowel movement but rather something along the lines of "the mother of all bowel movements." Truth be told, grain-eaters often have movements that empty out the entire descending colon, plus some from the transverse colon (perhaps totaling 12 to 18 inches) once daily. Transit time (from mouth to exit) varies from 16 to 22 hours in a healthy colon but for some can be up to seven days! The bowel movement should not be sticky (a possible sign of excess gluten) but instead easy to discharge and without the proverbial stink that can clear a room.

Believe it or not, that wickedly foul bowel odor is an indicator of poor fermentation in the colon. This olfactory assault is based on excessive fats, bad fats (trans fats, rancid fats, and so on), excessive sugar and animal proteins, and the time the food remains in the colon. A healthy colon will pass its entire contents within a 17 to 24 hour period.

Yes, all this bowel talk may sound uncomfortably vivid, but it's a fact of traditional whole foods eating. It also makes for memorable off-the-wall conversation at social gatherings.

Good deep sleep

The ability to quickly fall into a deep sleep and then awaken and spring to action is a sign of good health. But if you awaken feeling like you've been run over by an 18-wheeler, you're not getting the kind of sleep that results in a well-rested and energized body. Good sleep is one of the keys to strengthening immunity and fortifying your body to better cope with daily stresses. Ideally, sleep medication shouldn't be necessary; in a well-fed macrobiotic body, a couple of pre-bedtime yoga stretches and some deep breaths usually ensure that you don't have to count sheep. You may discover that six-and-a-half to seven hours is adequate and that you often awaken automatically, promptly, and ready to take on your day.

Eating late at night is a poor yet common strategy for falling sleep; although it can make you fall into a groggy slumber, it often results in endless dreaming, disturbed rest, indigestion (from over acidity), and often a fatiguing next day. A full sleep schedule of dreaming may sound entertaining, but it doesn't engender the restful sleep you need.

Emotional stability

The highs and lows of blood sugar can make you moody to both extremes; either you're feeling happy, positive, energetic, and whistling with energy, or you're depressed, negative, fatigued, and everything feels like an effort. The one commonly recognized benefit to eating whole complex carbohydrates is that they help to regulate blood sugar. Obviously, emotional instability can have many complex psychological and even neurological origins, but balancing your daily nourishment provides a strong foundation for creating emotional stability.

Cravings

Pay attention to your *cravings* — foods your body tells you to eat — because they happen for some very specific reasons. In many cases, cravings signal certain dietary imbalances that you can fix by eating regularly to maintain your blood sugar and reducing dietary extremes (eating less sugar, less animal protein, and minimal dietary salt). They can also tell you whether you're headed toward nutritional deficiencies.

Cravings can also have psychological and sentimental sources (such as "my dad used to buy me that type of chocolate"). Many people use certain foods as a sort of reward system or for emotional comfort. If you can remove the physical stimulus behind a craving, the craving often deceases or goes away entirely.

Physical flexibility

One of the marvels of a newborn is their natural flexibility. Their muscles seem so pliable and relaxed. Compare this with old age and the typical senior citizen's body that has lost not only its flexibility but also its resiliency and you have a strong contrast. Traditional Chinese medicine has long equated good health with physical flexibility. However, good flexibility doesn't come solely from habitual stretching — the way you eat can also influence your muscle, joint, and spinal health. Poor eating habits can increase your acidic body fluid profile, contributing to muscle hardness, but a balanced whole food macrobiotic diet minimizes those muscle acids. (See "Understanding the Acid and Alkaline Picture" later in this chapter for more on how food affects your acidic profile.) These effects — reduced muscular hardness, better immune resiliency, and a body more responsive to maintaining the benefits of being stretched consistently — mean more natural flexibility. Combine this macrobiotic diet with a regular yoga practice or sustained stretching for even better results.

Body pain

Pain, for all its inconvenience, is another way your body speaks to you. Most people relate to pain as an uninvited guest that needs to be handled symptomatically — with medication. Rarely do they question why they're in pain and what they can do to get rid of it and prevent it from returning. The quick fix of medication is occasionally necessary for pain that is difficult to manage (because this state can become an immune drain), but be sure to address the dietary issues behind your pain. On a dietary level, what aggravates this pain? Do certain foods contribute to internal inflammation, causing your muscles to expand and pressure sensitive nerves? Headache, lower backache, menstrual pain, muscle pain, and joint pain are some of the everyday pains that we take for granted and don't associate with faulty diet. Pain isolates you from life. Pain, for all its inconvenience, is another way your body speaks to you.

Memory

How's your memory? Do you have equal recall between short-term and long-term memory? Memory qualifies as a barometer of good health because it's an indicator of good circulatory flow within the brain and a circulation that isn't burdened by arterial plaque or the effects of blood sugar swings.

Relationship harmony

Our personal relationships reveal much about our ability to be vulnerable and expressive in the way we love and communicate. Relationship is the constant mirror that reminds us of our shortcomings and demands we adjust and harmonize ways of better relating. It forces us to think of others, become less self-absorbed, practice gratitude, and find the faith to be patient and the generosity to be loving and not critical. These are all qualities of good health. Good, stable, passionate, and enduring relationships share qualities of self-disclosure, gratitude, sacrifice, responsibility, and play, bringing out the best in each other and inspiring mutual growth.

Sense of humor

The ability to laugh at yourself and share laughter with others is a characteristic of good macrobiotic health. A humorless person is tense and finds it difficult to express joy and not feel self-consciousness. Ultimately, the ability to laugh requires strength and courage to surrender and abandon everything to the moment.

Life passions

Nineteenth-century German poet Christian Hebbel famously said, "Nothing great is ever accomplished without passion." Having a *passion for living* doesn't mean acting like a cheerleader on caffeine. It means having different interests (creative or challenging pursuits, goals, or other ways of sharing yourself with others) that you find meaning in and enthusiastically put your heart into. It is a barometer of health because it is another aspect of appetite. In fact, it encompasses a body, mind, and spirit appetite — a hunger to learn, to engage, to share, to inquire, to improve, and to challenge on every level of body mind and spirit.

The Food-Blood Connection

What happens to the food you eat? How does it provide the energy that creates growth and well-being? How does the food end up becoming a waste product? These common questions are best answered in their sequence of breakdown.

Some foods provide zero nutrition but are still critical to good health. One of the most important foods for its effect on your bowel physiology is fiber. You don't really absorb it, but its critical role is to expand within your intestine, brush along the walls of the intestine to help stimulate peristalsis and help clean and detoxify your intestines, promoting bowel regularity and better *absorption*.

One of the most sustaining and memorable analogies that I have about blood relates to a busy river. In fact, blood is often called "the river of life." At any given time, more than 5 quarts of blood circulate in the adult human body, comprising 7 to 8 percent of an individual's weight.

The historical importance of blood has had great cultural significance in many rituals, religious and otherwise. Different cultures thought blood contained mystical powers, and we are constantly reminded about the importance of this precious fluid by blood bank donation requests for life-giving transfusions. Blood analysis is one of the first barometers of health that gives physicians a clear picture of faulty chemistry that includes cholesterol levels, liver enzymes, circulating proteins, nutritional deficiencies, or infectious conditions.

Digestion is an amazing arrangement of alternating acid and alkaline secretions in each digestive stage: The mouth houses alkaline saliva; the stomach releases powerful acid digestive juices; the duodenum discharges alkaline bile salts (as does the pancreas in secreting its alkalizing enzymes into bile fluid); the small intestine has a mild acid secretion; and the large intestine secretes a mild alkaline fluid. Each of these processes is described in more detail in the following sections.

There's purpose in opposition! In this case, each stage serves to attract the maximum amount of secretion from the next, insuring better digestion and assimilation. Therefore, what you eat becomes part of the blood matter (or indigestible material, which you discharge as waste product).

Stage 1: Mouth

The journey begins in the mouth, where you chew food into smaller particles and where the mild alkalinity of salivary enzymes starts digesting the carbohydrates.

Stage 2: Esophagus

The *esophagus* (also known as the *food pipe* or *alimentary canal*) begins at the back of the throat and ends at the entrance to the stomach.

It produces wavelike muscular contractions that push food into the stomach and keep it from backing up into the mouth (which is always handy when you're eating with company). Food travels down the esophagus at the rate of 1 to 2 inches per second, so travel time from throat to stomach may be 5 to 6 seconds.

Stage 3: Stomach

The stomach resembles a hollow muscular bag that begins to contract and churn food into smaller particles for later absorption within the intestine. It's surprisingly small, usually measuring the size of an individual's cupped palms. The stomach can hold a little under 2 quarts (1.9 liters) of semi-digested food that can remain there for 3 to 5 hours. The arrival of food causes the stomach walls to release two types of digestive acids (approximately 1.5. pH) that help kill bacteria and other food-borne carrying germs as well as break down proteins. One of the reasons that these strong acids don't dissolve the walls of the stomach is because cover cells in the stomach walls secrete an alkaline mucus that protects the *epithelium* (stomach lining) against shear stress and acids.

Stage 4: Digestive secretions

The liver produces bile, and concentrations of bile are held in the gall bladder. *Bile* acts as an emulsifier or detergent, helping in fat digestion. When food is released into the duodenum, the gall bladder releases bile (containing alkaline salts) into the duodenum to help with fat digestion as well as digesting the fat-soluble vitamins A, D, E, and K. The pancreas also has alkaline enzyme secretions that help further digest remaining sugars to prepare the small intestine for their absorption.

Stage 5: Small intestine

The *small intestine,* a hollow tube that is approximately 8 feet long in newborns and grows from 12 to 22 feet throughout adolescence, has thousands of small finger-like *villi* (projections that contain an internal network of blood capillaries). The villi stick out from the small intestine walls and absorb food directly into the blood. They push anything they can't absorb (such as fiber) farther into the large intestine. The small intestine also secretes a small amount of mild acid solutions such as *sucrase, maltase, lactase,* and *peptidase* that help break apart sugars and peptide proteins for increased assimilation.

Most of the digestion happens at the beginning of the small intestine, where nutrients, vitamins, water, and residual minerals become absorbed by the digesting material called *chyme.* Almost 80 percent of the water you take in is absorbed within the small intestine. As soon as the intestine absorbs nutrients, they go through the cell wall into the capillary and directly to the bloodstream, where they're ferried to the liver for processing. The liver is like a country-to-county border crossing. Nobody gets in without being checked.

The liver also does a heroic job of processing out the by-products of toxic drugs and harmful chemicals. Generally, food remains in the small intestine for 5 to 6 hours.

Stage 6: Large intestine

As the chyme makes its way into the large intestine, also known as the *colon*, it's in the final stage of digestion. At this point, food isn't broken down any further. Instead, the colon absorbs vitamins produced by its resident bacteria. The large intestine also has an alkaline bicarbonate secretion that helps neutralize the acidity of undigested fiber. The function of the colon is to absorb fluid from the chyme and form the mass into a more compact and dry material. Then it's pushed through the intestine so it can be discharged from the bowel. The colon has a wider diameter than the small intestine, with a length that measures approximately 5 feet. The food matter moves through the colon for a period of 12 to 24 hours, depending on your condition and dietary fiber intake.

Understanding the Acid and Alkaline Picture

The body uses many different substances that each play specific roles in essential function and development: dozens of sugars, 22 amino acids, more than 100 types of minerals and trace minerals, and at least 40 different vitamin compounds. Although these unique substances have great diversity, they all share membership in either of two clubs: the acid club or the alkaline club.

This classification of acid and alkaline comes from basic biochemistry, which represents the acid and alkaline percentages of substances in terms of *pH* (potential of hydrogen) on a scale from 1 to 14. As you can see in the following pH scale, the more acidic a substance, the lower the pH factor; more alkaline materials have higher pHs.

Acid 1 2 3 4 5 6 **7** 8 9 10 11 12 13 14 **Alkaline**

Neutral materials have a pH of 7.

Here are some foods and their pH values:

- ✔ Water: 7.0
- ✔ Cow's milk: 6.6
- ✔ Pork/beef: 6.5
- ✔ Coffee: 4.9
- ✔ Cottage cheese: 4.6
- ✔ Beer/wine: 4.4
- ✔ Orange juice: 3.8

Opposites can neutralize each other, which is why a stomachache from excessive sugar or soda (2.9 pH) can be neutralized by a bit of baking soda with water (12.0 pH) or 2 teaspoons of activated charcoal in water — a common folk remedy for upset digestion that functions much like over-the-counter antacids.

In its optimum healthy condition, the blood needs to be slightly alkaline; virtually all of your essential physiological functions — from digestion, cardio, and respiratory function to immunity — need their internal environment to be slightly alkaline, except for the stomach's secretions. Nearly all of your cells and tissues hold ample amounts of alkaline matter such as minerals, oxygen, and bicarbonate. Combined, these elements within the cell contribute to establish a slightly alkaline pH that registers just over 7.0.

An alkaline condition gives us stronger resiliency to recover quickly from illnesses such as flu conditions, allergy reactions, colds, and sinusitis. Ultimately, our health and disease conditions in the body are determined by the degree of alkalinity or acidity in the body's tissues and fluids.

In the two minutes that it may have taken you to read the above two paragraphs, your blood completely passed through the hardest working organ in the business: your liver. The liver filtered your toxic wastes and acids from the bloodstream and also produced enzymes to help compensate and alkalize your blood.

Biochemistry explains that the blood pH must be regulated between 7.35 and 7.45 for optimum metabolic health. You can compare pH to the reading of a thermometer used to evaluate the body's temperature; several degrees above or below 98.6 degrees Fahrenheit is no cause for alarm. However, should your temperature elevate to 103 degrees (high fever) or fall to 96 degrees (potential hypothermia), this shows dangerous imbalances that can potentially turn fatal.

The body's blood pH is usually around 7.35 to 7.43; a low pH of 6.95 can result in a diabetic coma and eventually death. Conversely, an elevated alkaline pH of 7.7 may cause titanic convulsions and also result in death.

TECHNICAL STUFF

Our self-regulating acid balance system

Here's where your body comes to the rescue. To maintain a safe balance of acid and alkaline factors, the human body has eight basic automatic mechanisms that work diligently to keep you in balance and handle the onslaught of acid excess:

✔ **Phosphate/ammonia buffers:** The kidneys discharge excess acids or alkaline elements by way of the urine. A distinct ammonia odor in urine is often a sign of an overly acid system that can't neutralize those acids with the regular buffering elements and must rely on the strong alkalizing back up of ammonia to neutralize this acid excess. This may be why the men's rooms in sports stadiums reek of an ammonia odor — sports events usually offer lots of acid foods like sodas, hot dogs and burgers.

✔ **Protein buffers:** Cysteine, glutathione, taurine, and methionine circulate within the cells, lymph fluid, and blood plasma.

✔ **Fat buffers:** Low-density lipoproteins bind acids in the lymph, blood, and extracellular fluids. These acids are then flushed through the urine. One obesity theory suggests that if the elimination of these acids is hampered, the acids migrate into body cavities and inactive body areas (hips, buttocks, thighs, and abdomen) as storage materials, thus increasing weight.

✔ **Hormone buffers:** Aldosterone and antidiuretic hormone (ADH) are essential factors for maintaining alkalinity in the kidney.

✔ **Electrolyte buffers:** Sodium, potassium, and calcium circulate in the blood, lymph, and cellular fluids to bind acids and remove them through the urine.

✔ **Bicarbonate buffers:** These originate in the red blood cells and work in the kidneys, blood, lymph, and tissues to neutralize acids.

✔ **The exhalation process:** When you breathe out, you release acid waste products such as carbon dioxide and almost immediately feel a centered, calm alkalinity.

✔ **Water consumption:** Hydrating your body with good quality water helps to dilute excessive acids.

All this goes on automatically while you plan your next dessert! A body that constantly is in conflict with heavy acid loads winds up with corrosion to body tissue. Gradually, the acids work their way into random areas of the body's 60,000 miles of artery and vein pathways and have a dissolving effect comparable to acids poured onto marble.

Choosing the right foods for good pH balance

The three main macro-nutrients are carbohydrates, fats, and proteins. The following sections list the most common poor-quality sources from these food groups and list healthy alternatives as well.

Other acidic sources from the modern diet are the artificial chemicals most foods contain, as well as alcoholic beverages. I discuss these sources as well.

Carbohydrates

Carbohydrates include flour products (such as breads, muffins, cakes, and cookies), white or brown sugar, honey, maple syrup, chocolate, pastries, candy, ice cream, boxed breakfast cereals, fruit, fruit juice, barley malt, rice syrup, molasses, white pasta, refined grains, and many more.

- ✔ **Acid source:** *All* sugars produce acetylaldehyde and alcohol, sodas contain carbonic acid, and chocolate contains bromine. Sugar also promotes inflammation. For arthritics, people in constant low-level pain, or those who have any condition ending with the suffix *-itis* (meaning "inflammation"), simple and refined sugar is one food group worth restricting.

   Yes, you're thinking that chocolate is supposed to be so good for you, and indeed there are some healthful factors in organic-quality chocolate, but as mentioned earlier, it's reductionistic thinking that sees only parts to emphasize the good stuff. We have to examine the whole of a substance, and for some, the sugar and bromine factor combined might not be all that healthful.

- ✔ **Healthier varieties of carbohydrates:** Whole grains such as brown rice, millet, quinoa, barley, and so on, cooked with a pinch of sea salt (per cup) and well-chewed for best digestion.

Fat

Fatty foods include deep fried foods (fish and chips, French fries, fried chicken), salad dressings, tempura, dairy foods, meats (red and white varieties), trans fats, and so on.

- ✔ **Acid source:** One of the more harmful components that fatty acids break down into is *arachidonic acid*, known for its ability to promote inflammation and make red blood cells stick together (inhibiting oxygen flow). Studies suggest that this particular acid may lead to heart disease. Trans fats are also heart-damaging. Now banned in many cities, trans fats increase LDL (low-density lipoprotein cholesterol, commonly known as the "bad" cholesterol) while decreasing HDL (high-density lipoproteins, sometimes called "good cholesterol").

- ✔ **Healthier varieties of fats:** Cold-pressed organic oils such as olive, sesame, and flax, as well as nuts and seeds.

Protein

Red meat and red meat products (such as beef jerky, hamburgers, hot dogs, and sausage), chicken and chicken products (deep-fried nuggets, fried wings, and so on), pork and pork products (such as bacon and ham), and fish and fish products (like fish sticks) are all common sources of protein.

- ✔ **Acid source:** Excessive dietary proteins, especially from animal sources, are responsible for excesses of uric, nitric, sulphuric, and phosphoric acids, as well as surplus ammonia.

- ✔ **Healthier varieties of proteins:** Beans and bean products (tempeh, tofu, and so on). If you are a meat eater, a minimum amount of free-range, naturally fed organic meats can be supplemental but not act as a main protein.

Alcohol

Individual reaction to alcohol is variable, and the occasional drink should not pose a problem for most people. However, a Harvard University study of more than 89,000 women found that women who drank more than one drink a day had a 50 percent higher chance of getting breast cancer than those who never drank. And alcohol has its by-product consequences.

Alcohol increases uric acid in the blood (a problem in gout), generates acetaldehyde, produces liver-damaging free radicals, depresses testosterone, diminishes Vitamin B-1, and increases endotoxins that produce cytotokine release. All of these factors contribute to inflammation.

Food chemicals (additives)

The American artificial flavor industry introduces over 10,000 new processed food products each year for U.S. consumption. Nearly every one of these foods utilizes flavor additives, not to mention additional additives such as a variety of sugars, preservatives, dyes, aroma enhancers, and chemicals that influence texture and packing chemicals made up of plastic and resins, particularly for frozen foods.

Most of these chemicals have documented degenerative effects and may contribute to inflammation. Although many of these ingredients are actually slow-acting poisons, the position of the food and beverage industry and government health organizations like the FDA is that these poisons aren't actually poisonous, because humans "seem to have a small tolerance for minimal quantities."

Acid Source: Nitrates, food coloring, MSG, fluoride, chlorine, biosphenols, and artificial flavors such as FD & C red number 3 (or yellow, green, and so on) can contribute to inflammation in the body. Despite the promotion of flavoring companies, these are toxins and don't belong in the human body.

The hip fracture monster lurks

The *American Journal of Clinical Nutrition* recently cited a seven-year study conducted at the University of California — San Francisco that involved approximately 9,000 women. The study revealed that those afflicted with chronic acidosis were at greater risk for bone loss than those whose pH levels tested normal.

Researchers involved with the study assert that many of the hip fractures prevalent among middle-aged women were directly connected to excess acidity caused by a diet high in animal protein and low in vegetable fiber because their bodies were leeching calcium from the bones to neutralize acid pH levels.

Clearing up acid and alkaline myths

Whether you speak to a nutritionist, macrobiotic, raw food eater, physician, or chemist, the subject of acid and alkaline in regard to nutrition remains a fiercely contentious issue.

Who can you believe? The following should help clear up four misconceptions about the relationship of acid and alkaline to health and nutrition:

- **"Acid and alkaline foods make little difference in the body."** Regardless of what anyone (expert or otherwise) says, the fact remains that the antacid market made over $1.09 billion globally in 2007, and that market increases by 8 to 10 percent each year. In the U.S. alone, over 62 million people suffer from gastrointestinal problems such as acid reflux, heartburn, and intestinal distress from excess gas. Something is causing these problems, and it's not just visits from the in-laws. Eating habits most commonly create acid excesses that can cause distention, pain, deficiency, fatigue, and cravings. The biggest offenders are acid-heavy foods: simple sugars, excess proteins, excess fats, and so on. Over a long period of time, acidity is similar to rust — its corrosive quality destroys tissues, arteries, and veins, and it interferes with cellular activity across the board.

- **"The blood is never acid!"** True. The body's natural mineral buffering systems see to this almost instantaneously — but at the risk of flooding tissues with acids and diminishing alkaline reserves. The blood may never be even slightly acid for any substantial period of time, but the remaining nine gallons of additional body fluids are undoubtedly subject to acid residues from food and blood-sugar swings that result in inflammation or immune weakness. What the body goes through to maintain its blood alkaline balance is directly what compromises health.

✔ **"You can never eat strong acid-forming foods again!"** Initially, you need to experiment and see that a dietary change, such as a flexible multicultural macrobiotic approach, can make a difference. As you establish sensitivity, you find that you can broaden your diet to include better-quality types of your foods from the past. However, for the most part, you may happily find that you no longer crave them, that they taste unappealing, and that a little bit goes a long way when you do indulge yourself.

✔ **"Fruits and vegetables are alkaline."** Vegetables are in fact alkaline, but fruits contain varying amounts of sugar and end up becoming acid in the body.

Some argue that in the process of *titration* (a common laboratory method of analysis that burns food and analyzes ash content), fruits show a good degree of alkaline ash. However, what actually occurs in the body can't be duplicated in a lab, so this statement is misleading. In the body, simple sugars flood the body so quickly with glucose that the oxygen necessary for effectively burning and metabolizing the sugar is simply not abundantly available. The end result of this inadequate burning generates acidity. Additionally, when the sugar of these fruits ferments during human digestion, it produces an acidic ash.

Lumping fruits and vegetables together is akin to saying "I like carrots and wood chips" — they're two completely different substances and not compatible. Fruits can be very helpful to balance excess alkalinity, but on their own their acid profile demands enjoyment in moderation, not as a staple food. Often, fruits eaten with major meals may cause quick digestive fermentation that results in gas.

Balancing your acid and alkaline chemistry

As traditional wisdom goes, the hallmark of good health has always been moderation.

You can look at the larger picture of acid and alkaline by keeping your diet close to the middle of the acid/alkaline scale, relying on the principle foods of whole grains, vegetables, beans, sea vegetables, fruits, oils, and perhaps some limited animal protein. If you eat this way, you can enjoy good-quality small indulgences without worry or fear. Table 4-1 illustrates this scale. Most of your diet should come from the Low Alkaline and Low Acid categories.

Table 4-1	Alkaline and Acidic Foods		
High Alkaline (Small Amounts)	Low Alkaline (Principle & Secondary Foods)	Low Acid (Principle & Secondary Foods)	High Acid (Special Occasions)
Sea Salt	Sea Vegetables	Grains	Fruit
Miso	Green Vegetables	Breads	Sugar
Soy Sauce	Root Vegetables	Beans	Vinegar
		Fish	Alcohol

In counseling vegetarians, I've noticed their dietary emphasis is generally more on the acid side, with excessive amounts of raw food and fruits, oils, spices, nuts, honey, flour products, and juices, but with very little or no dietary salt.

For someone just coming from the standard modern diet of plentiful animal protein and sugar, this may be a good transition for a short while, but in the long run, it can be debilitating. The balance that a vegetarian may need in this case is less emphasis on sweets and concentrated sweets (honey, sweet syrups, and so on) and more emphasis on whole grains, beans, some cooked foods, the inclusion of alkaline fermented foods such as sauerkraut and miso, or just using a bit more salt in the diet. This switch can make a radical positive difference within days, particularly with energy levels, libido, mood, and sleep quality.

Many past cultures used a small volume of an alkaline substance when preparing grain to help neutralize the grain's mild acidity, making its acid compounds easier to tolerate and the hull softer for its passage. The Japanese often used a small piece of seaweed when cooking rice; in northern Japan, they sometimes used a small mineral stone (quartz tachycte, or black obsidian) in the water when cooking rice so the rock minerals would diminish acids. The American Indians often used wood ash (charcoal) in the water when cooking corn, and in Mexico, it was common to use limestone when making flatbreads. All of these customs somehow intuitively knew the value of balancing acid dietary factors.

Chapter 5

Macro Boot Camp: Nutrition in a Nutshell

* *

In This Chapter

▶ Embracing carbohydrates

▶ Putting protein in its place

▶ Focusing on fat

▶ Complementing your diet with sea salt, supplements, and herbs

* *

In this chapter, I give you some dietary bottom lines for carbohydrates, fats, and proteins, and I provide practical suggestions for reducing cravings and making healthier choices to balance and secure your individual nutritional needs.

I also help you make informed decisions about supplements, herbs, and quality salt, all of which contribute to your overall health.

Getting Comfortable with Carbs: Overcoming Carbo-Phobia

When people decide that they're going to go on a diet, they often eliminate carbohydrates from their meals right off the bat. Then they drop pounds and declare it's all because they stopped eating those evil carbs. Usually folks lose weight by virtue of simply lowering caloric intake and eliminating sugar, but their mistake is a common one: the tendency to classify all carbohydrates as a no-no ingredient for succeeding in weight loss.

I call this problem *carbo-phobia,* and the misunderstanding is promoted by the media, self-styled nutritionists, plain old ignorance, and fear.

Of the three macronutrients, carbohydrates are needed in the largest amounts. Conservative nutritional estimates claim that 50 to 65 percent of the total calories that you take in should be derived from carbohydrate sources. Here are seven reasons carbohydrates have such superstar status:

✔ They are the main source of fuel for your body.

✔ They are burned most efficiently as a fuel source.

✔ They are required by your central nervous system, brain (your brain runs almost entirely on glucose and can't use fat or protein for its energy needs), muscles (including the heart), and kidneys.

✔ They provide glucose to all of your body's cells and tissues for energy.

✔ They are required for intestinal well-being and waste discharge.

✔ They can be stored in your liver and muscles for future energy needs.

✔ They can be found in whole grains, grain products, beans, vegetables, sea vegetables, fruits, nuts, and seeds.

Simple versus complex carbs

The common mistake most people make is to lump all carbohydrates into the "it makes me fat" category — when, in fact, carbohydrates have dramatically different effects in your body. Although all carbohydrates are made up from sugars of different types, the two main categories are called *simple* and *complex*.

✔ **Simple carbohydrates** are composed of one or two molecules of sugar. They're immediately sweet to the taste. The burning of simple sugar in your body is similar in intensity to the burning of newspaper in a fireplace: quick and rapidly spreading heat. Then it burns out, and you have plentiful ash.

✔ **Complex carbohydrates** are a composed of long strands of simple sugars. A single starch molecule can contain anywhere from 250 to 1,500 individual sugar molecules. Complex sugars initially taste bland. As a complex sugar is well chewed, the saliva begins to break down the long chains, and the taste becomes noticeably sweet. Complex sugars have a slower burning efficiency in your body, comparable to putting logs on a fire; they burn slowly, consistently, and evenly. They are an enduring heat.

The simplest sugar, *glucose,* elevates blood sugar quickly, while the elevation curve of complex sugars is more gradual. Whole grains (whole wheat, brown rice, barley, and so on) ground into flour are now called *grain products* (bread, pasta, muffins, cookies, and the like). As a *particle* of grain — despite being from a whole grain source — flour is more quickly absorbed, easily elevating blood sugar. This is the opposite effect from whole unbroken grains, which give a slight raise to the blood sugar. More extreme blood sugar highs and lows can create mood swings, fatigue, and strong cravings for sweets and salted food; therefore, you have less control over your health when your blood sugar is jumping all over the place.

Someone eating a large percentage of sugar frequently craves more fat in her diet, such as nuts, nut butters, butter, salad dressing, and cheese, because it feels more stabilizing in her body and slows the rise of blood sugar.

However, if that person were to eat more complex sugars, her craving for sugar and fat frequently becomes minimized, making dietary change less of an effort.

Table 5-1 clarifies complex and simple carbohydrate classifications. Each sugar category has its refined and unrefined products. On the whole, it's best to eat the bulk of your carbohydrates from the *unrefined complex carbohydrates* category, with smaller amounts of *refined complex carbohydrates*. For pleasure foods or sweet cravings, make healthier choices from the *unrefined simple carbohydrates* category. Unrefined complex carbohydrates have the most stabilizing effect on blood sugar. In being slowly broken down, they provide maximum endurance energy.

Table 5-1		Simple and Complex Carbs	
Simple Carbs (Like Burning Newspaper)		*Complex Carbs (Like Burning Logs)*	
Refined (Quick Rise)	*Unrefined (Gradual Rise)*	*Unrefined (Stabilizing)*	*Refined (Gradual Rise)*
White flour	Fruits	Brown rice	Breads
White sugar	Agave nectar	Whole oats	Pasta
Brown sugar	Honey	Millet	Crackers
Beet sugar	Maple syrup	Quinoa	Rice cakes
Corn syrup	Molasses	Buckwheat	
Sucanat	Barley malt	Teff	
Date sugar	Rice syrup	Whole wheat	
Maple sugar		Rye	
Turbinado sugar		Beans/legumes	
Dextrose		Vegetables	
Fructose		Sea vegetables	
Evaporated cane juice			

Discovering the benefits of whole grains

You've seen the cereal boxes and heard the advertisements about certain foods that have "whole grain goodness" or are made with "natural whole grains;" you've probably heard the television commercials barking about some new fiber supplement "made from whole grains," and no doubt, you've seen a dozen glossy magazine covers touting "No More Carbs! Lose Weight Now!"

Is there any truth to this? Partially. *Macronurients* are essential nutrients needed in large amounts (hence, "macro") for growth, metabolism, and other biochemical functions. The basic three are carbohydrates, fats, and proteins. Fiber is a type of carbohydrate that your body can't break down. As a result, it passes through your digestive tract, attracting toxins and stimulating waste removal.

Diets with insufficient fiber set the potential for the development of chronic constipation, and hemorrhoids and the risk of colon cancer. Conversely, diets with whole food fiber have been known to reverse heart disease and diabetes, lower cholesterol, and help obesity.

Among the many health benefits to eating whole grains, six can be considered essential.

- ✔ **Whole grains help sustain blood sugar.** You get a gradual rise that doesn't create hormonal havoc with insulin or pancreatic secretions. This creates more endurance, energy, and mental calm.

- ✔ **Whole grains reduce fat and sugar cravings.** Eating a food that helps stabilize blood sugar and provides energy helps reduce sweet cravings as well as cravings for fatty or oily foods.

- ✔ **Whole grains help reduce internal toxins.** Dietary fiber can bind estrogens within the digestive tract. It also helps by adding beneficial gut bacteria to the intestines, which help with nutritional absorption.

- ✔ **Whole grains promote bowel regularity.** Indigestible whole grain fiber swells in the intestine, stimulating the movement of intestinal contents and ensuring a more adhesive and thorough bowel discharge with regularity.

- ✔ **Whole grains contain vitamins B and E.** Many of the B complex vitamins are held within the bran of whole grain; niacin, pantothenic acid, vitamin B6, vitamin E, riboflavin, and thiamine (B1). Essential for good immunity and protection from diseases such as pellagra and beriberi, whole grains increase cardiac strength, can help reverse type 2 diabetes, improve DNA health, enrich the quality of body tissues, help combat depression, support red blood cell development, and introduce thousands of phytochemicals to help you stay healthy and fight disease.

▸ **Whole grains reduce cholesterol.** A number of studies have cited whole grains as being responsible for protecting the heart. Phytoestrogen compounds and antioxidants in whole grains are thought to be the factors behind lowering cholesterol and the risk of heart disease.

Debunking the "grain is bad for you" myths

For thousands of years, agricultural societies cultivated grains from common grasses that grew abundantly. So we've had hundreds of generations to get our digestion primed for grains. Yet, two arguments frequently come up among the anti-grain people. Generally, these people have horns, breathe smoke through their noses, and hate the thought of chewing anything you have to cook, but there is some meat on their contentious bones, so I briefly look at their claims in the following sections.

Claim 1: There's "harmful" phytic acid in grains

Grains, grain products, and even soy foods contain "harmful" phytic acid in the bran of the grain, which can bond with key minerals such as calcium, magnesium, iron, copper, and zinc and prevent their absorption in the intestinal tract.

Yes, this is true for some. *Phytates* are phosphorus compounds found in cereal grains, legumes, nuts, seeds, and various soy foods, and they block the uptake of important minerals, specifically zinc. In truth, despite all the yelling and finger pointing by anti-grain and anti-soy concerns, this would only be a problem if people exclusively consumed large amounts of phytates, such as soybeans or wheat bran. However, the phytic acid levels that exist in macrobiotic plant-based whole foods are really not high enough in phytates to cause such extreme problems.

Are artificial sweeteners okay?

Artificial sweeteners are highly toxic products have no place in a whole foods natural diet. Documented studies provide volumes of evidence of the harmfulness of these substances, and that alone should discourage the use of these non-foods, which were created strictly for profit and without any concern for human health.

The best barometer for testing these products should be your own taste sensitivity. Do you really think they taste okay? If so, you may have forgotten what real food tastes like. Try eating a whole foods diet for three weeks to restore the taste of real sweetness to your taste buds and then try some artificial sweetener. You'll instantly see for yourself.

Soaking, sprouting, or fermenting the grain before cooking or baking can neutralize this acid and allow nutrients to be released for absorption. The soaking process not only neutralizes acids but also breaks down the starches and difficult-to-digest gluten. You can soak the grain in an acid medium, such as lemon juice or water with a little bit of vinegar. Adding a healthy pinch of sea salt to the grain cooking water also reduces acidity, thus adding to the digestion factor.

Of all the grains, brown rice, millet, and buckwheat are more easily digested because they naturally contain fewer amounts of phytates than other grains.

However, the old adage that every front has a back applies here: The flip side of the phytate issue is that there are some overlooked benefits to trace amounts of phytates. Some studies have shown that phytates actually *prevent* the formation of free radicals, maintaining a safe level of mineralization in the body. Phytates also play an important role in cellular growth and can isolate and remove excess minerals from the body.

Physician and nutrition author Stephen Holt suggests that phytates shield people from dangerously high levels of iron. Additionally, some studies attribute phytates to halting the growth of cancerous tumors, because phytates can bind with minerals that feed tumors.

Claim 2: The gluten in grain is bad for you too

Grains contain gluten, which for some people is difficult to digest and can put a crippling burden on the entire digestive system, instigating reactors with allergies, celiac disease, chronic indigestion, and yeast overgrowth.

Familiar grains that contain gluten are wheat, rye, and barley. The jury is still out on oats, but for most, they don't seem to be a problem.

Some of the best grains that don't pose a problem to celiacs or those predisposed to gluten intolerance are brown rice, brown/white basmati rice, wild rice, millet, buckwheat, quinoa, amaranth, and teff.

Meet and greet some vegetables!

The three vegetables that account for nearly half of the total amount of vegetables typically consumed in the United States are

- ✔ Potatoes, typically consumed as chips and fries
- ✔ Iceberg lettuce (one of the least nutritious varieties of lettuce), typically added to sandwiches or used in house salads
- ✔ Canned tomatoes, presumably from a national obsession with pizza and pasta

Sour news on fructose

The average American often begins her day with a glass of orange juice, followed by some cereal sweetened with high fructose corn syrup (HFCS). Lunch and dinner might include a soda with canned soup or pasta sauce sweetened with HFCS. Dessert might be some ice cream or cookies also likely to be sweetened with HFCS, bringing the possible consumption of this unnatural sugar to more than 80 grams per day.

HFCS is extremely soluble and mixes well in many foods. Because it's inexpensive to produce, sweet, and easy to store, it's used in a wide gamut of foods, including bread, food sauces, bacon, beer, and even "health products" like protein bars and "natural" sodas.

Pure fructose doesn't come from fruit. It's an extract from corn and is far from "good for you." HFCS contains no enzymes, vitamins, or minerals and robs the body of micronutrient storages. Research indicates that fructose interferes with the heart's use of important minerals such as magnesium, copper, and chromium. Among other consequences, HFCS has been implicated in elevated blood cholesterol levels linked to the formation of blood clots. It can also inflame the intestinal lining of those with even mild IBS symptoms. Additionally, fructose has been found to inhibit the action of white blood cells so they lose their capacity to defend the body from harmful foreign invaders.

Originally, fructose was recommended to diabetics because it's absorbed only 40 percent as quickly as glucose, causing a modest rise in blood sugar. However, research on other hormonal factors has demonstrated that fructose actually *promotes* disease more readily than glucose. Although glucose is metabolized in every cell in the body, all fructose must be metabolized exclusively by the liver. The livers of animals fed large amounts of fructose revealed fatty deposits and cirrhosis, similar to problems that developed in the livers of alcoholics. Because the liver metabolizes it, fructose doesn't cause the pancreas to release insulin as it does normally. Fructose converts to fat more than any other sugar, which is one reason Americans consuming HFCS gain weight.

Make HFCS a must-avoid ingredient in your choice of sensible nourishment.

One study found that 42 percent of Americans ate daily portions of cookies, cakes, pies, or pastries, but less than 10 percent ate dark leafy green vegetables every day. Throw in some bread and approximately 30 teaspoons per day of refined sugar, and this constitutes the daily carbohydrate volume for millions of Americans.

Vegetables are a vital part of any diet and offer a world of beneficial *phytochemicals* (*phyto* is Greek for "plant"), which are biologically active compounds that keep the body strong and resilient. Many phytochemicals have properties that protect our cells from free radical damage as well as anticancer protection.

There are literally hundreds of pytochemicals, and nutritional research has only touched the surface of vegetable healing potential. One of the most researched phytochemical groups is *phenolic* compounds. This group includes *flavonoids, monophenols,* and *polyphenols*. They are associated with protection from and treatment of heart disease, hypertension, cancer, diabetes, and others.

Vegetables can be categorized three ways:

- ✔ **Green leafy vegetables:** Hands down, these veggies win the "most nutritious" award. Greens like kale, collards, and broccoli are a rich source of nutrients, far beyond what is available in meat — and at dramatically lower costs. Rich in chlorophyll, which nourishes red blood cells, green leafy vegetables are also a superior source of alkaline minerals, which help neutralize acid-laden diets. A complement to any animal protein, leafy greens are a calcium solution for those who prefer not to depend on meat or animal products.

- ✔ **Root vegetables:** Dense and compact, root vegetables are essentially plant roots that are eaten as vegetables and are great sources of vitamins and minerals. Root vegetables are known to produce warmth and nourishment during colder and more challenging seasons.

  Many traditional cultural medicines believed roots helped repair reproductive systems and the bronchi leading into the lungs. Common medicinal roots include ginger, ginseng, turmeric, and arrowroot.

  Some varieties of root vegetables, such as carrots, onions, parsnips, and white radishes, have a delicate sweetness that can be brought out with varying cooking times and are helpful for sweet cravings. Burdock, popular throughout Japan, is now available in many large natural food markets. It is known for a slightly bitter taste, but has great healing capacity and is popular with sweet vegetable combinations (carrots and onions) as well as in hearty vegetable stews.

- ✔ **Ground vegetables:** Vegetables that grow low to the ground are the liaison between roots and greens. They tend to be nourishing to the organs found in the middle of the body (liver, spleen, pancreas, kidneys, stomach, and so on). Veggies in the squash and pumpkin family are examples, as well as cabbages and cauliflower. Ground vegetables also offer unique sweet tastes.

  Cabbage has amazing versatility. It can be shredded and made into sauerkraut or a variety of fermented dishes; its leaves can be steamed and used as pouches for different vegetable stuffing and are popular with other sweet vegetable combinations, such as carrots and onions.

A word about the nightshade family of vegetables

The *Solanaceae* family of plants, which includes nightshade vegetables, has been highly cultivated for food over the last 150 years. This group includes potatoes, tomatoes, eggplant, cherries, peppers (sweet peppers and chili peppers, but not black pepper), paprika, tobacco, and petunias. Some plants of this family have distinctive medicinal value, while some are poisonous. The good news is that the risk of becoming seriously ill from eating potatoes, tomatoes, eggplant, or peppers is relatively small. However, for susceptible individuals, the symptoms these vegetables can produce make it worthwhile to avoid these foods as an initial experiment for your healing.

Nightshade vegetables contain solanine, which is a chemical that makes too many nightshade foods unsuitable for many people, especially those already prone to joint pain or inflammation. Solanine is also a calcium inhibitor and consuming it may promote mineral imbalance, adding to joint pain and swelling. It can also cause diarrhea, headache, vomiting, and heart failure in sensitive people, based on the severity of their exposure.

An American horticulturist, Norman F. Childers, developed the theory during the 1940s that nightshades may aggravate arthritic symptoms. Childers found that eliminating foods of the nightshade family cured his own arthritis and researched his theories into his 90s. He believed that eating nightshade foods results in a buildup of chemicals (glycoalkaloids) as well as steroids that could cause inflammation, muscle spasms, pain, stiffness, and bone weakening.

Many arthritis patients complain about pain and inflammation in their joints after consuming nightshade vegetables. The best way to check your sensitivity toward nightshade vegetables is to avoid them for an entire month while refraining from all sugar and eating macrobiotically. This time away from sugar and nightshades will regulate your health and sensitivity. After this month of eating simply, introduce nightshades back into your diet and note any pain or joint sensitivity. This process can help you determine which particular nightshade worsens your condition.

Fruits: The pleasure of sweet — at the right times

For many, macrobiotics was thought to be a diet that didn't permit eating fruit. In the early days, fruit was eaten only on special occasions. People believed that, despite being natural and wholesome, fruits contained simple sugar, and although they didn't instantly elevate blood sugar in the same way that refined sugar did, they still had a net acid effect. Their sugars also had an exaggerated response on people eating whole foods. In excess, fruit sugar could produce fatigue, inflammation, and weaken mineral stores. Eating too much fruit, particularly fruit juices, can elevate triglyceride levels — a type of fat in the blood that can increase your risk for heart disease.

Today, fruit is suggested as a source of natural sugar, but this depends on your health. If you suffer from loose bowel, fatigue, anemia, cancer, sugar cravings, poor memory, unsatisfying sleep, or have any kind of infectious condition, it may be wise to reduce or eliminate fruit temporarily and see how quickly your body responds to a whole food diet of grains, vegetables, beans, and some sea vegetables. Complete your meal with a bit of hot tea, often a satisfying way to conclude your meal.

Fruit is also best when eaten alone and not on top of a meal. One of the things that I tell natural food restaurant owners who consult with me is that if they encourage their patrons to try their desserts, they should do so considering what the patron had for dinner. If a patron has a meal of grains, beans, vegetables, and soup, and then sloshes down a fruit dessert on top of it, the likelihood of getting indigestion or gas is highly probable. Then, as they're leaving the restaurant and wishing to discreetly relieve themselves, they're usually thinking, "Man, I won't be coming back here for a while." Fruit often ferments the rest of the meal's contents because it digests quickly, while other more complex sugars are still being broken down.

Here are a few additional concerns about fruit to keep in mind:

- ✔ For some, the additional amount of sugar in tropical fruits may warrant reduced amounts.

- ✔ Fruit juices are concentrations of sugar minus the fruit fiber; so with a glass of juice, you're getting many fruits. An ordinary glass of orange juice can come from four oranges! That's too much sugar and too much acid.

- ✔ Fruits can be eaten a number of ways: fresh, cooked, or dried. However, a couple of handfuls of deceptively innocent dried fruits may fill a basket if they were fresh.

Sea vegetables: Kelp yourself grow healthy

Sea vegetables, marine algae also known as *seaweed,* are the super-foods of the ocean. Nutrient dense and rich in minerals and trace minerals, extracts of sea vegetables are found in nearly every type of prepared food — puddings and salad dressings to ice cream, breads, and even cheeses. The most popular way of using sea vegetables was as a thickener or recipe stabilizer. However, for hundreds of years, costal and inland cultures have harvested and eaten a variety of sea vegetables as a regular part of their diets.

Containing nearly ten times the amount of choice minerals over land vegetables and with high amounts of iron, iodine, magnesium, calcium, and potassium, sea vegetables are an essential in a whole foods macrobiotic eating plan — especially if you have a sweet tooth or decided to eliminate or reduce animal protein.

However, these nutrient-packed vegetables can help restore your health by supplying elaborate vitamin and mineral matrixes. Some of the comparison figures are astounding:

- Kelp has at least 125 times more iodine and 7 times the magnesium as garden vegetables do.

- Dulse, a seaweed common to the North American East Coast, is more than 25 times richer in potassium than bananas and contains more than 175 times the potency of beets when compared to iron values.

- *Nori,* that dark green seaweed wrapper sold in rectangular sheets and wrapped around what we know as sushi, has Vitamin A content equal to carrots and double the protein of certain meats.

- The black stringy seaweed called *hiziki* contains more than 14 times the calcium as whole milk and is far easier for your body to absorb.

Sea vegetables are a handy way to acquire *folate,* which has been shown to reduce colon cancer risk and also helps break down *homocysteine,* a chemical that has recently gained attention from cardiovascular researchers who associate high levels of this chemical with stroke and heart disease.

Studies have documented that sea vegetables have isolated components that lower blood pressure, prevent arteriosclerosis, and fight tumor growth. They are also known for their anti-inflammatory effects and have been shown to help in reversing high blood pressure and skin conditions, such as psoriasis and eczema.

Because they're packed with certain nutrients, eating too many sea vegetables, for some individuals, can result in an excess of iodine, risking the possibility of a hyperactive thyroid. A small amount of different seaweeds three to five times weekly can be a healthy addition for almost any diet.

Sea vegetables can be soaked briefly in water, chopped, and added to many dishes to enhance vegetable dishes, stews, salad, soups, or even noodle recipes. Do they taste fishy? Some do and some are an acquired taste, but when you begin to eat them frequently, you'll find them tasty and satisfying. Table 5-2 lists common sea veggies and their uses.

Table 5-2	Frequently Used Sea Vegetables
Sea Vegetable	*How to Use*
Agar	Vegetarian alternative to gelatin for desserts
Arame	Mild sea veggie used as a side dish
Dulse	Used in soups, side dishes, and salads
Hiziki	Strong tasting sea veggie used as a side dish
Kelp	Sea veggie powder frequently used as a condiment
Kombu	Used most frequently as a stock ingredient
Nori	Used to wrap sushi, as a condiment, or in soups
Sea lettuce	A soft textured sea veggie used in salads
Spirulina	Algae powder used as a whole food supplement
Wakame	Popular sea veggies used in soups

Figuring Your Body's Protein Needs

Our Western dietary habits are so entrenched with animal meats as principle foods that the image of meat automatically appears when people hear the word "protein." In less affluent societies, the principle protein is usually of the vegetable variety. Usually, that means beans or products made from beans, such as tofu, tempeh, or fermented bean products popular throughout Asia, such as miso or its byproduct, soy sauce (also called *tamari*). On the average, the standard American diet contains more than 55 percent animal products.

Proteins are considered the building blocks of our human material. Found throughout muscles, tendons, organs, and blood, protein also makes up hair, skin, and nails.

Why we need protein

We need protein for

- Immune function
- Repairing tissues

- ✔ Manufacturing essential enzymes and hormones
- ✔ Energy when carbohydrates are not available
- ✔ Growth (critical for children, teens, and pregnant women)
- ✔ Preserving lean muscle mass

Protein is made up of long chains of amino acids, which are key factors in most of the processes and functions of the body. Most hormones, red blood cell hemoglobin, the antibodies of the immune system, and all enzymes have protein as a central component. Because your body is constantly making new proteins and because you don't store amino acids in the same way that you do fats, you require an almost daily supply of protein.

Amino acids contain carbon, hydrogen, and oxygen, just as is found in carbohydrates and fat. Of the 22 amino acids required to maintain good health, 8 are known as "essential amino acids" and can only be obtained from food. Other amino acids can be manufactured in your body from different substances. Additionally, some toxic substances such as urea are made as byproducts and must be eliminated by the kidneys. Ultimately, excess protein ends up creating greater waste loads for your kidneys to eliminate.

You don't have to eat meat to get protein

The best sources of essential amino acids are whole grains, beans, vegetables, sea vegetables, nuts, seeds, and fruits. The common protein sources of meats and dairy foods contain other substances that can lead to a number of health problems, including coronary heart disease. Even broccoli contains protein. In fact, there's more protein in 100 calories of broccoli than 100 grams of steak! Table 5-3 compares some animal and vegetable proteins.

Table 5-3	Comparing Proteins (Per 3.5 oz serving)	
Food Source	*Protein (grams)*	*Cholesterol (milligrams)*
Red meat	24.9 gm	92 mg
Chicken	26.9 gm	107 mg
Fish	26.7 gm	41 mg
Brown rice	8.0 gm	0 mg
Tofu	8.1 gm	0 mg
Beans	8.2 gm	0 mg

The macrobiotic perspective on animal protein has no firm ruling. The idea is to re-create your health and sensitivity and discover your own limitations, what works best for your health, and what doesn't. Animal protein is never recommended as a principle food, and whether it should be included in your diet — to any extent — depends not only on personal preference, but your condition and health goals.

If you have high cholesterol, diabetes, or heart disease and want to change these conditions, avoiding all animal protein and saturated fats is essential for your healing. If you are oriented toward regular spiritual practice, it may be a refreshing experience to go without for as long as you can, for the value of seeing how this affects your demeanor, energy levels, meditation quality, and so forth. On the other hand, if you've made a quick dietary transition from the standard American diet to a whole foods macrobiotic approach with no animal protein and find yourself frequently tired or having consistent cravings for meats, putting a small amount back in as a transition link may be helpful.

Although it may not be an ideal choice of food for some, you should respect the fact that some of people don't fare well with strong restrictions from animal protein. Surely, we can all dramatically reduce our volume, but it should always remain a personal choice.

How much protein do we need?

Traditional Western nutrition has a long history of teaching that plant proteins are of a lesser quality than animal proteins. This was because it was believed that the essential amino acids weren't present in plants in proportions that were ideal for human requirements.

For a while, it was suggested that vegetarians always consume grains and beans together, thereby getting what was thought to be the optimum requirement with each meal of complementary amino acids. However, in the last 25 years, further research has proved that diets based solely on plant proteins can be wholesomely adequate and offer recommended amounts of all essential amino acids for adults within the course of a day's meals, as opposed to attempting to balance every meal with grain and bean combinations.

Despite what you hear in the media about our seemingly bottomless protein needs, the truth is that the human body actually needs very little protein for optimum functioning.

The current recommended daily allowance is 0.8 grams of protein per kilogram of body weight, about 44 grams for a 120-pound female and around 55 grams for a 150-pound male. This amount isn't written in stone, but recommended. The bottom-line assumption, without the charitable "safety factor" that nearly doubles the minimum requirement, is about 0.5 grams per kilogram per individual, per day. However, the average American habitually takes in more than 100 grams of protein daily — an amount that could result in debilitating long-term consequences.

Some studies suggest that the minimum requirement to prevent the loss of lean body mass is only about 35 grams of protein, which amounts to about 1.25 ounces of protein per day for the average individual. Keep in mind that a very active individual may require more. This low amount can easily be met from plant-based foods — where protein in varying amounts can always be found.

According to the recommended daily allowance, minus the safety margin, you should have approximately 10 percent of your total calories as protein, approximately 50 to 60 grams of protein daily.

Most plant-based foods, with the exception of fruit, provide a minimum of 10 percent of calories from protein, with vegetable greens contributing nearly 50 percent. Most plant-based diets contain as much as 40 to 60 grams of protein daily. This should be ample protein for your needs.

Problems with excess protein

I maintain that the typical Western diet is too rich in protein, especially animal protein. If that's the case, what are the consequences of too much protein? Here are a few:

Waste product creation

When protein is metabolized, due to its nitrogen and sulfur content, it can't burn cleanly. Toxic byproducts from these elements must be eliminated through the kidneys, adding additional burdens to kidney and liver function.

Elevation of insulin levels

When you eat protein, just as insulin has to process sugar, it also has to process protein. In *The Good Carbohydrate Revolution,* authored by Terry Shintani, MD, MPH — a physician supporting a whole food dietary approach — he writes that enzymes in the digestive system break protein down into amino acids, which are absorbed into the bloodstream. The sudden elevation of amino acids signals the pancreas to produce insulin in order to bond with the amino acids and escort them into the cell structure, just as it does sugar.

Protein may not stimulate sugar levels to rise; however, its increase within the blood demands more insulin from the pancreas. Some studies have shown that protein stimulates the need for insulin, in certain cases, more than sugar. The caution here is to not think that protein is an adequate substitute for whole carbohydrates in order to control pancreatic overload.

Calcium loss

The increased risk of osteoporosis is another overlooked problem from protein indulgence. A protein molecule, being a long string of amino acids that resembles beads, is digested by being broken apart so the amino acids can enter the blood. Instantly, the blood goes beyond a safe acid range. To neutralize this potentially dangerous excess, it needs alkaline minerals, such as calcium.

The body is now forced into an immediate balancing act. When sulfur-laden amino acids are introduced into the blood from animal proteins, they're routed through the kidneys, where they are reduced into sulfuric acid. Because this byproduct is dangerously acidic to kidney tissue, the body withdraws calcium out of the bloodstream and discharges it into the kidneys to neutralize the sulfuric acid. Now, to replace the calcium in the bloodstream, the body extracts it from your bones. Ultimately, the more protein consumed, the more calcium sacrificed from your bones.

Excessive fat/saturated fat and cholesterol in animal protein

High fat intake has long been known to be the cause of many conditions that aren't the inevitable consequence of aging: obesity, diabetes, heart disease, excessive clotting, cholesterol plaque, and connections to breast, prostate, and colon cancer. Some meat products are actually higher in fat than they are in protein: hot dogs, 75 to 83 percent fat; steak, 55 to 65 percent fat; and chicken thigh (excluding the skin), approximately 48 percent fat. The concern for saturated fat is in how it elevates LDL, also known as "bad" cholesterol, increasing heart disease risk proportionately.

A common misunderstanding about cholesterol, considering that it's found in every cell of animals, is that lean meats have as much cholesterol as fatty meats. Traditionally, although there were very few strict vegetarian cultures, most never ate the volume of meat that we do today, typically using it as a condiment, flavoring agent, or small side dish, as opposed to a principle food.

Quality concerns

Other concerns arise with a diet high in animal protein, such as the effect hormones given to animals have on hormonal diseases; gout, a disease resulting from excess protein; pollutants found in meats from the environment and chemicalized feed; as well as parasites and numerous infectious diseases that often contaminate meat.

These concerns are basically an argument of quality; however, the argument of excess — from fat, cholesterol, and too much protein — can orchestrate its own havoc. Plant proteins pose very little risk and also provide necessary fiber.

Beans: A healthy, affordable protein choice

Browsing at a local outdoor Mexican market while in Central Mexico, I noticed more than 15 varieties of beans on a display table; large beans, medium-sized beans, small beans, flat beans, fat beans, colorful beans, dull-colored beans, speckled beans — the choices were plentiful. The man behind the stall table told me that some beans were best as side dishes, others as flour, some for soups, and others most suited when combined with grain.

Typically, beans are soaked overnight with a slice of carrot or ginger in the water, and then the soaking water, along with the carrot, is discarded the following morning before cooking, because the water contained the starches responsible for gas. Then the beans are boiled in fresh water, and this water, after coming to a rapid boil, is also discarded. Again, fresh water is added, and the beans are brought to a second boil and then cooked in this water for 2 to 7 hours, depending on the dish and type of bean.

Beans can enhance different dishes: Add a sprinkling of cooked chickpeas to a salad; cook some beans with onions and spices for a side dish; create a puree dip for chips or as a spread on tortilla or chapatti; combine them with rice or any other grain, like the famed New Orleans dish, red beans and rice; use them as a main ingredient; add them to any soup recipe; bake and serve them with vegetables in a casserole dish; roast some beans (frequently done with chickpeas) for a satisfying crunchy snack.

Legumes

Beans are a part of the legume family, which includes peas and peanuts. Here's a list of common legume family members:

- Adzuki beans
- Black beans (turtle)
- Black-eyed peas
- Black soy beans
- Chickpeas (also known as garbanzo)
- Fava beans
- Great northern beans
- Kidney beans
- Lentils (red, brown, and black)

- ✔ Lima beans

- ✔ Mung beans

- ✔ Navy beans

- ✔ Pinto beans

- ✔ Split peas (green and yellow)

Bean product alternatives: Tofu and tempeh

There are also a number of bean products other than legumes to consider in a healthy diet. A couple of excellent examples are tofu and tempeh.

Tofu is staple food, eaten in small quantities throughout Asia for the past 2,000 years. Tofu is known for its good nutrition and culinary versatility. It has a cheese-like quality and is laboriously made by curdling "milk" made from boiled soybeans with a natural coagulant. It's notorious for its bland taste, but tofu blends with and absorbs flavors from other foods. Rich in B vitamins and a vegetable protein source, tofu is often portrayed as a meat substitute. Although it has many advantages, tofu's phytoestrogens have become a concern in some research as substances that may feed cancers. Some research has even linked excessive amounts of tofu to dementia.

However, this is a typical Western obsession: We are introduced to a healthy food and then discover 896 ways of eating it. Ever order miso soup from a Japanese restaurant? You'll only see a couple of cubes in the soup doing a backstroke. You don't see huge slabs of it served as a side or main dish, and you won't see soy milk used as a replacement beverage for milk. More is not always better. So now we have this nutritional backlash where many nutritional researchers are saying, "Soy is bad!" Yes, perhaps — if you eat it every ten minutes. But traditionally, it was used very sparingly. In such volume, tofu, I believe, can be a very healthy addition of bean-related protein to your diet.

Originating in Indonesia, where it's still eaten regularly, *tempeh* is a press cake of dehulled, cooked soybeans that have been mixed with a vegetable culture and usually incubated for two days. It qualifies as a naturally fiber-rich and easy-to-digest fermented food full of protein, calcium, iron, B vitamins, soy isoflavones, monounsaturated fats, and *saponins* (soap-like foaming chemical compounds). It contains no cholesterol and has a coarse, chewy quality that offers a welcomed variety of texture to meals. Frequently, it is marinated (in lemon juice, soy sauce, or rice wine) and then baked or fried and used in stews sauces, wraps, soups, or casserole dishes. Sliced thin and baked, it offers a satisfying crunchy taste.

Avoiding a trip to the bean complaint department

Hands down, the biggest bean complaint is what I call "The Cowboy Syndrome," better known as acid indigestion, an air attack, to break wind, a fart, or to offer a tooter. Frankly, by any term, it's all the same: a rude indicator that your food combinations, volume, or acid intake needs to be adjusted. It's not just an odor problem; in most cases, that's secondary. It's an indicator that your digestion is compromised.

Most gases emitted from the body are mixtures of ordinary environmental gases such as oxygen, nitrogen, carbon dioxide, and methane. The mixture depends on many different factors, but chiefly relates to food digestion. Common gut bacteria that produce hydrogen and methane can also contribute to the problem. Supposedly, bacteria feed on partially digested foods and, based on chemical compatibility, release gas during the digestive process of fermentation.

My personal experience attributes these lower eruptions to poor food combinations or several other factors in the list that follows. Become conscious of these and you'll enjoy good digestion and feel better.

- ✔ **Use sea salt when cooking beans:** Add sea salt when the beans are four-fifths cooked. Use ½ to ¾ teaspoon of sea salt per cup of dry beans (1 cup of dry beans makes 3 cups of cooked beans). Cooking the salt allows it to bond with a starch called *raffinose,* which is found in grains, beans, and vegetables, to reduce or eliminate gas factors.

- ✔ **Remove dairy products from your diet:** For many deficient in the enzyme *lactase,* dairy foods can cause gas, especially in combination with whole grains and fibrous vegetables.

- ✔ **Control overeating tendencies:** The common practice of overeating tends to increase acidity and intestinal fermentation. Eating before bed and to excess is a surefire combination toward producing some very memorable music.

- ✔ **Avoid simple sugar and grain combinations:** Mixing lots of fruit with your oatmeal or having a glass of fruit juice with your rice and vegetable meal is one of the most common mistakes people new to whole food diets make. Some people are even sensitive to grain and bean combinations. Desserts should not go on top of your meal. Wait a bit. Have some tea or maybe take a brief walk, but piling something sweet right on top of a meal is a recipe for disaster.

- ✔ **Watch your bean volume:** Don't try to make up for lost bean time and pile them high on your plate. Begin with a small volume and gradually work your way up to slightly bigger volumes over a period of weeks or months.

- ✔ **Chew as if your life depends on it:** Digestion begins in the mouth, particularly with carbohydrates (beans are also a carbohydrate), which use alkaline enzymes in your saliva to initiate the first stages of digestion.

- ✔ **Avoid mealtime tension:** Becoming upset or emotionally distraught negatively influences your digestion. When you don't feel present at meals, you rush and forget to chew.

✔ **Cook certain foods thoroughly:** Foods from the *cruciferous family* (cabbage, greens, and broccoli) need more heat for better cell wall breakdown, a touch of sea salt, and thorough chewing for maximum digestion.

If you follow these recommendations and still find yourself with a bit of gas, you can relieve your discomfort with natural home remedies. Many cultural folk medicines recommend alkaline medicines to reduce acidity and buffer any excess. Some of those remedies are *umeboshi plums,* a tart apricot-like fruit that is pickled in salt for six months; *charcoal powder,* usually taken with water; and *baking soda,* often dissolved in a glass of water.

Protein production from a global perspective

From a global perspective, relying on bean and bean products as a vegetable source of protein is not only more healthfully beneficial, but more compassionate to our earth than depending on animals as a staple protein source. The production of beef and other animal protein consumes vast amounts of natural resources, such as water, fossil fuels, and topsoil, and pollutes our air and water at the same time.

According to the Water Education Foundation, 2,464 gallons of water are required to produce 1 pound of beef in California. This is the same amount of water that you'd use to take a seven-minute shower daily for six months. In contrast, 25 gallons of water are needed to produce approximately 1 pound of wheat. The U.S. Geological Survey says that 40 percent of fresh water used in the United States in 2000 was used to irrigate feed crops for livestock. Only 13 percent was used for domestic purposes, including taking showers, flushing toilets, washing cars, and watering lawns. Either transitioning to a plant-based diet or minimizing the amount of meat in your diet is by far the most important choice you can make to preserve water.

It requires more than 50 grams of grain to create just 1 gram of edible beef protein. We remove animals from their natural habitats and feed them foods that contain large amounts of herbicides, pesticides, petroleum, and artificial fertilizers. Even the gross amount of feedlot waste creates its own pollution problems. Animal waste lowers the pH of our water (making it more acidic) and contaminates our air; and the gases emitted contribute to global warming.

Emphasis on the value of fish as a protein source is depleting vast numbers of species and making us more dependent on *aquaculture* — fish farming — which has grown into a billion-dollar industry. Approximately 30 percent of all the fish consumed annually are raised on these farms. Most fish farms are rife with pollution, disease, and suffering, specifically from parasitic infections, diseases, and injuries. This comes from tons of fish feces, antibiotic-laden fish feed, and diseased fish carcasses. Most aqua farms squander resources; it can require nearly 5 ponds of wild-caught fish to produce to spawn just 1 pound of farmed fish.

The single most important act you can do to protest these industries is switch to a macrobiotically oriented plant-based diet.

Sensible Suggestions for Dietary Fat

There's fat in a carrot! And even in brown rice! That most foods have some degree of fat indicates its importance in our daily diets.

In order of priority, here are four factors that determine your fat needs:

- **Degenerative conditions:** If you have cancer, heart disease, or any other disease aggravated by fat, it's wise to keep your fat content fairly low.

- **Your current body weight:** If your current body weight is on the heavy side, your fat intake should be limited. Excess weight predisposes you toward being at risk for any number of diseases, including cancer, heart disease, and diabetes. On the other hand, if your body weight is slim, you may require more of certain kinds of fats (monounsaturated, specifically) in your daily diet.

- **How much fat you've had in the past:** If you've eaten high amounts of fat in the past, gradually transition to a lower-fat diet to enhance your health and potential for avoiding disease.

- **Your current nutritional status:** Any deficiency problem, either mineral or essential fatty acid, or absorption problem signals that you may need to pay more attention to dietary fat.

Although fats are often the instigators behind many diseases, including obesity, some fat is essential for survival. Although the percentage of recommended fat varies widely depending on whom you listen to, you need fat in your diet for a number of reasons:

Fats in food . . .

- Prevent essential fatty acid deficiency.

- Allow your body to absorb fat-soluble vitamins (A, D, E, K, and carotenoids).

- Provide you with energy.

- Enhance flavor and add texture to keep food from being bland and dry.

- Remain in the stomach longer, making meals more satisfying.

- Aid your body in producing *endorphins* (natural chemicals in the brain that produce pleasing feelings).

Fat in your body . . .

✔ Offers backup energy if your blood sugar falls too severely.

✔ Adds cushioning, protecting bones and organs from shock.

✔ Is used as a building block for a variety of body chemicals from hormones to immune function.

✔ Insulates your skin from excessive cold and heat.

✔ Maintains the health of cell membranes and ferries nutrients across them.

✔ Normalizes growth and development.

When you lack fat, the following can happen:

✔ You may lose your hair.

✔ Your body weight decreases.

✔ Growth is diminished.

✔ You tend to bruise.

✔ Your wounds heal more slowly.

✔ You may miss menstruation cycles.

✔ Your skin becomes dry and scaly.

✔ You don't tolerate cold as well.

✔ You may have frequent cravings for protein or overeat.

Getting to know your fats

Research has shown is that it's not only the *amount* of fat but the *type* of fat you consume that matters. The following are types of fats you encounter in your diet:

✔ **Monounsaturated fats:** These fats remain liquid at low temperatures and are found in many vegetable oils (olive, peanut, canola). Monounsaturated fats lower total blood cholesterol by lowering LDL cholesterol, but not lowering HDL cholesterol.

✔ **Polyunsaturated fats:** These fats are also liquid at room temperatures and are found in some vegetables oils (sesame, corn, safflower, sunflower, soybean). They also exist in fish and fish oils, which have been shown to decrease triglyceride levels. Polyunsaturated fat can lower HDL cholesterol, as well as total cholesterol, but it also lowers HDL, so limiting this type of fat is suggested.

✔ **Saturated fats:** Usually solid or semi-solid at room temperature, these are unhealthy fats that encourage the body to produce more cholesterol, which, in most cases, raises blood cholesterol levels. Saturated fat also stimulates the production of LDL cholesterol, also known as "bad" cholesterol.

✔ **Trans fats:** Commonly known as *hydrogenated fats,* trans fats were devised as a money-saving tactic by the food industry to increase product stability and shelf life. In this process, hydrogen atoms are added to make fats more saturated, turning liquid oil into stick margarine or shortening. Trans fats have been banned in most retail products because they contribute to the risk of heart disease.

Here are a few other fat-related terms you should be familiar with:

✔ **LDL:** Low-density lipoproteins are a type of fat protein that transports cholesterol and triglycerides from the liver to peripheral tissues, keeping cholesterol within the bloodstream. An excess of cholesterol carried by LDL leads to plaque buildup along your artery walls. LDL is known as the "bad" cholesterol.

✔ **HDL:** High-density lipoproteins enable fats to be transported within the bloodstream. HDL can remove cholesterol from artery walls and transport it back to the liver for excretion or to be used by the body. This is why HDL cholesterol is known as "good" cholesterol. An elevated level of HDL has been shown to protect against heart disease. Regular exercise helps to elevate HDL levels.

✔ **Triglycerides:** These chemicals are the main form of fat in foods. They are produced within the body and stored as a fat from any excess calories from any food group. Alcohol can also elevate triglyceride levels. A high triglyceride level isn't always a risk factor for heart disease. However, the risk increases if combined with other risk factors.

✔ **Omega-3 fats:** This is a unique *essential fatty acid (EFA)* of polyunsaturated nature that you can't manufacture in your body. They have been shown to reduce the clotting of blood platelets, thereby lowering the risk of arterial blockages and heart attacks. Some vegetarian sources are olive oil, walnuts, and flax seeds. Some fish with high levels of omega-3 fats are salmon, albacore, mackerel, sardines, herring, trout, and tuna. Bottom feeders (mackerel) and very large fish (tuna) generally accumulate mercury, a toxin, and are best avoided.

✔ **Omega-6 fats:** These fats are polyunsaturated and considered EFAs, but they're not made in the body, so food is the only source. Most people consume these fats with regularity. Omega-6 fats include fatty acids such as *linoleic* and *arachidonic* acids. Excess intake of omega-6 fats has been linked to heart disease, asthma, arthritis, diabetes, ADHD, depression, and certain forms of cancer. Omega-3 and omega-6 are recommended in proportions of a much higher ratio of omega-3 to omega-6. The average American diet provides more than ten times the recommended amount of omega-6.

Table 5-4 summarizes the types of fats you can consume.

Table 5-4	Classifying Dietary Fat		
Fat Type	*Sources*	*State at Room Temperature*	*Effect on Cholesterol*
Monounsaturated	Olive oil, sesame oil, flax oil, peanut oil, canola oil, nuts, avocado, whole grains	Liquid	Decreases LDL, increases HDL
Polyunsaturated	Fish, whole grain, cereals, corn, safflower oil, nuts, seeds, bananas	Liquid	Decreases LDL, increases HDL
Saturated	All animal fats: meat poultry, fish, dairy products; chocolate, coconut, processed and fast foods	Solid	Increases LDL, increases HDL
Trans fats	Margarine, vegetable shortening, hydrogenated vegetable oils, deep-fried foods, most fast foods, and commercially baked products	Solid or semi-solid	Increases LDL, decreases HDL, elevates triglycerides

Figuring your fat needs

You actually require very small amounts of dietary fat. Although the modern diet supplies more than 40 percent of its calories in fat, you can get by with 15 percent of your total calories derived from fat. A macrobiotic lifestyle encourages a low-fat diet, suggesting that with a higher degree of whole foods, you need less dietary fat. For transition diets, I recommend getting 20 percent of your calories from fat, gradually reducing to 15 percent. Dramatic arterial plaque reversals have been seen with diets in the 10 percent range.

How sugar can change into fat!

Sugar eventually affects every organ in the body.

In digestion, it's stored as a form of glucose (called *glycogen*) in the liver. However, the liver only has approximately 60 to 80 grams of storage, so its capacity is limited. As a result, daily sugar consumption can make the liver expand much like a balloon.

If the liver is filled, the excess glycogen returns to the blood in the form of fatty acids. These acids are then distributed to the most inactive areas and more fatty areas of the body, such as the abdomen, thighs, buttocks, and breasts. When these areas become filled, excess then is attracted to active organs such as the heart and kidneys. Eventually, this excess diminishes the organs' functioning, and their tissues degenerate and turn to fat.

Naturally, the entire body is influenced by the degeneration. As a result, blood pressure problems develop, circulation and lymph systems weaken, and immunity suffers.

On a whole foods diet that includes whole grains, vegetables, beans, sea vegetables, and fruits, it's much easier to reduce fat cravings naturally. In addition to consuming small amounts of nuts as a snack or condiment and using 1 to 3 teaspoons of oil — depending on how many will be eating — in a daily sautéed dish, you'll reduce or eliminate your for additional fats.

Your overall cholesterol level should be around 150 for maximum cardiac health. The famous Framingham Heart Study, so named for the Massachusetts city where it was started 1949, discovered after 30 years of monitoring that not a single person with a cholesterol level below 150 mg/dl had a heart attack.

Eliminating or reducing fat cravings

Fat is a natural part of our dietary makeup, but strong cravings for fat can indicate a dietary imbalance. Look to see if any of the following reasons, individually or collectively, may be the cause of your fat cravings.

✔ **Avoid poor-quality carbohydrates:** When your diet lacks the complex sugar of whole grain, you may crave fat, whether it be something fried, nuts, nut butters, or animal protein. Refined carbohydrates make blood sugar erratic, whereas fat can have a more regulating effect.

✔ **Reduce bread or flour products:** Eaten your toast dry lately? It's not the most pleasing experience. When I stopped eating dairy food in my late teens, the only substitute that would satisfy my toast and butter cravings would be toasted bread with some kind of nut butter, such as peanut or almond. When I go to an Italian restaurant, I no longer test myself. I don't ask for a bread basket while I'm waiting for my order. Otherwise, I'll inhale the entire basket and pour olive oil on every piece. It adds up, too. Reduce the amount of flour products you consume, and you may see your fat craving drop as well.

✔ **Limit comfort food:** There's something satisfying about the texture of creamy desserts. The most satisfying creamy comfort foods tend to be a mix of fatty and sweet, such as pudding, mashed potatoes smothered in butter, ice cream, and so on. Comfort food cravings have a more psychological basis than physiological. You may have positive associations that you relive when you enjoy comfort foods, or you may find refuge in a sensory world that helps you tune out current stresses. Although there can be some therapuetic value in all of this, unhealthy ingredients can weaken immunity and foster depression, worsening your state after you've finished your treat. Try to re-create some of your favorite comfort foods with healthier ingredients. Same principle, less toxicity.

✔ **Get some protein:** In cases where you may lack protein, particualrly during a dietary transition, one of the most common cravings is for fat, because fat seems to be a dietary equalizer, creating a sense of fullness and extended time for digestion. Eating small amounts of beans, bean products, or some animal protein (optional) can reduce this craving.

✔ **Get fanatical about fermentation:** An old Chinese doctor whom I once studied with used to claim that fat cravings resulted from intestines that didn't have adquate amounts of beneficial bacteria. Eating small amounts of fermented foods helped restore better bacterial conditions that would quickly reduce cravings. Sauerkraut, pickles, and miso diluted into a vegetable soup are good sources of quality fermentation.

✔ **Try supplements:** If you're craving fats all the time, your body may be trying to overcome a lack of fatty acids. In this case, if a dietary adjustment doesn't seem to change the cravings, supplementation may be a more immediate and concentrated way to acquire those needs.

✔ **Get enough salt:** Sometimes when you crave fatty foods like chips or french fries, you're really looking for dietary salt as opposed to more dietary fat. Yes, your body often talks to you through cravings, but sometimes the message is in another language!

Suggestions for Sea Salt, Supplements, Herbs

There are some very black-and-white opinions on sea salt, supplements, and herbs. The following sections attempt to find the middle ground and explore these options so you have a basic understanding of how they can enhance your diet.

The benefits of sea salt

Salt is essential for life — you can't live without it. Unfortunately, most of us don't realize the dramatic difference for what passes as "regular salt" (the standard refined variety) and salt that has been sun-dried (solar evaporated) directly from the ocean — not mined from the earth. The difference is dramatic. (See the "Why sea salt and not table salt" section for more on this.)

According to the U.S. Department of Health and Human Services New Dietary Guidelines, sodium intake is recommended to be below 2,300 grams daily, roughly 1 teaspoon. One study cites Americans as consuming five to ten times as much sodium as they require — approximately 3 to 3.5 teaspoons daily!

If you're average, you need less than 1.5 grams of sodium each day to keep your system working well. This comes out to approximately ½ to ⅔ of a teaspoon daily. Culinary traditions teach that when salt is added during the cooking process, the salt in the food helps the body better absorb the food's nutrients.

Healthy sources of sea salt include

- Sea salt: Yes, you can buy sea salt right in your grocery store.
- Naturally fermented soy sauce
- Miso soybean paste
- Naturally fermented sauerkraut

Why sea salt and not table salt?

The table salt that passes for salt today is worthless. Stop buying it. It's mass produced, refined, heated to 1,200 degrees (thereby altering the natural chemical structure of the salt), and then flash-cooled. Table salt is 99.5 percent sodium chloride and 0.5 percent chemicals, such as mosture absorbents, sugar, and iodine.

Commercial salt producers add the following to "improve" salt:

- **Potassium iodine:** This chemical is added due to fear of goiter, because iodine is critical for forming thyroid hormones.

- **Dextrose**: Because the iodine is volatile and oxidizes in the presence of light, simple sugar is added to stablize the iodine.

- **Sodium bicarbonate:** The combination of potassium iodine and dextrose makes salt turn a dull purple, making it less marketable. So sodium bicarbonate is added as a bleaching agent for the salt, making it bone-dry and sterile in the process.

- **Sodium silico aluminate:** This chemical coats the salt crystals to ensure the salt granules don't stick together in humid conditions.

Sea salt is made by a natural solar evaporating process of sea water, asssuring that the larger salt crystals will still have their valuable trace minerals (such as silicon, copper, calcuim, and nickel) intact. Solar-evaporated sea salt typically contains at least 84 buffering elements that help to protect our bodies from the harsh effects of pure sodium chloride.

These days, the need for putting iodine in our salt supply is questionable. For most people living in developed countries, even those living a good distance from the sea, developing goiter isn't as common as it used to be. The rationale for iodizing salt is that, because iodine levels vary in most foods, the addition of iodine offers a margin of safety. If iodine is a concern, the addition of fish or sea vegetables, combined with a varied whole food diet, should offer sufficient iodine. Some foods that contain excessive levels of the minerals manganese and cobalt can interfere with thyroid function, causing a greater release of iodine.

Signs that you need salt rehab

Are you getting too much salt in your diet? Or are you not getting enough of the right kind of salt? Watch for these symptoms:

- **Thirst:** Salt = thirst. We've all experienced this. It's the best neutral medium for dilution. If you're thirsty all the time, consider making a major cut in your salt.

- **Irritability:** The constricting effect of salt and its effect on your nervous system, possibly due to lowered blood sugar, stand as a possible indicator of excess.

✔ **"Dark eyes:"** Oriental folk medicine suggests darkened eye orbits, particularly in the area below the eye, as well as the inner corner of that area toward the nose, reveals weak adrenal glands. Among the many different stimulants (sugar, caffeine, and the like) and lifestyle habits (staying up late, chronic exhaustion) responsible for this darkened coloring, salt can be another factor.

✔ **Overeating:** Excessive salt can increase your cravings for sweet food or for overeating, presumably because you may be trying to avoid sweet food and compensating by eating more volume — "stuffing" yourself, as it were. Often, reducing salt and salt products has quickly shown clients that their cravings for food volume may be based simply on eating too much salt.

✔ **Facial or ankle swelling:** For some individuals, the swelling of ankles and hands or puffiness around the eyes shows a tendency toward kidney exhaustion and a need for better quality and reduced salt.

✔ **Sweet food cravings:** A union made in food heaven: salt and sugar! The more salt you consume, the greater your desire will be for some type of refined or simple sugar. Conversely, the more sugar you consume, the more salt you'll crave. This seesaw of salt and sugar is the basis of fast-food menus: Have a burger (protein) and fries (fat), and then finish it off with a milkshake or apple pie (simple carbohydrate).

✔ **Need a drink?** Alcohol is a concentrated source of fermented sugar, so its effects are more exaggerated. Often a smart bar owner will offer free salted snacks (nuts, chips, popcorn) to patrons. The more of these snacks patrons consume, the more likely they'll order more drinks.

Selective supplement strategies

Does it matter where your nutrients come from, as long as you're healthy? Some people believe in "better living through chemistry." These folks believe that taking supplements can compensate for faulty food plans, inadequate soil, stressful lifestyles, or conditions in need of nutritional and immune repair.

On the other hand, food fanatics — or advocates of specific dietary plans — believe that we can get all the nutrition we need from the food we eat. We can still rely on healthy diets, even if they include foods from pesticide-laden soils (even if they have now switched to organic), chemically treated water that nourishes our food, junk food ingredients that have found their way into many natural foods, not to mention the consistent influence of poor air quality, toxins in our water supply, and the daily grind of emotional stress and a general angst that pervades city living.

It's a rapidly aging cliché, but that it has even become a cliché is evidence of its truth, and that is: "You are what you absorb!"

The vitamin balancing myth

In light of all that science is constantly discovering about the body, it seems a bit simplistic to think that you can take some pills to compensate for your ills or make up for lost nutrients. Many supplements don't respond in our metabolism in the same way that food breaks down. Here are a few examples:

- ✔ Prolonged use of zinc can cause a copper/iron deficiency and upset the sodium/potassium balance. Too much zinc often causes the identical symptoms of zinc deficiency, such as fatigue, hair loss, reduced resistance, inflammation of the prostate, and vitamin D deficiency.

- ✔ Too much copper and iron creates a vitamin C deficiency, while an excess of vitamin C, when tissue levels of copper are insufficent, can show up as symptoms of vitamin C deficiency.

- ✔ Taking iron for prolonged periods of time can cause anemia, because iron needs copper to be properly utilized. A lack of copper can cause iron to accumulate within the tissues instead of the hemoglobin molecule.

- ✔ An excess of calcium can lead to a phosphorus and magnesium deficiency. Often the symptoms of these nutrient deficiencies are identical to those of a calcium deficiency. Taking additional calcium results in greater magnesium loss. This can cause an increased sodium retention and eventually, possible vitamin A decifiency.

- ✔ Excesses of boron and iron negatively influence your vitamin B2 levels. At the same time, takling too much of vitamin B2 can cause a deficiency of B1.

There are those in the anti-supplement community who conclude that supplements are a way to create expensive urine. They suggest that your body will use what it needs and discard the rest. But things may not be that simple.

How are you supposed to know what's best for you and how to avoid such imbalances? How can companies claim that everyone needs to take *their* product? Because something is "clinically proven" doesn't mean much when you consider the difference between what goes on in lab-controlled conditions compared to your dynamic internal workings.

If all of the info in this section is giving you a headache, you're not alone. The fast and ever-changing world of supplement research can be overwhelming. However, some people don't have the absorption capabilities that others have and may require a greater concentration of nutrients. Sometimes this can stimulate their bodies to work more efficiently. The followings sections offer some guidelines related to supplement use.

First, change your way of eating!

The best advice I can offer before you spend all kinds of money on supplements is to first try dietary change. From this you can assess what you may be lacking. You have to be extremmly deficient to come out deficient on a blood panel, but they can give you a broad picture of your blood deficiencies and excesses, liver activity, cholesterol, kidney function, and immunity.

If you introduice supplements without changing your diet, you may go three steps forward with supplementation and eight backward with a faulty diet. Your body isn't designed to consume and use isolated nutrients.

The benefit of eating whole foods is

- ✔ You get a full complement of nutrients, such as vitamins, minerals, and antioxidants, and not just one specific nutrient.
- ✔ Food nutrients are naturally balanced the way Mother Nature intended, so they don't conflict with digestion, absorption, or your metabolism.
- ✔ It's safer to take food nutrients, and they also taste better.

So which supplements should you take?

Here are some specific nutrients that have showed to improve certain aspects of health:

- ✔ **General supplement use:** Take a multimineral and multivitamin preferably food-source based
- ✔ **Special health enhancers:**
  - Awashaganda
  - Beta glucan
  - Co-Q10
  - Curcumin
  - Fruit pectin
  - Ginseng
  - Green tea
  - Lipoic acid
  - Mushrooms (reishi, maitake, cordyceps, coriolus)
- ✔ **Hormonal supplements:**
  - DHEA
  - Melatonin
  - Pregnenolone

Allow your body time off from supplements

You should give your body one to two days of recuperative time every week if you take daily supplements. Do *not* take supplements every day. Give your body a rest, keeping it in a state of change, by declaring your weekends supplement free (or choose one or two other days).

If you are on prescribed medications, this advice does *not* include pharmaceutical meds recommended by your physician. I'm only addressing nutritional supplements

Although it's best to fine-tune your sensitivity by eating well for several weeks, I've recommended some general supplements to clients who were weak or deficient as a way to show them how to make a quick change in their condition. Often, prompt and noticable results inspire and motivate people.

Healing with herbs

The medicinal benefits of herbs have been recorded and handed down from numerous cultures for thousands of years. Written records from Native American, Egyptian, Hebrew, Roman, Persian, and African folk medicine practices show that herbs were a foundational part of illness prevention and treatment.

Many pharmaceutical industry formulas were based on powerful herbs whose chemicals were isolated and standardized into what we now know as *medications.* Herbalists rebut the use of medications with the claim that herbs have a more powerful and balanced effect when used in their whole, natural forms.

Most herbs have a gentle and subtle effect on your health. My own experience has seen that people eating plant-based diets tend to be more sensitive to the healing effects of herbs and can sustain those results.

As with supplements, the important point to remember about herbal support for your health is that herbs are exactly that: support. A faulty diet sabotages the well-intended effects of herbs, so allow them to work together.

Common herbs that have a definite place in health maintainence and healing include aloe vera, astragalus, burdock, dandelion, black cohosh, calendula, cat's claw, cayenne, chamomile, cinnamon, comfrey, corn silk, dong quai, echinacea, elder, eucalptus, fenugreek, flax, garlic, ginger, ginseng, ginko, golden seal, gotu kola, green tea, horsetail, hydrangea, kava kava, kuzu, lavender, licorice, milk thistle, mustard, myrrh, nettle, oat straw, olive extract, pau d'arco, peppermint, red clover, red raspberry, rosemary, sage, slippery elm, tea tree, thyme, tumeric, valerian, wild yam, wintergreen, yellow dock, yerba mate, and yohimbe.

The gamut of available medicinal and nutritional support from herbs can't possibly be done justice in a small chapter section. In its larger application, herbal treatments involve extracts, powders, teas, infusions, tinctures, plasters, poultices, compresses, salves, ointments, and creams.

Try to purchase herbs that have a "certified organic" label on the packaging. Many states now have certification programs that are run under federal guidelines.

Calcium, osteoporosis, and the dairy industry hype machine

Calcium keeps our bones and teeth strong and aids muscle contraction. It helps our blood clot, nerves to relay messages, and keeps our heartbeat regular. However, the widespread emphasis of calcium as the solution to osteoporosis assumes that this rampant condition is one of calcium deficiency. Almost daily, in television commercials and print media acting as proxy for the dairy industry, we are being told that calcium from dairy sources is the magic bullet, despite a wealth of evidence to the contrary. What the commercials conveniently fail to point out is that the body absorbs only 30 percent of milk's calcium and that osteoporosis is quite common among milk drinkers.

The average daily calcium that a South African consumes is anywhere from 185 miligrams to 205 miligrams. Compare this to the African American daily average of 1,000 milgrams. Yet, perplexing as it seems, the hip fracture rate for African Americans compared to South African blacks is nine times higher! The dairy industry pays dietitians, researchers, and physicians to endorse dairy products, spending over $300 million annually to keep their products in the public eye.

Nowhere in the world is dairy consumed in the high proportion that it is in Western countries such as the United States. But believe it or not, most of the world's population does not experience the high rate of osteoporosis that Americans do. In some Asian countries, where dairy intake is fairly low, fracture rates are dramatically lower than in the U.S. and among Scandinavian populations, where dairy is consumed heavily.

In reviewing 34 published studies from 16 countries, Yale University researchers discovered that the countries with the highest rates of osteoporosis, including the United States, Sweden, and Finland, were those in which the populations consumed the high percentages of meat, milk, and other animal foods.

So from where is calcium being leeched in order to produce this situation? According to recent research, osteoporosis is more of a condition of gross calcium *loss.* Calcium is being leeched from the body due an excessive and consistent acid-based diet, which draws minerals from your body's bones and tissue to neutralize potentially dangerous levels of acidity. Considering our high-protein habits, caffeine intake, sugar, and alcohol use, we need to recognize that the solution to the problem of osteoporosis lies not in eating more dairy but in reducing the acidity of our diet.

Chapter 6

Whole Food Templates: Customizing Your Food Plan

. . . .

In This Chapter

▶ Avoiding foods that compromise your health

▶ Picking a macrobiotic diet

▶ How to get maximum absorption from what you eat

. . . .

*U*ltimately, what you digest and absorb is as important as what you eat. Beyond the mechanical urge to fill your stomach and satisfy your appetite, what you eat, how you eat, and how you can maximize absorption work together to create your health.

I this chapter, I outline four healthy and balanced eating plans. You can choose the one that's right for you and customize it to fit your needs. Creating your own dietary plan ensures that you can follow and refine it as you become increasingly sensitive to which foods work for your body and lifestyle and which ones don't. At the same time, knowing how to maximize digestion is the key to better absorption. This chapter offers practical recommendations for personalizing an eating plan so you can benefit from consistency while minimizing cravings for foods that don't support good health.

I end this chapter with essential information about increasing your ability to absorb nutrients from your food and avoiding a gaseous side effect of changing your diet.

Designing a Macrobiotic Diet to Fit Your Needs and Lifestyle

To personalize a dietary approach, you have to be clear about how much time you can devote to re-creating your health. This process requires educating yourself, planning, preparing food, and cooking. This section lets you choose a beginning dietary template that you can customize to your lifestyle and health goals.

The reason that most diets fail is because they are presented with limited options for change and as static templates — a one-size-fits-all proposition.

The macrobiotic approach I detail in the following sections differs from the standard macrobiotic diet template in that it is a bit more flexible in its percentages of recommended foods. It is also a temporary template that you can experiment with to determine how you feel with this kind of dietary change. As you become more familiar with these new foods and begin to eliminate some of your previous foods, you'll find a new sensitivity that will guide you to adjust and further refine your dietary needs.

First things first: Avoiding "no-no" foods and changing some habits

During your experimental period, you need to steer clear of foods on the "no-no" list and observe some simple lifestyle habits. Following these recommendations can produce prompt and positive dramatic changes in your health in a matter of weeks, if not days.

The experimental period of adopting your macrobiotic diet is similar to giving your car a tune-up. Imagine that you're tuning a car that you've neglected for a long time. You change the plugs, oil, distributor, battery cables, and the timing. However, your work doesn't end there. You must test drive it and listen carefully, putting the car through its paces to evaluate your work. In the case of switching to a new way of eating, you tune and condition your body through a transition to a dietary template that matches your lifestyle and commitment level. After several weeks, you do a test drive to evaluate how everything is working. This tells you how to proceed.

The sections that follow present some basic suggestions to help you adopt your new lifestyle.

Twelve foods to avoid during your experimental period

In attempting to change the way you eat and obtain the most positive results, you need to limit foods that

- ✔ Contribute to inflammation
- ✔ Cause blood sugar swings
- ✔ Increase cravings

Foods that contribute to these conditions also sap your energy, disrupt bowel regularity, destabilize your blood sugar, and prevent you from falling into a deep sleep. You don't have to swear off "no-no" foods forever, but you'll experience favorable results during your experimental period if you temporarily restrict them from your diet. As you fully embrace the macrobiotic lifestyle, these foods may have an occasional place, socially and otherwise, but you do yourself no favors if you consume them regularly.

Here's my list of "no-no" foods:

- ✔ Any food containing white, brown, or any other refined sugar
- ✔ Fruit juice
- ✔ Milk, cheese, cream, butter, ghee, yogurt, and ice cream
- ✔ Refined oils
- ✔ Caffeine
- ✔ Alcohol
- ✔ Recreational drugs
- ✔ Medications (with some exceptions for current prescriptions)
- ✔ Heavy use of spices
- ✔ White rice and white flour
- ✔ Foods containing chemicals, preservatives, dyes, and insecticides

Twelve lifestyle changes to improve your health

Your daily health program should also include the following 12 lifestyle suggestions that can make a significant difference in your health and well-being:

- ✔ **Try to get a minimum of a half hour of brisk walking, indoor biking, or swimming daily.** Tell yourself it's only a 15-minute walk in one direction. (Of course you have to come back, but this may be an easier way to frame it.)

- ✔ **Reduce the volume of food that you consume and eat more frequent meals.** Try eating four meals a day, instead of the traditional three. This isn't a forever recommendation, but it can help produce positive results more quickly.

- ✔ **Don't eat for a minimum of three hours before going to bed.** However, that doesn't mean you should go for six hours without eating, because doing so lowers blood sugar and makes sleep difficult. Sleep is for rest, not digestion.

- ✔ **Try to retire before midnight and rise early in the morning.** This allows you to experience a deeper and more restful and nourishing sleep.

✔ **Make mealtimes more of a ritual.** We usually perform rituals with more attention and respect. Clear your table, sit with good posture, take your time, give thanks for all the factors that have brought you the food that will nourish you, chew your food, take some breaths, and enjoy this time.

✔ **Scrub your body daily to aid lymph flow.** You can use a brush, damp cloth, or gourd loofah. Take five minutes out of your day to help your detox system. (Chapter 5 explains how you can improve your lymphatic health.)

✔ **Try to wear cotton undergarments, limiting the amount of artificial fibers that you wear close to your skin.** This also applies to bed linens, towels, furnishing, and lighting. Make these eco-friendly and as natural as possible.

✔ **Spend a little time in nature at least once a week.** I find that a daily bike ride through a nearby park invigorates me and has a calming effect. At least once a week, walk barefoot through the grass, sit against a big tree beneath the coverage of foliage, and bask in nature. Find ways of regaining your sense of wonder and awe for the miracle of life.

✔ **Keep your home clean and orderly, especially your kitchen.** There's nothing more uninspiring than a dirty kitchen with a sink full of dishes.

✔ **If possible, choose gas over electric cooking.** The belief is that natural is best and supports better energy flow throughout the body. Microwaving foods on a regular basis isn't recommended. Try also to limit the use of electricity close to the body, such as electric blankets, shavers, toothbrushes, close exposure to televisions and computers, and so on. After a time away from significant exposure to electricity, you'll feel a difference and find ways to minimize your exposure.

✔ **Assess the products you use for kitchen cleaning, hygiene, and self-care.** You'll be surprised how many ingredients don't support your health or immune system. Seek out natural solutions. Everything you put on your skin eventually enters your liver, causing it more work, storage, and potential danger.

✔ **Keep large green plants throughout your home to enrich the oxygen content of the air.** Even in cold weather, opening a window permits better air circulation and removes any sense of energetic room stagnation.

Transitioning from your old diet to a macro-healthy one

The popular question that everybody seems to be eternally asking is: "What's good for _____?" Fill in the blank; it may be any health concern: minerals, a specific condition, more energy, joint pain — any number of things. However, the first thing to think about should not be "What's good for X condition" but

"What's *not* good for *X* condition." After you find out what's aggravating the condition, you can treat it.

For example, for arthritis pain, supplements such as glucosamine and condroitin are being recommended. In the last several years, television commercials have appeared with older, white-haired spokespeople recommending this supplement for seniors. Even in commercial pet food, you see these supplements being added and advertised on their packaging as good for your doggy's bone health.

But what you don't hear are warnings about what we are currently eating on a daily basis that weakens or destroys bone health. You don't hear the commercials recommending that seniors abstain from excessive protein, refined flours, dairy products, caffeine, sugar, or artificial sugars because they weaken mineral reserves, foster inflammation, and result in accumulative bone loss. At the same time, you never hear dog kibble manufactures saying, "This is just a corn flour product with meat scrap flavoring and a bunch of artificial supplements — a completely unnatural pet food that does not support pet health." In general, food marketing focuses on the "What's good for *X*" issue.

One of the easiest ways to transition from your old diet to a new, healthier diet is to do in a comfortable gradient — without the cravings! That can be done more successfully, not with willpower but rather with food exchanges that make the transition easier. See Table 6-1 for my recommendations.

Table 6-1	Food Exchanges
Standard Foods	*Modern Multicultural Macrobiotic Foods*
Red meats	Reduce volume and frequency of red meats. Gravitate toward white meats. Eat more vegetable protein sources (beans, bean products).
Dairy products	Reduce or eliminate dairy foods. Increase vegetable oils, nuts, and seeds. Take more mineral source foods (green vegetables and sea vegetables).
White breads, enriched breads, pasta, muffins, and so on	Try whole grain cereals, whole grain bread, and whole grain pasta.
Canned and frozen vegetables	Minimize the use of frozen vegetables and eat fresh vegetables (organic if possible) instead.
Refined sugar and sweetened desserts	In moderation, eat fruits, juices, natural jams, and cookies with natural sweeteners such as agave, barley malt, rice syrup, maple syrup, and honey.

(continued)

Table 6-1 *(continued)*

Standard Foods	Modern Multicultural Macrobiotic Foods
Soda pop	In moderation, give fruit spritzers (fruit juice and carbonated water) and try.
Coffee and caffeinated beverages	Try a gradual caffeine reduction. You can drink black and green teas, as well as herbal and grain teas.
Alcohol	You can drink the occasional natural beer or spirit. Or try nonalcoholic beer.

Considering supplements as an aid in your dietary change

In an ideal macrobiotic world, you wouldn't need supplements — you would get everything your body needed from the food you ate. But this is the real world, and the debilitating foods that we've eaten previously (coupled with other habits that negatively influence our health) have led me to recommend using supplements for a brief period of time, or at least until a person becomes more accustomed to the macrobiotic diet.

For people who come into a macrobiotic diet with conditions of fatigue or anemia, diets dependent on stimulants such as sugar and caffeine, or a fast-paced lifestyle, I may recommend using supplements for a temporary period of 1 to 2 months before gradual easing off. The following list describes a few supplements I often recommend:

- Enzymes can often help with digestion when taken after a meal.

- A probiotic (beneficial intestinal bacteria) taken with some regular fermented products (such as miso or sauerkraut) can help people with absorption problems, digestive sluggishness, or anemia.

- A combination of enzymes, probiotics, and a general multisupplement is helpful for people that have been on medications (including antibiotics).

A 5/2 (five days on, two days off) supplement regimen — preferably using supplements made from whole food sources — can make the macrobiotic transition easier. Those off days are important because they keep the body in a state of change, so it doesn't get mechanically accustomed to concentrated nutrients all the time.

Four Dietary Templates: Which One Is for You?

Becoming macrobiotic means redefining your relationship with food. You need to consider not only how you eat, but also what you eat and how you shop, cook, and plan meals. The choices you make are roads that lead to your specific goals.

The question you must answer is: What kind of commitment are you prepared to make to improve your health? Do you want to dabble in these changes or make major changes? Do you have support around you? Can you find the time to trade in old nonsupportive habits for healthy ones?

When I first began following macrobiotics, it was presented to me and others as "the diet," a one-size fits-all template. Any variation usually meant, to our rigid way of thinking at the time, that you weren't macrobiotic. In truth, macrobiotics was presented with some margin of flexibility, but as youthful fanatics who wanted to do everything perfectly, most of us took the recommendations literally. After many years as a counselor, I discovered that if I offered someone a plan that they didn't perceive as doable — whether because of their lifestyle, self-discipline, or social circumstances — it often triggered an all or nothing reflex. The client would either try to follow the plan exactly as outlined or shelve the entire thing and rebelliously eat the worst.

As I continued counseling, I began to recognize the profile of someone who was ready for major lifestyle changes and who was not. Usually, some stressful fact was the trigger behind their change: They hit bottom emotionally and needed to take better care; they were sick or afraid of getting sick; they were in pain and had no success with any other program; they had new love and sudden motivation to take better care; or they had just arrived at a place in their life where they wanted change. I found that when more flexible guidelines were presented, most clients had the best overall results. The success factor was in getting people to eat better more consistently, instead of offering them a rigid template that they couldn't follow consistently.

Ultimately, you have to be realistic yet still consider the need for self-challenge. Some days, you have to follow the plan mechanically for the value of seeing what kind of result it can produce. Often, within days, I've heard clients comment how radically different they've felt; they've experienced increased energy, deeper sleep, better bowel function, more mental clarity, and so on. Your body's reaction will tell you whether this change suits you, and you'll figure out how to control your health and well-being.

I present four dietary templates here:

- ✔ The New Multicultural Macrobiotic Template
- ✔ The Convenience-Food Eater's Template
- ✔ The Macrobiotic Weight-Loss Template
- ✔ The Macrobiotic Healing Diet Template

There is no single right way to take on a macrobiotic diet, but only a way that is suitable for your particular condition, will, and circumstances.

If you try an introductory method that's not so restrictive, you quickly find yourself motivated to experiment with a stricter template to see quicker benefit. Suddenly you have the impulse to take better care of yourself. Most of us began macrobiotics in the late '60s and early '70s by being frightened that we'd be poisoning ourselves with any foods outside that strict template. We'd eat well during the day, chew every mouthful countless times, and in the evening sneak off to the deli and inhale cheesecake or whatever looked sweet. This experience made me realize the need to suggest a next step for clients and not a dramatic leap. Conversely, some people may need a more extreme leap so they can see more immediate results and experience the power of food.

The four templates are introduced in the following sections, and Table 6-2 at the end of the chapter gives you a handy reference with the guidelines for all of them so you can compare them side by side and take away the important info at a glance. Take a look and decide for yourself which one may work for you.

The New Multicultural Macrobiotic Template

This template can serve as an easy introduction for your first macrobiotic adventure. It suggests less grain and more vegetables than the standard macrobiotic templates of the last 40 years, includes some raw foods, and is a bit more permissible on fruits with small amounts of animal protein if these items have played a big part in your previous diet. Just be sure to limit fruit to two daily servings, preferably at least 30 minutes after a meal. This adjusted template makes the plan more practical, less foreign, and more appetizing by offering a greater variety of dishes. The prevailing philosophy behind this template is that it is far healthier to be consistently eating generally well than eating an overly strict regime that you end up going on and off of, especially because the tendency when you go "off" is to go right for sugar and refined foods. Figure 6-1 shows the New Multicultural Macrobiotic Template with primary foods shaded in gray.

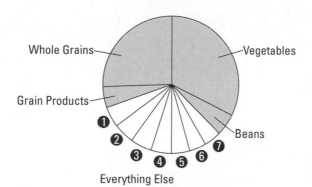

Figure 6-1:
The New
Multi-
cultural
Macrobiotic
Template.

Everything Else Percentages
1. WYW: Small amounts of whatever you want
2. Beverages: Herbal, plant, and grain based
3. Swing percentage: More grains or vegetables
4. Oils, nuts, and seeds
5. New foods: Experiment with sea plants, fermented foods, etc.
6. Animal proteins (optional, or add more bean, grain, or vegetable if desired)
7. Seasonal fruit

The Convenience-Food Eater's Template

Most people face an overwhelming daily schedule of balancing work with family, personal interests, exercise, food preparation, eating, education, recreational time, and rest. They've lost the meaning of food's value, and most know little about the powerful and transformative effect that balanced food offers. People well-suited to using this template are always on the go and are looking for quick energy foods to save time.

I began to use this template for people who told me that they didn't have time to cook. Although this transition can still help you feel better, positive results may take longer; however, if this template is most suitable for your chosen lifestyle, by all means, adopt it. If you have to use precut store-bought vegetables, frozen foods, canned beans, and boxed grain with shorter cooking times, make it work. Often, clients doing this plan find inspiration to go deeper because of the quick positive changes they notice in energy levels, sleep quality, bowel function, and a greater sense of calm.

The essence of this plan is to introduce some grains and vegetables into your daily diet. Other foods that you've previously eaten a greater percentage of also should be reduced. For example

- Bean protein helps with reducing animal protein.

- Using a bit more oil, nuts, and seeds helps with reducing the desire for dairy food.

✔ Fruits help with sugar reduction and are a healthier and less concentrated sweet choice.

✔ Allowing yourself healthier versions of frozen and canned choices can make a positive difference initially and still cut corners when you're crunched for time.

With this template, you do the best you can while still educating yourself about your choices and how food nourishes. As you see progressive changes, you'll find more inspiration to venture further and experiment with more commitment — when you're ready. Figure 6-2 shows you the Convenience-Food Eater's Template with primary foods shaded in gray.

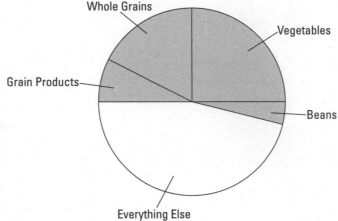

Figure 6-2:
The
Convenience-
Food Eater's
Template.

The Macrobiotic Weight-Loss Template

Some people immediately lose weight when they switch to a general macrobiotic template. However, others find it difficult to lose pounds. Although they seem to maintain and reap most of the advantages of a healthier diet change, their body stubbornly clings to fat reserves. Usually the person has eaten lots of dairy food, oils, flour, and meat and has had an inactive lifestyle. Sometimes these people, specifically women, tend to have low thyroid activity. In the language of body types, this type usually describes an *endomorphic* individual.

If this describes you, or if you want an accelerated weight-loss plan, the Weight-Loss Template may be the plan you need to start with. Here are the highlights of this template:

✔ It emphasizes a larger percentage of vegetable fare and reduces grain consumption.

✔ It suggests refraining completely from flour products, if possible.

✔ The emphasis of onion (red and brown onions, leeks, scallions, chives, shallots, and radish family vegetables) helps reduce fat accumulations and has a favorable diuretic effect on the body.

✔ Small concentrated protein sources eaten twice a day, along with some dietary oil used in cooking, make meals more satisfying. It also limits the tendency to overeat. Protein can exert a slight diuretic effect, helping you to lose weight through fluid loss.

✔ Light use of sea salt is recommended: a pinch in the grain or a sprinkle of soy sauce ($^1/_2$ to $^3/_4$ teaspoon) in the vegetables.

Finally, the effect of consistent activity brings better circulation and toxin removal to the entire body. Figure 6-3 illustrates this template with primary foods shaded in gray.

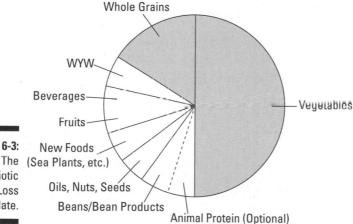

Figure 6-3: The Macrobiotic Weight-Loss Template.

The Healing Diet Template

A *healing diet* is a food-and-lifestyle plan that supports the body as it attempts to heal itself. There are no miracle nutrients or natural magical bullets that do it all for you. The first thing you need to do is to make sure your diet and lifestyle aren't aggravating your condition. Secondly, see whether your approach covers the following four points.

✔ Your diet should offer good nutrition.

✔ The foods you eat should help strengthen your natural detox functions: the eliminative organs (liver, kidneys, intestines, and skin). Their natural detoxing ability is channeled through your daily bowel and urinary discharge, exhalations, emotional expression, movement, and sweat.

✔ Your diet should help to regulate blood sugar, avoiding swings that contribute to diseases, cravings, and moodiness.

✔ Your diet should help to strengthen your biggest ally in healing — your immune system.

These are the most important factors of the Healing Diet Template. What is different about this template is that it suggests a slightly higher percentage of whole grain and omits concentrated sweeteners and all simple sugars.

Food is best if made fresh and not frozen or canned. Thorough chewing and eating small amounts of fermented foods ensure good digestion and improved absorption.

This template assumes that you *think of your food as medicine*, so you shouldn't dwell on what you may be missing and would like to indulge in. It's about healing and the need to do it in a focused, strict way for the benefit of seeing your body's honest reaction.

A variety of nutraceuticals can help bolster immunity, aid the liver, support adrenal function, and provide solid nutrition. These nutraceuticals may include maitake, shiitake, and reishi mushrooms, astragalus, ashwagandha, milk thistle, melatonin, chlorella or algae products, trace minerals, ginseng, various herbs, whole food source multivitamins and minerals, and so on.

Figure 6-4 illustrates this template with primary foods shaded in gray.

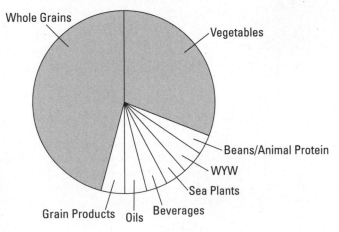

Figure 6-4:
Diet
Template.

Looking at the dietary templates side by side

The four templates are designed to offer broader appeal and most specific recommendations to those new to macrobiotics or those who want to refine their practice. Some may be more interested in weight-loss, healing, or even dabbling as their time permits. Table 6-2 lets you compare the parameters of each template so you can decide what works for your situation. Here are a few terms that will help you navigate the table:

✔ **Principle Foods:** The essential foods that provide your nutritional basics and make up your main dietary percentages. You could live on these exclusively if you had to.

✔ **Secondary Foods:** The foods that supplement your diet and enhance principle foods. You eat these foods daily but in smaller amounts.

✔ **Pleasure Foods:** The special foods you allow yourself to enjoy in small amounts. I usually call this section of your diet the *Whatever You Want* (WYW) percentage. If you are eating to heal yourself, take this percentage only rarely.

✔ **Swing Percentage:** The idea of a swing percentage is to take more of what appeals to you, not so much due to taste but instinct.

Table 6-2	Macrobiotic Dietary Templates			
	The New Multicultural Macrobiotic Template	*The Convenience Food Eater's Template*	*The Macrobiotic Weight-Loss Template*	*The Macrobiotic Healing Diet Template*
Principle foods				
Whole grains	20 to 30 percent	15 to 20 percent	15 to 20 percent	45 percent
Grain products	5 percent per day (1 to 2 slices of bread or servings of pasta)	5 to 10 percent per day (2 to 3 slices of bread or servings of pasta)	Minimum, according to craving	5 percent per day (1 to 2 slices of bread or 2 servings of pasta)

(continued)

Table 6-2 *(continued)*

	The New Multicultural Macrobiotic Template	The Convenience Food Eater's Template	The Macrobiotic Weight-Loss Template	The Macrobiotic Healing Diet Template
Vegetables (greens, roots, and ground varieties)	35 percent	25 percent	40 percent	35 percent
Beans or bean products (tempeh, tofu, so on; canned or dried)	5 percent	5 to 10 percent in soups, spreads (hummus), bean burgers, so on	5 to 10 percent in soups, spreads (hummus), bean burgers, so on	5 to 10 percent
Secondary foods				
Fruits	5 to 10 percent, according to sweet cravings	5 to 10 percent, according to sweet cravings	5 to 10 percent, according to sweet cravings	On occasion
Beverages (Grain-based teas, herbal teas, vegetable juices, and so on)	As desired — especially hot tea after meals.	As desired — especially hot tea after meals.	Have up to a cup of hot or warm non-caffeinated tea after meals. This has the effect of stopping the appetite.	As desired — especially hot tea after meals.
Vegetable oils, nuts, seeds, and limited dairy products	5 to 10 percent	5 to 10 percent	5 to 10 percent	1 to 2 teaspoons of vegetable oils, nuts, or seeds; NO dairy products
Reduced animal protein (Fish is preferable)	5 to 10 percent *(optional)*	10 to 15 percent	5 to 10 percent *(optional)*	Once or twice weekly, if craving *(optional)*

	The New Multicultural Macrobiotic Template	The Convenience Food Eater's Template	The Macrobiotic Weight-Loss Template	The Macrobiotic Healing Diet Template
Swing percentage	Additional percentage of whole grains or more vegetables, according to your needs			
New foods (Sea plants or fermented foods — sauerkraut, pickles, miso, and so on)	Devote a small percentage of your dietary template to exploring new foods	Devote a small percentage of your dietary template to exploring new foods	Devote a small percentage of your dietary template to exploring new foods	Try small amounts of sea plants as a side dish two to three times a week
Pleasure foods				
WYW: Whatever You Want	Enjoy the best quality, and control the volume of what you eat	Enjoy the best quality, and control the volume of what you eat	Best to have "treat" foods during the day so that they don't negatively influence sleep	Use fruit or other quality treats for sweet cravings

You Are What You Absorb!

We spend a good portion of our lives processing organic matter. We consume food, which then travels through various digestive stages designed to reduce its size and extract its goodness simply for the purpose of sustaining us. It's very simple, really: If you stop eating, you die. So it now becomes a matter of absorbing the most nutrients from what you consume in order to thrive, not just survive.

The word *digestion* refers to the way you break food down in your stomach, within the duodenum (an extension of the stomach), and the small intestine. Words that generally describe how nutrients make their way into your body are *assimilation* or *absorption*. Absorption occurs within the stomach (for sugars) and small intestine (everything else). Good absorption is based on many factors, some of which are how well you chew; your mood (which influences digestive secretions); good nutrition; an appropriate amount of fermented food in your diet (which enhances intestinal bacteria); and a diet of reduced fat and acidity.

Digestion begins with your senses as soon as you think about, see, and smell food. Chemical reactions prepare your body to digest what you're about to eat so you can absorb nutrients. Juices flow, saliva accumulates, and your digestion receives messages to prepare enzyme secretions for end-stage digestion.

However, the first physical stage of the digestive process begins in the mouth, with its teeth, musculature, and salivary enzymes. The simple and mechanical act of chewing breaks the food apart, allowing more of its surface area to be introduced to the alkaline enzymes present in your saliva. This prepares the food for further breakdown by the strong stomach acids.

Mastication made easy: Just chew it

Stemming from the Greek word *mastikhan,* which means to "grind the teeth," *mastication* is the process of "positioning the food between teeth and tongue so that it can be mashed and crushed as a primary digestion stage" — so reads a technical book on mastication and swallowing. As a primary stage of digestion, mastication, also known as chewing, can be considered the ultimate digestive aid.

Why we aren't chewing enough

With the increased consumption of sweets, dairy foods, and animal proteins, most people have become lazy chewers because the salivary enzymes have little effect in breaking down such foods. Of the three basic macronutrients (carbohydrates, fat, and protein), carbohydrate digestion starts in the mouth, where enzymes in our saliva go to work.

The breakdown of proteins and fats begins in the stomach and the upper part of the small intestine. Proteins and fats are broken down by stomach acids or bile salts, which are produced by the liver and stored by the gall bladder.

Adding to this tendency toward jaw lethargy is the fact that refined, fatty, and high-protein foods often have little texture or taste after a few chews. If held in the mouth for long, their additives may create an unnatural and unpleasant aftertaste and acrid odor that rises into the nasal passage. As a result, most people have developed the unconscious habit of moving their food to the back of the palate and swallowing it before it's thoroughly chewed.

Mechanical digestion is nearly as important as chemical digestion. They work together.

The widespread preference for diets heavily laden with meat, dairy products, and sweets is accompanied by an equally widespread insensitivity to discerning whole food quality and subtle tastes. Many people's sensory receptors have become dull and confused — they can't imagine eating a bowl of oatmeal without the addition of some kind of sweetener. They find it unthinkable to have something bland in their mouth that demands work to produce a sweet taste.

Chewing enables you to distinguish the refined and fake from the whole and real. Salivary enzymes can digest as much as 30 to 40 percent of starches before food even reaches the stomach. Here's the key to figuring out what you're eating: Real food should become tastier and naturally sweeter the more it is chewed and mixed with saliva. And relaxed chewing enables you to enjoy the whole spectrum of taste and aroma by allowing the throat to open up.

The irony of the trend to consume more whole foods is that although we're changing the quality of the food we eat, we're still maintaining poor chewing habits left over from our old eating system. Forget gulping — that's for barnyard animals. Chew your food because your stomach doesn't have teeth!

Here are my seven secrets for effective chewing. Go ahead; try them at your next meal:

- **Control your inner pig:** Put less on your fork, spoon, chopstick, or shovel. People often put so much in their mouths that they become overwhelmed with saliva and swallow to avoid choking. Remember to put your eating implement down after each mouthful. When you load up that utensil and keep it waiting close to your mouth, you create a subtle pressure to rush through the mouthful for the next bite. Take a short break between mouthfuls. "Chew more, eat less" as an old adage goes.

- **Do the grind:** The human jaw is unique in its ability to move in different directions. You can chew up and down, as well as side to side. I once lunched with a Japanese folk medicine professor and observed him chewing thoroughly but quickly, as opposed to my up-and-down, laborious chewing-the-cud style. I asked him about it, and with a smile he imparted his personal wisdom: "Don't be a cow. The human jaw goes many directions. Make chewing a quick motion. That is the best way."

- **Isolate saliva:** Ever eat taffy? As a child, I loved rolling, squeezing, and concentrating it in my mouth to extract all that sweetness from the treat before swallowing the liquid and then mashing the taffy for more. You'll find a similar technique helpful when you eat whole grain.

  When you begin chewing, your mouth secretes an abundance of saliva to initiate digestion. On impulse, we usually swallow the entire mess, wondering how any more chews could be possible. But it is possible, and the secret is to isolate the saliva, just like you'd do with taffy or hard candy.

As the fluid gathers, isolate the food to one side and use your cheek muscles to draw the liquid back and swallow. Then continue working on the food.

You can chew something forever with this technique, and although it may sound ridiculously technical, it can feel very natural after a couple of times. You end up tasting the food in ways that you never had and appreciating the subtlety of distinctive taste and flavor. In the process, you also develop flattering cheek muscles to go with your slim, vital figure.

✔ **Take a breath:** To facilitate good breathing, which promotes calm meal-times and better digestion, you must take full, calming breaths with long, gentle exhalations as you eat.

✔ **Don't count your chews:** Contrary to what you may have read in some macrobiotic books about chewing until your eyes cross, don't focus on a specific number of chews. In fact, I usually recommend that clients *not* count chews, but instead "chew brilliantly well at only one meal weekly." By designating one meal per week where you focus on chewing, you become more aware of when you're not chewing during other meals, and you automatically chew more efficiently. Counting chews often leads to obsessive, boring meals and an alienating sense of self-righteousness. If anyone suggests you count each mouthful, tell 'em to get a life.

✔ **Avoid drinking iced beverages with meals:** Drinking with meals can dilute salivary enzymes as well as stomach enzymes and hinder diges-tion. If you're eating a whole food diet low in salt and sugar (liquid trig-gers), you may find that thorough chewing satisfies your craving for liquid during a meal. A little hot tea, slowly sipped after a meal, is a satis-fying way to complete the meal.

✔ **Practice mindful chewing:** A pilot study at Indiana State University found that mindfulness, including specific instructions to slowly savor the flavor of food and become aware of how much food may be suitable, helped to reduce eating binges by 75 percent. Savor every bite; enjoy the flavors, textures, and fragrance of your meal. Make your meal table orderly and beautiful with nice cutlery, distinctive plates or bowls, and fresh flowers. Lose the newspaper, television, and noisy company as meal partners. Instead, create an atmosphere that is comforting with dimmed lights, soft background music, and several candles. Creating fewer distractions in your environment while making the mood more relaxing is a habit that encourages more satisfying meals, better digestion, and a deeper calm.

Clearly, most of us can do a little better in the chewing department. When clients ask me, "What do you put on your cereal?" my response is remarkably simple: "My teeth!"

The most important quality that you can bring to your eating is to be present with what you're doing. Taste your food, savor it, feel it nourishing you, and develop a sense of gratitude for your food, your senses, and the miracle of transforming your health.

Natural absorption support: Avoiding the ill winds of digestive gas

Any material on digestion needs to include the reality of one possible consequence of not digesting adequately: gas. This unsavory byproduct is especially important to mention because I suggest frequently including beans and bean products (notorious gas-producers) into your diet. The problem with gas is not just the obvious inconvenience of its embarrassment but also the fact that it indicates poor digestion and acidity.

Sometimes, during the first several weeks or months of switching over to a whole foods diet, you may experience intermittent gas because of beginner's mistakes: You may overeat, make poor food combinations, eat too fast, and so on. However, you can prevent gas by taking a few measures:

- **Avoid overeating.** People often attempt to compensate for what they lack by gorging themselves. Perhaps you need a bit more oil in your diet, or maybe you should be eating more frequently or consuming a greater variety of textures and tastes. Eating too much rather than addressing specific dietary needs produces increased acidity and hinders digestion, creating gas.

- **Chew thoroughly.** Digestion begins in the mouth (see the "Mastication made easy: Just chew it" section earlier in this chapter). Chew small amounts thoroughly and really taste the essence of your food. Thorough chewing initiates digestion in the mouth, making it less likely for you to have gas-causing food combination problems in later stages of digestion.

- **Don't mix liquids and solids.** This mix can dilute nutrition and make it more difficult to chew because it increases your impulse to swallow food before you've chewed it properly. It also results in feeling less satisfied after a meal.

- **Avoid frequently eating refined sugar.** Eating refined sugar compromises digestion because its digestion requires more minerals, which the blood pulls from tissue fluids, bones, and anywhere else it can get it. In most cases, the resulting acidity can cause flatulence.

- **Be mindful of food combinations.** Drinking juice (a highly concentrated sugar) with food that is complex sugar (as in whole grain, vegetable, or bean) and needs to gradually break down into simple sugar initiates a fermented mess that frequently results in gas.

✔ **Eat more slowly.** Rushing through meals (like many do so they can get to dessert) can create poor food mixtures that result in gas or digestive discomfort. Ideally, you want to wait 15 to 20 minutes before diving into dessert after a meal, so that your digestion gets a head start before it has to deal with the simple sugars in that pie.

✔ **Cook with sea salt.** This alkalizing addition to food improves digestion and partially neutralizes acidity. Here are some recommended amounts:

- A pinch per cup of whole grain before cooking

- A pinch (or a teaspoon of natural soy sauce) in a skillet of water-fried or sautéed vegetables toward the end of cooking

- $1/3$ to $1/2$ teaspoon per cup of dry beans cooked from scratch, added about $4/5$ of the way through the cooking

✔ **Include fermented foods in your cooking.** Fermentation, one of the oldest and most economical methods of producing and preserving foods, is used to create essential foods in many regions of the world. The fermenting process enhances flavor, improves nutritional value, and provides helpful microorganisms that increase beneficial gut flora. Experiment with sauerkraut (a great addition to the bean product tempeh — also a fermented product); umeboshi (a tart and tasty addition to salad dressings); miso (wonderful as a hearty soup bouillon paste); brine pickles (easy to make from cucumbers or any other vegetable); and kimchi (fermented cabbage). For some people, a reputable *probiotic supplement* (one that provides beneficial intestinal bacteria) can help with replacing bacterially deficient colons.

✔ **Enjoy peaceful meals.** Mealtimes aren't suitable occasions for debates, business talk (unless it's a business meal), or conflict resolutions. Any stressful situation can cause your digestive secretions to become inhibited or less efficient, leading to gas. Make light conversation, chew well, and use this time to truly nourish yourself for what lies ahead in your day or evening.

✔ **Take digestive enzymes.** Some people with compromised digestion fare better with enzyme support. You can find a number of digestive enzymes available at natural food markets. These supplements are usually plant-based enzymes (usually taken right after meals) that help break down food more effectively in the stomach for better absorption. Don't confuse digestive enzymes with probiotic supplements, which contain beneficial bacteria to help with absorption.

✔ **Move!** A light walk taken after a meal is a ritual in many cultures for good reason: It increases circulation, helps digestion (which may mean less gas), enhances oxygenation, and promotes increased vitality.

Part II
Healing the Macrobiotic Way

The 5th Wave
By Rich Tennant

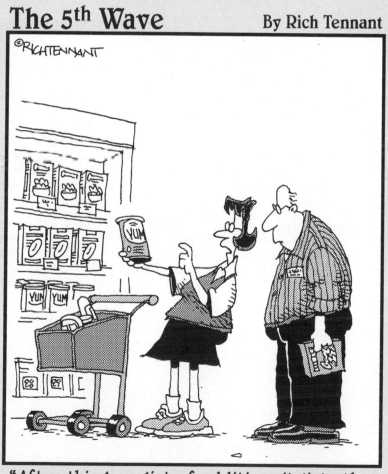

"After this long list of additives it lists the expiration date. Does that pertain to the product or the person who eats it?"

In this part . . .

Healing ourselves from degenerative disease or acting as our own advocate to prevent sickness requires that we understand all the factors that influence good health. This section addresses the broad concept of healing in practical and do-able terms, including suggestions for healing common diseases. It also explains what to avoid in order to sustain good health. Finally, this section reveals the factors that are behind extraordinary healings and how we can marshal body, mind and spirit to achieve health renewal.

Chapter 7

Laying the Groundwork for Macrobiotic Healing

*H*arry visits his doctor and points to nine different places on his body. "Doc," he moans, "I can't stand it anymore. I got pain in almost every area I touch. What's wrong with me?" The puzzled doctor promises a complete work-up and asks him to return the following week. At their next appointment, the doctor says, "Harry, after lab work and X-rays, I discovered the source of your problem. You have a broken finger."

This chapter is designed to give you the information that Harry should have had: how the body works, what makes it thrive, and how it heals. Improving your health begins with education. You should understand the power of nourishment, know what doesn't support your health, and be aware of available alternatives. I also explain the stages of illness and how your body begins to heal. Finally, you read about how to maintain your lymph system.

Recovering Our Health: Recognizing the Stages of Illness

Recovery, from the Latin word *recuperatio,* means to regain anything lost, usually relating to health or strength. Being able to maintain and recover your health requires that you know what direction your health is headed. This section presents the stages of illness, which reveal different levels of physical, mental, and spiritual sickness.

Every physical, mental, and spiritual illness belongs to one of the seven levels I explain in the following sections. Today, illness has become so commonplace that people practically take for granted that having some of these symptoms is "normal" — an inevitable consequence of aging. Or they blame a mysterious illness on genetics, viruses, stress, or maybe their mothers-in-law. Although these reasons can sometimes be a *part* of the problem, the truth is far simpler and rarely farther than your kitchen cabinets and refrigerator. Recovering good health isn't a complicated mystery. The first step is to understand how lifestyle and diet can make a significant difference.

Looking at the larger picture, all symptoms of a physical, mental, or spiritual illness branch out from the same root — an unbalanced body, mind, and spirit.

Empowering yourself with some basic knowledge about how the body works and what it needs is the first step to recovery. Experimenting with dietary change and remaining open and willing to confront the challenges of everyday life is the next step. This can open the door to a deeper sense of meaning and purpose. This is the real beginning of *macro-bios:* a great life.

Stage 1: Fatigue

Although it's natural to feel tired after an extensive workout or long day, a general and constant feeling of physical and mental fatigue can be an early indicator of a developing sickness or health imbalance.

Additional symptoms are muscular tension, frequent urination, excessive sweating, temporary bowel irregularity, and periods of feeling overheated or chilled. You may even begin to feel less mental clarity and a dulling of your perceptive abilities.

Recovery factor: Regaining more energy and clarity can occur rapidly — sometimes in a few days to a week. Taking time for relaxation, good sleep, whole food, and regular exercise can do wonders in a very short time.

Stage 2: Pain and suffering

The most common reaction to physical pain is to take a pill to alleviate symptoms of illness. For emotional pain, people invariably opt for something to numb their feelings. But simply treating the symptoms ignores the cause.

This stage is characterized by frequent aches and pains, muscular discomfort, cramps, shortness of breath, irregular heartbeat, mild inflammation, fever and chills, and restricted range of motion. Mentally, you may experience frequent depression, worry, and a growing feeling of insecurity.

Recovery factor: In most cases of mild pain, you can reverse these symptoms within a period of several days to several weeks. You may need to modify your diet, confront emotional concerns, get adequate sleep, focus on health education, and exercise regularly.

Stage 3: Blood disease

Stage 3 is one of chronic symptoms. The quality of your blood determines the health of your body's cells, tissues, organs, and ultimately body systems. Conditions such as high and low blood pressure, ulcers, anemia, nutritional deficiencies, more advanced forms of inflammation, skin disease, and numerous other conditions are influenced by your blood quality. More advanced mental conditions can appear as nervousness, hypersensitivity, timidity, and a tendency to feel mentally fragmented.

Recovery factor: Addressing these conditions can take from one week to four months, depending on individual considerations. As in Stage 2 (see the preceding section), adjusting your diet, modifying concentrated nutrient support, confronting emotional concerns, getting plenty of sleep, understanding your health, and exercising regularly can usually help or reverse these conditions if diligently practiced.

Stage 4: Emotional conditions

Eventually, this progressive slide into poor health can affect your emotions, leading to mood swings, anger, constant depression, anxiety, frustration, despair, or apathy. These conditions are mostly based on your blood's nutritional quality, as well as its hormonal levels, good circulation, and regulated blood sugar levels. In time, you may find yourself feeling more fearful and using more caution when facing new challenges or surroundings. You may also become more defensive or combative. And as you lose mental flexibility, your body becomes more rigid and hardened.

Recovery factor: Change often takes from two to four months. These changes require a healthy and balanced diet of whole foods, concentrated nutrient support, regulated blood sugar, consistent exercise, early-to-bed sleep, meditation, health education, emotional support, and a stronger emphasis on reconsidering your values and meaning.

Stage 5: Organ disease

As your health continues to be influenced by poor nutrition, inactivity, and emotional stress, the quality and functioning of your organs and glands begin to deteriorate. This results in structural changes in organs, growths, poor hormonal regulation, and malfunction of the body's systems. Conditions that reflect organ disease include diabetes, atherosclerosis, stone formation, cancer, and many other types of sicknesses. The mental extremes show up as chronic stubbornness, prejudice, narrow-mindedness, extreme rigidity, and self-delusional thinking.

Recovery factor: A longer period of several months to one year is necessary to overcome these conditions. Those who recover usually tend to be exceptional individuals who commit to renewing their health, often by redefining all aspects of their lives. Therapies may include eating a balanced diet of whole foods, concentrated nutrients, taking herbs, learning more about good health, exercising daily, seeking professional and familial emotional support, and meditating. Faith and hope also play starring roles in this get-well drama.

Stage 6: Nervous disorders

More advanced physical and mental conditions develop in Stage 6 when problems in Stage 5 aren't addressed. These may include paralysis or more extreme mental conditions, such as schizophrenia and paranoia. At this advanced stage, physical and mental coordination is noticeably limited.

Recovery factor: A period of six months to several years is required to reestablish health. People who have overcome these types of disorders have completely changed their lives to embrace a healthy environment. Their exceptional healing is the result of quality and balanced whole food, herbal or (in some cases) supplemental support, regulated blood sugar, and the elimination of dietary extremes such as refined sugars, alcohol, reduced fats, and animal protein. Professional emotional support, as well as encouragement from family and friends, consistent exercise, contact with nature, and continued education, also has a role in healing at this advanced stage.

Stage 7: "Spiritual" disease

Often referred to as *arrogance*, *"spiritual disease"* has traditionally been considered the most developed form of sickness, even though the previous stages may not have been experienced and these individuals may appear healthy. This condition affects most people's lives in some way as selfishness, vanity, egocentricity, self-pride, exclusivity, and so on.

People with this condition suffer from their arrogance, impatience, and intolerance, even though they appear successful. They often lack faith, hope, and joy, and their ability to freely love is almost always compromised by their judgments. This common condition affects much of the world socially, as well as within ideologies.

Recovery factor: It can take several years to a lifetime to change to a more grateful and natural quality of life. Sometimes arrogance can be instantly cured by a profoundly emotional or spiritual experience or in the face of difficulty, the death of a loved one, or failure. Recognizing ignorance and discovering a deep sense of gratitude can present the beginning of renewed health and a harmonious spirit.

Four Elements of Dietary Healing

Four health strategies act together to form the foundation of a macrobiotic healing program. These strategies help to strengthen the body's ability to defend, regulate, and cleanse itself, while maintaining fortified health.

These four elements of dietary healing constitute the blueprint for establishing a good health foundation. The power of balanced whole foods, one mouthful at a time, offers a critical key for transforming our health and the health of generations to come.

Improving nutritional health

Whole grains; a mixture of root, ground, and green vegetables; legumes; sea vegetables and fruits; quality vegetable oils; and nuts and seeds can fortify your blood while rejuvenating your health. However, improving nutritional health doesn't simply mean eating what's good for you but minimizing the refined food, excessive fats, sugars, and animal proteins as well. Check out Chapter 5 for more on nutritional health.

Minimizing the amount of acidic foods that you consume preserves the body's alkaline mineral status. Concentrated food supplements and herbs can also contribute to your well-being when taken with a healthy dietary program.

Regulating blood sugar

A flexible macrobiotic diet can help regulate blood sugar because of its high complex carbohydrate percentage, mostly coming from grains, beans, and vegetables. Complex sugars gradually release their broken sugar compounds into the blood, creating moderate highs and lows instead of the extreme blood sugar spikes that occur with foods high in refined sugar and make your hormones run wild.

Foods that spike blood sugar can spur inflammation. Inflammation is now considered a bigger threat to your heart than high cholesterol levels. Inflammation is usually the body's response to infection or tissue damage, and it can be *local* (occurring in a particular part of the body) or *systemic* (occurring across an entire system). Inflammation is the *-itis* in arth*ritis,* bronch*itis,* col*itis,* gastr*itis,* and sinus*itis.*

Although many conditions can cause inflammation (genetics, environment, and so on), one of the most overlooked reasons is faulty diet and irregular blood sugar patterns. Head to Chapter 8 to read more about how macrobiotics can help you regulate blood sugar.

Fortifying immune function

The state of *natural immunity* (from the Latin *immunitas,* meaning freedom from disease) is accomplished by the still-mysterious immune system that, strangely enough, has no major organs of its own yet is composed of many types of microscopic cells and molecules that exist throughout the body. With watchful senses, the cells and molecules stand guard to protect you from anything foreign that could pose a threat to the body.

Good health depends on an immune system that's in premium condition. Immune function is unobtrusive when it's running smoothly — it's quiet, efficient, and fiercely protective. However, knock out the immune system, and a young person can suddenly look aged and worn. Scientific research has shown that it takes only 100 grams (a glass smaller than 4 ounces!) of carbohydrates from glucose, sucrose, honey, or orange juice to suddenly deactivate the toxin-eating ability of the white blood cells. They actually become temporarily paralyzed when a large amount of simple sugar enters the system, and your immunity becomes compromised when these cells can't protect you.

A macrobiotic diet combined with daily exercise and adequate rest is one of the best ways to strengthen your immunity. Chapter 8 gives you more details on boosting your immunity through macrobiotics.

Strengthening your body's detox ability

What you take into your body as nourishment, what you breathe in with the air, and what your skin's pores absorb must go through an elaborate process of breakdown, storage, and discharge. The hard-working internal filtering factories responsible for detoxifying your body are the liver, kidneys, skin, intestines, lungs, and lymph systems. What you store depends on the condition of these organs, the blood quality, the flow of blood and lymph fluid, as well as how much fat you hold (toxins can hide out for decades in body fat).

A macrobiotic diet minimizes your exposure to most food toxins. Some of the traditional foods recommended have been shown to absorb toxins and discharge them via the bowel. Additionally, as you become accustomed to eating balanced whole foods, your elimination organs become stronger, allowing you to consistently detoxify through natural channels without discomfort.

Nourishing Yourself with Movement

For many people, the word *exercise* is synonymous with *work*. With the full-time business of a job and family, who needs *more* work? Comedian Martin Mull summed up many people's attitude toward exercise: "The trouble with jogging is that the ice falls out of your glass."

Exercise, at whatever level you're comfortable with, works best if you consider it a priority — an essential part of your self-healing regime and an additional way you nourish yourself. Not *finding* the time means not *making* the time. If you adopt a healthier diet and lifestyle, you will sleep less and have more energy, and then exercising no longer becomes a matter of finding time.

Ultimately, you must understand the value of exercise and then plan for it through regular scheduling and a bit of discipline. You find time to sleep and eat, so exercise should be no different. In time, the positive difference you feel as a result of exercise will reinforce your attitude toward it. You'll want to maintain the natural state of well-being that exercise provides.

Enjoying the benefits of regular movement

You may suddenly get the urge to lie down at the mere mention of the word "exercise," but its value is worth emphasizing: Regular exercise increases energy, helps maintain strength, improves will, decreases tension, and lends a solid feeling of renewal that nourishes the spirit. And that's only for starters!

The hallmark of health has always been moderation, and so it is with exercise. Consistent exercise, to a level that does *not* stress, is the best practice.

One of the ways exercise improves general fitness is by providing the muscles with an increased flow of energy. Good exercise stimulates twice the amount of a starch called *glycogen* that is stored in the liver and muscles. Glycogen is an athlete's primary fuel. If enough glycogen is stored in the muscles, it doesn't have to be dispatched from the liver. This is one reason athletes have stronger endurance and stamina. At the same time, exercise helps to detoxify the body by promoting the removal of carbon dioxide and other waste products from body tissues to the bloodstream and, ultimately, to the eliminative organs.

Here are some of the amazing physical benefits of regular exercise:

- ✔ Lowers your blood pressure
- ✔ Strengthens your heart
- ✔ Improves oxygen levels in your blood
- ✔ Improves your circulation
- ✔ Reduces blood fat levels
- ✔ Relieves depression
- ✔ Increases your ability to handle stress
- ✔ Improves your appearance
- ✔ Enhances your self-esteem
- ✔ Helps deepen your sleep
- ✔ Helps stabilize your blood sugar levels
- ✔ Helps manage your weight
- ✔ Oxygenates and strengthens your lungs
- ✔ Keeps your bones strong
- ✔ Increases your muscle strength
- ✔ Boosts your metabolism rate
- ✔ Reduces your cancer risk
- ✔ Provides more energy and endurance
- ✔ Improves your mental clarity and ability to focus
- ✔ Improves your complexion
- ✔ Helps you live a longer and more vital life

Now, if someone offered you a safe little pill that gave you all of these benefits for just a dollar a day, would that be appealing? Well, such a pill doesn't exist. Yet, for a brief investment of 20 minutes daily, you can receive all of these benefits by simply putting one foot in front of the other and moving!

Don't wait for the impulse. Forget about waiting until you "feel like it." If you want these benefits, make a commitment, grab that bike or those walking shoes, and face your daily challenge.

Making the best exercise choices

First and foremost, exercise puts you back *into* your body, providing a centering effect that stabilizes your thinking and creates calmness. The natural vitality that exercise brings can be refreshing, confidence boosting, and healing.

Most people are overwhelmed by their exercise choices: weight lifting, walking, jogging, rowing, cycling, swimming, yoga, rebounding, T'ai Chi, tennis, dance, stretching, isometrics, stair climbing, and on and on. No doubt, the choices are plentiful. Understanding the benefits of different exercises will help you choose according to your needs. I explain the basic four types of exercise in the following sections.

Strength training

Strength training is the process of exercising with progressively heavier resistance to build or retain muscle. Strength training requires the contraction and movement of muscles, as in weight lifting, but requires no extended demand for oxygen as some other exercises do. Strength training benefits skeletal muscles and bones with minimal advantage to your heart, blood vessels, and lungs.

Unless you perform regular strength exercise, you lose up to ½ pound of muscle every year after age 25. Muscle is considered very active tissue with high energy requirements. Even during sleep, your muscles are responsible for more than 25 percent of your calorie use.

Stretching

Stretching is an essential element of any exercise program. It increases physical performance, decreases the risk of injury, increases blood flow, distributes nutrients to the joints, increases neuromuscular coordination, reduces soreness, improves balance, decreases the risk of low back pain, and reduces muscular stress.

Anaerobic

The word *anaerobic* means "in the absence of oxygen." Anaerobic exercises are fueled by the energy in your muscles. Examples are sprints, dashes, tennis, short walks, recreational biking, weight lifting, and so on. Because there are rest periods and the movement isn't sustained, the workout doesn't create a large enough demand for oxygen to offer full cardiovascular benefits. Anaerobic exercise benefits bones, joints, metabolism, and energy levels.

Just plain fun activities

The following activities are not sustained or vigorous, so they fail to sufficiently burn calories or condition the heart and lungs. However, they still have obvious benefits, such as improving muscle tone, relieving tension, and improving circulation, as well as being competitive and fun.

- ✔ Baseball
- ✔ Bowling
- ✔ Football
- ✔ Golf
- ✔ Softball
- ✔ Volleyball

Aerobic

Aerobic exercise is the most beneficial to the heart, lungs, and circulatory system because its repetitive movements involve large muscles in a rhythmic motion. For an exercise to be aerobic, it must be sustained for at least 20 minutes, causing elevated heart and lung rates — but it shouldn't be so strenuous that you can't maintain it. Walking, jogging, cycling, aerobic dance, swimming, skating, and stair climbing are popular forms of aerobic exercise. Nonstop, active yoga (power yoga, as opposed to the traditional stop-and-start hatha yoga) can be aerobic if the movement is continuous.

For maximum aerobic benefits, your movement with aerobic activities should be consistent and brisk. The test of going into *oxygen debt* is to see if you can talk while exercising (you may want to have a partner beside you so you don't get funny looks). If you can talk while moving, you're not in oxygen debt and you'll know how much more to increase without going into debt. You know you're in debt when your breath suddenly feels very labored or short and the words cannot come out in an easy flow. This is usually called the *talk test*. Maintaining this level of exercise for 20 minutes offers many aerobic benefits and you end up forcing your body to adapt to this change. A longer period of strenuous exercise increases the supply of oxygen to the body's cells.

If you have had a period of inactivity, begin your exercise program gradually. Consult your medical practitioner to make sure you choose the kind of exercise that is right for you.

Motivating yourself to exercise

Motivation to exercise works best if it is something that you program yourself to do with firm commitment. Rarely do you really *want* to leap up out of a warm bed and push your body into exercise mode first thing in the morning. One way to motivate yourself is by remembering the value of exercise. You don't have to like it, but do remember that your mind and body need it.

Exercise should be something you look forward to doing, not something you need Herculean force for just to put on your running shoes. Use exercise as a focusing meditation by concentrating on your breathing or devoting your walk to sorting out an issue in need of a resolution. Bring along an MP3 player and listen to your favorite upbeat music, motivational recordings, or something inspirational.

Consider exercise as a way to become physically inspired and to reconnect with your inner healer, even if it's only a brief walk in the park.

Native Americans have an interesting perspective on longevity. They believe that each soul is allotted a specific number of beats for its particular lifespan. When one reaches that ultimate figure, it returns to Mother Earth. During exercise your heart temporarily speeds up to accommodate your body's oxygen needs. However, at rest in a well-conditioned body, your heart naturally slows to a lower pace. This is why athletes have a very low resting pulse. Because exercise, reduced stress, and healthy eating ultimately slow the heart, you can choose to extend this earthly visit with regular exercise.

Becoming a Lymph-O-Maniac

You're not alone if you don't know anything about your body's lymph system. Our associations with the word *lymph* are generally negative, such as when we hear that someone's cancer has spread to the lymph nodes. However, according to Gerald Lemole, MD, a professor of surgery and 35-year veteran of thousands of heart operations, "There would be far less heart disease and far fewer heart attacks if people took care of their lymphatic systems." In the following sections, I explain the lymphatic system and how you can maintain it.

What the lymphatic system is and how it works

The *lymphatic system* is the circulatory system of our immune system. Considered the "river of life," we have more lymphatic fluid in our bodies than blood and more miles of lymphatic ducts than blood vessels. Lymph fluid is a colorless, watery fluid that contains plasma and white blood cells. This efficient system sweeps toxins from around our cells, filters out germs, and, in cleaning our blood, ensures that toxic substances reach the liver for cleansing and then exit to kidneys for elimination.

This intricate system of lymph vessels weaves through our bodies, intertwined with our blood vessels. Along these vessels are *lymph nodes,* fibrous, mesh-like tissues populated with cells that catch and destroy invading germs. The nodes act as a filtration system that keeps the ultra-small particles of bacteria from entering the bloodstream. You're probably familiar with the glands (they're actually nodes) in your neck that swell when you have the flu, but those are just a few of the hundreds of lymph nodes scattered throughout your body.

If your lymph flow is weak, the toxins stay in your nodes and vessels longer. According to Dr. Lemole, when your lymphatic system is inefficient, you are at a higher risk for inflammation and hardening of the arteries *(atherosclerosis)*. Without adequate movement to stimulate lymph flow, the cells are left stewing in their own waste products and starving for vital nutrients that they need. This situation can contribute to many degenerative conditions and advance aging.

How to improve your lymphatic health

The blood has the hardest working organ in the business on its side: the heart. Its constant beating provides the pressure that supports our circulation. However, the lymphatic system has no real pump to force fluid through the vessels. The secrets to optimum lymphatic health are keeping the fluid moving and keeping your lymph ducts open.

You can move lymph through the following activities:

- **Massage:** The friction of some forms of deep tissue massage that focus on the lymph areas of the neck, chest, groin, and abdomen actually pushes lymph.

- **Exercise:** Exercise is good for lymph because the contraction of muscles moves lymph fluid through its vessels and into the nodes, where detoxing occurs as resident white blood cells eat anything that doesn't belong.

- **Repetitive deep breathing:** The lungs actually act as a bellows mechanism, stimulating the fluid to move upwards toward the neck. The simple act of a full inhalation and exhalation creates a dramatic pressure within the chest cavity that amplifies the bellows effect to promote strong lymph flow.

- **Using a mini-trampoline or rebounder:** Rebounding is reported to increase lymph flow 15 to 20 times. Most of all, like the natural instinct of kids jumping on a bed, rebounding is FUN! The mini-trampoline subjects the body to gravitational pulls ranging from zero at the top of each bounce to two to three times the force of gravity at the bottom (depending on how high you're rebounding).

✔ **Alternating hot and cold temperatures (sauna with a cold water dip):** Personally, I advise my clients to do this every time they shower! Make sure to first increase the hot water as much as you can comfortably tolerate. Then, just as you would walk into a cool ocean and experience the temperature gradually as the water level increases up your body, hold the shower head, turn the water to slightly cool and aim it at your feet, gradually bringing it up the length of your body. Finish with a towel rub and notice how alive you feel!

✔ **Dry skin brushing:** This is a swift, powerful, and easy way to help the natural detox process by moving lymph and improving circulation.

Because of its significant benefits, dry skin brushing warrants further explanation. The skin is the largest organ in the body and is responsible for one-fourth of the body's detoxification each day, which makes it one of the most critical elimination organs!

Dry skin brushing is popular in European and Asian spas, as well as many healing treatment centers throughout the world. The Russians, Turks, Scandinavians, Koreans, and Japanese have used this treatment for centuries. Here are some of the immediate benefits of dry skin brushing:

✔ Accelerates toxin elimination

✔ Stimulates blood flow and circulation

✔ Reduces cellulite

✔ Enhances lymphatic flow

✔ Exfoliates the skin and removes dead skin cells

✔ Offers anti-aging through cell regeneration

✔ Helps skin remain toned, moist, and supple

✔ Strengthens immunity

To perform dry skin brushing, all you need is a natural bristle brush, skin mitt, vegetable gourd brush *(loofah),* or even a coarse washcloth — and 5 to 10 minutes.

Here's how to perform the dry skin brushing technique:

1. **Using your brush, mitt, or washcloth, briskly brush or rub the sides, tops, and soles of your feet, moving upward toward your calves, in small circular motions.**

   It is thought to be more beneficial to brush from the extremities toward the core of the body in a circular motion.

2. **Brush the sides, fronts, and backs of your calves and around the knees and thighs.**

   Avoid brushing over bruises, cuts, or irritated areas.

   For the underside of the thighs, a two-handled long loofah can be used more vigorously.

3. **Work your hips and buttocks (great for a cellulite treatment!), as well as the entire abdomen in large and small circles. Then continue on by doing your chest and sides of the ribcage.**

4. **Gently brush around the breasts and the middle of the front ribcage where many lymph nodes are concentrated.**

   Always brush gently over sensitive areas. With consistent practice, your skin will become more resilient and endure more vigorous brushing.

5. **Even though it's hard to reach, don't forget to rub your back.**

   For this area, you may find it easier to use a stick brush or a long loofah. Holding both ends of a folded hand towel may also work.

6. **Raise one arm up and brush from your hand down toward your armpit before moving to the other arm.**

   Many nodes are also concentrated around the armpit, so be thorough in this area.

7. **Complete your dry skin brushing routine with small circular brushing or rubbing around your neck and shoulders.**

   The stick brush or long loofah also works well on the shoulder area (drape the loofah over your shoulder and hold one handle in front and one behind your back to rub) and is easier to manage than the mitt or washcloth for this particular area.

Try skin brushing on dry skin before a shower or bath, particularly in the morning. Washing will help get rid of the impurities that result from the brushing action.

You may be wondering, "Why not just do the brushing in the shower with some soap, and get it all done at once?" Brushing wet skin causes it to stretch and is not as effective for exfoliation as brushing your skin when it's dry.

Chapter 8

Macrobiotic Healing from the Inside Out

This chapter examines illness from a larger perspective than just treating symptoms. Western medicine has developed amazing technologies for symptomatic treatment, and this approach to medicine plays an important role in health care for crisis management and emergency situations where immediate treatment is required. Still, we need to incorporate in our lives some preventive strategies and maintenance efforts that support recovery. This chapter addresses those concerns.

If we compare cultural eating habits with our modern diets, we can see how food refinement has blossomed into its own food category, one that many people blindly follow without question. I had a recent conversation with a taxi driver who volunteered that he had high blood pressure when he found out that I was a health writer. I talked about dietary change that could help him and he waved it off, saying, "I take one pill a day and it all works fine." As long as we harbor the illusion that we are "taking care" of our problems with pills, we become dependent on their use and victims of their side effects.

This chapter shows how our modern diet causes illness, and I explain how a macrobiotic approach can help prevent illness.

Understanding the Limits of Symptomatic Medicine

You're driving in your car on a long, lonely stretch of scenic highway with no houses or gas stations for miles. You settle in and find a relaxing medium among the scenery, your random thoughts, and the hypnotic hum of the engine.

Suddenly, the "check engine" indicator lights up. You panic until you realize that you have a fat roll of electrical tape in your glove compartment. You grab the tape, tear off a small piece, and cover the light. It's no longer visible. The problem is solved, right?

Wrong, of course. All you've done is cover up the light.

Another example: You have a nasty sinus infection. You're in pain, your voice sounds like it's sneaking out of your nose, and the area from your cheeks to your brow feels like it weighs 100 pounds. You arrive at your physician's office seeking relief. He prescribes medications to handle the inflammation. You take the medicine and feel better.

It may lull you into a false comfort that the symptoms are no longer there, but is the infection really cured? Was the cause addressed? Did the physician inquire about your immunity? Was diet discussed? Did he ask about your exercise habits, sleep patterns, or unresolved stresses? Usually within the scope of a six-minute office visit, this can't be done. Most likely the treatment focused on the sinus inflammation, and the doctor wrote a prescription for intranasal steroids, decongestants, or expectorants. This addresses the symptoms, but it fails to answer the question of how you developed the infection in the first place or how you can prevent future occurrences.

Sometimes we *need* to take care of symptoms, so modern medicine has its place. Yet, as the macrobiotic principle "The bigger the front, the bigger the back" relates (see Chapter 3 for more on this concept), you pay a price with modern medicine in the form of potential side effects from medications, radiation, or surgery. The more dramatic the therapy, the greater the potential for side effects.

However, there's also an emotional price. You risk becoming dependent on medical practitioners to "fix" you, following exactly what they say and neglecting the larger picture of self-healing. This is not an empowering position, nor does it lead to long-term health. The problem with the medical system is not the system itself but the way in which it presents itself as the only and most effective way to treat sickness.

Understanding the way food influences blood sugar, hormonal regulation, tissue fluid acidity, tumor growth, immune function, and inflammation is a more sensible, cost-effective, and foundational way to rebuild health. Sometimes it may be necessary to use Western medicines to buy time, but don't delude yourself by thinking that taking care of symptoms is a solution. Your symptoms are your body talking to you. This requires careful listening.

How the Modern Diet Causes Illness

Traditional, whole food meals are nutrient dense and prepared in healthful ways, sometimes with vegetable oils used sparingly. The high-fiber, low-fat nature of whole foods reduces the risk for heart disease, hypertension, stroke, diabetes, obesity, and certain types of cancer. Research consistently proves this theory.

An abundance of information from medical and nutritional resources supports the benefits of a complex-carbohydrate, whole food diet and suggests that many diseases on the rise today can be attributed to the modern diet of high fat, high sugar, and excessive animal proteins.

Much of the food industry that we've come to trust interacts with government, the medical profession, and the scientific community to show a superficial concern for our nutritional needs. However, it produces deficient, chemically laden foods that don't support human health.

At no time in history did we ever take in the volume of artificial substances that we do today and tolerate it as "nourishment." However, many people have become so used to these foods that our taste buds can no longer distinguish the fake from the real.

If you look back at the eating patterns that humans evolved with over time, which is the topic of the next section, you see that the excesses of the modern high-fat, high-sugar, and high-protein foods can cause illness (I address the effects of these foods in the "Uncovering little-known inflammation sources" section later in the chapter). What we're eating now isn't what humans are supposed to be eating.

Historical food patterns

The last 5,000 years of cultural food history shows that most people were nourished by a starch-centered diet. Worldwide, there are more than 40,000 varieties of rice! In some regions of the world, grain, beans, and a variety of vegetables were primary staple foods.

These varied cultures in diverse geographical areas had in common a dietary template of principle foods in the complex carbohydrate category, such as whole grains, grain products, vegetables, beans, sea plants, fruits, and small quantities of animal-source foods.

Most people didn't suffer from the common diseases found in affluent societies today. Long-lived individuals within populations such as the Hunzakuts (northern Pakistan), Vilcabamba (Ecuador region in South America), and Abkhazians (Caucasus Mountains of Soviet Georgia) may have exaggerated their ages, but what countless researchers have agreed on is that these groups' senior populations are hearty, at least into their 90s, with strong bones, energy for manual work, and positive dispositions.

Research about the health habits of traditional societies revealed four commonalities:

- ✔ Leanness
- ✔ Natural complex carbohydrate–based diet
- ✔ Low cholesterol
- ✔ High activity level

When the Industrial Revolution rolled in during the early 19th century, major changes in manufacturing, transport, and agriculture began to spread throughout Europe, North America, and eventually the world. This was a major turning point in human society that suddenly influenced every aspect of daily life.

Prior to this time, people ate mostly grains and vegetable-based foods with small supplements of animal protein and animal byproducts. For the average person, animal protein was relegated to the odd animal bones added to the community pot of stew or a particular holiday feast during which an animal was sacrificed and consumed by everyone.

Although diets varied depending on where people lived, most of these healthy cultures unknowingly followed macrobiotic principles; they ate fresh, seasonal foods, little or no animal products, and no processed foods. They hiked up slopes to harvest foods, cultivated vegetables, and picked fruits. They didn't participate in formal exercise but rather lived a life filled with activity.

There is a simple sociological and historical consideration as to what defines real food for health. The ingredients for good health should be available and affordable to everyone, not just the privileged few who can afford rich foods or exotic supplements. Combining the diets of less affluent societies with modern technology can help us regain our sensitivity and optimum health.

Excess, not deficiency, causes modern-day illness

Carbohydrates, fats, proteins, calcium, phosphorous, magnesium, selenium, zinc, and other trace elements, as well as vitamins, are all required for human health and growth. Nature has provided these necessary raw materials for our needs in virtually every diet followed by traditional societies around the world.

However, the irony is that most of the diseases affecting affluent societies don't come from aging or nutritional deficiencies but from excess amounts of dietary components such as protein, fat, and sugar, as well as toxins from animal feed, pesticides, herbicides, preservation, and dye chemicals.

An example of this excess-versus-deficiency problem can be found in Eskimos, who have the highest dietary calcium intake of any population in the world — above 2,000 milligrams per day from fish bones. Their diet also ranks as one of the highest, worldwide, in protein — up to 400 grams per day primarily from fish. Globally, they also have the highest rate of osteoporosis (a loss of bone density).

The problem may appear to be a calcium deficiency, but the important question is: What are we eating on a daily basis that is leeching our calcium storages? For most cases of calcium deficiency, the problem is not deficiency but *gross calcium loss*. This occurs when the protein content is extremely high. When acid residues in protein break down, this acidity must be neutralized with minerals from the bones and body fluids. This occurs automatically and protectively to help the body maintain critical levels of blood alkalinity, because the blood must remain slightly alkaline. Therefore, the blood reacts to this balancing need at the expense of your bones, tissue, and cellular fluids. It's the wisdom of the body.

Many diseases may symptomatically appear to be related to deficiency, but if you address only the deficiency and not the cause (in this case, excess), the body still remains depleted.

Sickness is *not* the inevitable consequence of aging. It's aging *accelerated* by deficiency. Big difference.

The first step in healing is to take a "macro" view of your diet and lifestyle and identify your dietary extremes in order to focus on restoring more balance to your eating plan. Your excesses may include

- Excess food volumes
- Excess amounts of grain products (flour, pasta, crackers, and so on), fats (dairy foods, oils, nuts, nut butters, and so on), or animal proteins (meats, meat products)

> ✔ Excess stimulants (refined sugars, syrups, juices, fruits, and so on), caffeine (teas, coffee, sodas, over-the-counter medications, and so on), salt, or spices
>
> ✔ Excess stress beyond your body's toleration point
>
> ✔ Excess alcohol

The important thing is to not focus on only one area. You may take five steps forward covering your nutritional needs but eight steps backward through the damage from diet and lifestyle excesses. It's always about balance.

Although excesses dramatically influence health, deficiency concerns shouldn't be ignored. Your body needs essential fatty acids, intestinal bacteria support, digestive enzymes, B-12 supplements, and other vitamins and minerals (B-complex vitamin group, calcium, magnesium, zinc, selenium, and so on), and sometimes your body can't absorb these nutrients from dietary sources, thereby creating a deficiency.

The good news is that the body, if treated properly, can be very forgiving, despite how we've challenged it.

Looking at Illness from a Macrobiotic Perspective

Healing common diseases and conditions macrobiotically means looking at illness from a holistic perspective. It also requires that we discover natural and nontoxic ways to halt pain, strengthen immunity, regulate blood sugar, and make stresses more tolerable.

It's not just about taking special remedies, undergoing surgery, taking medications, or applying assorted therapies. Although these can aid healing, the core of healing must embrace a body, mind, and spirit approach. This requires an honest assessment of your imbalances in every area of life and a willingness to challenge these imbalances with determination and faith.

First you must activate your internal detox function. "Garbage in, garbage out," as they say. Reducing your intake of "garbage" so you're no longer contributing to the problem is the first step of healing. Understanding how you discharge internal toxins and how problems develop from an overburdened system is essential for healing.

Understanding the physical process of illness

The physical process of illness can be classified into two general categories: discharge and accumulation. Discharge and accumulation affect your health in different ways: Where discharge primarily affects your *condition,* accumulation (through degeneration) weakens your *constitutional* health, thereby shortening your lifespan.

Discharge

Often confused with sickness, *discharge* is the body's natural attempt to balance itself by throwing off, or discharging, its toxin load. This can occur internally (as pain, acidity, discharging of mucous, and so on) or externally (as in a skin condition that comes from the inside to the surface). Discharge happens when you habitually consume more food or food nutrients (carbohydrates, fats, proteins, and so on) than you can efficiently use or take certain dietary extremes that your body can't metabolize.

Usually it's wise to not interfere with most discharge conditions, unless they're acute, such as accompanied by a rising fever. However, after the excess is discharged, the symptoms typically disappear. Eating balanced food during this process can help you remain resilient while strengthening the body's self-healing abilities. Most discharge conditions shouldn't be considered an actual sickness but rather a physiological adjustment.

Examples of discharging are allergies (hay fever), coughs, lung phlegm, sneezing, achy joints, headaches, runny nose, watery eyes, skin blemishes or diseases, body odor, excessive perspiration, constipation, diarrhea, menstrual problems, low-grade fevers, recurrent infections, and so on.

Another example of discharging is tonsillitis, which develops when an inflamed lymphatic system attempts to localize the toxins that have entered the body, usually through poorly balanced food choices. The fever associated with tonsillitis is the body's way of burning off this excess.

Accumulation

Here's the frightening backside of discharge: If your eating habits are consistently unbalanced, the body becomes locked in a continual discharge process. Eventually, your ability to discharge becomes compromised, requiring the body to isolate the excess and store it internally in order to continue functioning. This is the first stage of *accumulation,* giving origins to fibroids, cysts, stones, polyps, tumors, and assorted systemic growths.

According to macrobiotic theory inspired by many traditional folk medicines, the accumulation begins in the peripheral locations of the body, favoring areas that have close proximity to the outside, such as the sinus cavity, inner ear, bronchi and lungs, kidneys, bladder, intestines, skin, and prostate gland. In the female body, the breasts, vagina, and uterus are also key accumulation areas. Eventually these regions can become common sites of infection or harbor the growth of different masses.

The psychological equivalent to a physical accumulation is mental accumulation — suppressed feelings or unexpressed emotions that hide behind passivity and indifference. Long-term suppression often evolves into distorted attitudes, fragmented thinking, depression, and eventually physical sickness.

Degenerative disease results when the body's organs and function begin to deteriorate. This type of illness indicates that the body's self-regulating mechanism is overwhelmed or dangerously depleted. This eventually causes structural and functional changes, which may include hormonal imbalance, tissue buildup, heart disease, cancer, and multiple sclerosis.

Some forms of degenerative illness develop when cells start decomposing into primitive, precellular forms. Cells are initially formed by the aggregation and fusion of countless bacteria. But when the reverse process happens, it's usually called an *infectious* disease.

Even though a degenerative disease can become life threatening, it's really the body's way of coping and adapting to more extreme and consistent abuse. The body is forced to protect itself by creating structural changes.

Uncovering little-known inflammation sources

If you've ever jammed your finger, sprained your ankle, or scraped your knee, you're familiar with inflammation. The accompanying redness, swelling, and pain are signs of inflammation. *Inflammation* (from the Latin *inflammatio*, meaning "to set on fire") is the activation of the immune system in response to infection, irritation, or injury. Your body uses inflammation to protect itself, to remove harmful invaders, and to begin the healing process for the affected area.

Anytime you see the suffix *-itis* in reference to a medical condition, this word ending indicates inflammation, such as colitis, sinusitis, pancreatitis, bronchitis, and so on.

Researchers are now linking inflammation to a growing array of chronic illnesses. Inflammation can involve every cell in your body and may be at the root of some of the deadliest diseases of the 21st century, including heart disease, diabetes, cancer, and Alzheimer's. Emerging research also links chronic inflammation to allergies, asthma, digestive disorders, hormonal imbalances, lupus, Graves' disease, fibromyalgia, osteoporosis, and neuro-degenerative disease. Individuals who tend toward anger, hostility, and depression have also shown increased systemic inflammation, putting them at risk for heart disease and numerous other conditions.

Macrobiotics has long recognized that inflammation plays a central role in disease and aging and that controlling and reversing inflammation is critical to balanced health. Although chronic inflammation may be a relatively new idea to conventional medicine, it's old hat in the traditional medicines of India and China. And while Western science hasn't worked out every step in the biology of chronic inflammation, we already know a great deal about how to reduce inflammation to promote health.

Inflammation from simple sugars and insulin swings

From a dietary perspective, the biggest culprit in causing abnormal inflammation is the standard American diet of heavily processed convenience and packaged fast foods. Simple sugar foods such as refined white sugar, brown sugar, corn syrup, agave syrup, barley malt, rice syrup, and molasses elevate blood sugar, creating an insulin release along with free radicals that result in oxidized fats. When oxidized, the fats form plaque deposits in the walls of your arteries, leading to a number of diseases. Research shows that a diet high in refined sugars and excessive refined flours can lead to heart disease and type 2 diabetes.

Insulin swings in the blood also increase stored body fat and the release of pro-inflammatory chemicals, which cause cell damage and accelerated aging. Although honey and fruit juice don't immediately raise blood sugar, they can still promote inflammation because they are simple sugars.

Inflammation from meats and fat consumption

Unhealthy fats used in preparing and processing commercial foods, especially trans fats and saturated fats, contribute to inflammation. Processed meats, such as lunchmeats, hot dogs, and sausage, contain chemicals such as *nitrites* that are associated with increased inflammation and chronic disease. Saturated fats are also found in meats, dairy products, and eggs. Although these foods provide valuable vitamins and minerals, our bodies really don't need the extra saturated fat. Trans fats are also included in this category. Most of these foods also contain fatty acids called *arachidonic acid,* and although some arachidonic acid is essential for your health, too much of it worsens inflammation.

Inflammation from nightshade vegetables

Nightshade vegetables, including potatoes, tomatoes, eggplant, and peppers, contain a chemical alkaloid called *solanine.* Florida horticulturist Norman Childers, PhD, discovered that by eliminating these foods he cured his rheumatoid arthritis. Although Childers's theory — that long-term consumption of the alkaloids in nightshade vegetables inhibits collagen and cartilage repair — has never been clinically proven, many patients have found relief from inflammatory and arthritic symptoms when they've eliminated these foods. But not everyone reacts to nightshades in the same way. If you tend to have inflammation or arthritis, avoid these vegetables for several weeks to determine whether this applies to you.

Inflammation from food additive chemicals and colorings

Food additive chemicals, such as nitrites, benzoates, and MSG, are known to exaggerate inflammation. Food colorings that give food an inviting appearance can also be harmful and toxic for the liver.

Inflammation from food allergies and gluten proteins

Certain food reactions can stimulate an allergic response in which the immune system releases massive amounts of chemicals, including *histamines,* to protect the body. These chemicals can trigger a cascade of allergic symptoms that affect the respiratory and cardiovascular systems, the gastrointestinal tract, and skin. Allergic reactions have a variety of symptoms, including mouth and tongue swelling, shortness of breath, cramps, diarrhea, mouth tingling, skin breakouts, and more. The most common allergy trigger foods that foster inflammation are wheat, eggs, nuts, fish, soy, dairy, corn, shellfish, and chocolate.

Celiac disease is a condition in which an individual can't tolerate gluten proteins found in most wheat products and instantly develops inflammatory symptoms. The core culprits are wheat, rye, barley, and commercial buckwheat.

Inflammation from herbs

Some herbs, such as echinacea, ginseng, reishi, and astragalus, may be too stimulating to an already overactive immune system. This can result in inflammation.

Halting and reversing inflammation

Some research has shown that fatty acids, often found in fish, nuts and seeds and their oils, and fruits and vegetables can help prevent inflammation. But again, the main concern should first focus on the dietary factors that aggravate inflammation. High protein, excessive fats (trans and saturated fats), too many simple sugars, excess alcohol, food chemicals, and some nightshades all play their part in creating inflammation and the conditions that evolve from this reaction.

A macrobiotically oriented diet of grains, beans, vegetables, and fruits in moderate volumes, combined with optional small amounts of animal proteins, is the best insurance toward halting and, in many cases, reversing inflammation.

Approaching immunity problems

In the 1980s, a popular game called *Pac-Man* featured a quick-moving little video creature that gobbled up invading ghost-shaped attackers. Pac-Man would roll along, engulf an entire ghost with his large mouth, and voilá, enemy vanquished!

Simple game, simple strategy — and strangely similar to the general workings of your immune system. Immune cells occupy every part of the body — the eyes, nostrils, skin, lungs, and lining of internal organs. When your body is healthy, immune cells stand guard 24/7, protecting you from foreign invaders that threaten your well-being, such as bacteria, viruses, dietary toxins, free radicals, chemical pollutants, oxidation, poisons, and even cancer cells. When these invaders are found, the immune cells disable them, just like Pac-Man did, with an army of white blood cells.

The organs and tissues that make up the immune system (from the Latin *immunitas,* meaning "freedom from disease") are the lymph nodes and vessels, spleen, bone marrow, thymus gland, and tonsils. Some immune cells guard the lining and blood vessels of specific organs, while others circulate through the body by means of the lymph fluid looking for action. The lymph fluid circulates within a separate network from the circulatory system and consists of a pale, thick fluid made chiefly from fat and white blood cells. With many of the immune cells headquartered in lymph fluid, they are almost always on alert status to be dispatched to the site of a threat.

Far in advance of getting noticeably sick, the body usually broadcasts telltale signs that your immunity is being compromised. These signs are unique to you and based on your constitution, diet, and lifestyle. The most common signs are allergies, headache, skin rashes, joint pain, a cough, cold or flu, fatigue, stress intolerance, postnasal drip, asthmatic reactions, a need for more sleep, and so on.

Your immune system uses the nutrients from your daily diet to heal your body as you sleep. This is usually why when you go to bed with a light injury or cut, it is noticeably improved when you awaken the next morning. A standard macrobiotic recommendation for improving immunity is to be in a deep sleep before midnight to ensure deeper and more healthful rest. This principle is in keeping with an old folk wisdom saying: "One hour before midnight is worth two hours after midnight."

Flip through any health magazine and you're bound to notice numerous ads claiming you can *boost, enhance, increase, stimulate, strengthen,* and *activate* immune function with *clinically proven, innovative, cutting-edge* technology and *revolutionary* supplements or herbs. Although many verifiable reports have been made on the immune enhancement of certain supplements and herbs, the primary question to consider is, "What factors weaken immunity?" Because recovering immunity is the basis of real healing, you first must change negative habits that decrease immunity. The macrobiotic perspective is to first look at the larger view before attacking a deficient symptom by attempting to "boost" it.

The following sections detail the factors that *negatively* influence our immune function.

Exposure to free radicals

Oxidation, the formation of highly reactive oxygen molecules, also known as *free radicals,* can cause our own molecules to break up and lose electrons. This break-up causes the beginning of cell and tissue decay in your body. When this happens, scar tissue can form, which eventually replaces the functional tissue of different organs.

If this occurs in the arteries, hardened plaques appear to attach themselves to the artery wall (a process known as *atherosclerosis*). This condition usually accelerates to create the possibility of a heart attack or stroke; if it occurs in the brain, conditions such as Parkinson's disease or Alzheimer's can develop. Free radicals also can cause cell mutation, the basis of cancer. Oxidants seem to be everywhere in the environment: cigarette smoke, chemical pollutants, industrial pollutants, sunlight exposure, ultraviolet rays, dietary fats, and food chemicals. Your body absorbs these harmful radicals through air, food, and water.

Consciously reducing your exposure to these irritants keeps your immunity from being burdened. *Antioxidants*, compounds that neutralize oxygen radicals, from plant sources can boost your immune reactions and act as cancer-prevention elements.

Lack of sleep

Sleep, like oxygen, is highly underrated. As a matter of fact, sleep is not only abused but also taken for granted and typically appears last on our priorities list. The growing list of disorders related to sleep and immune dysfunction is making us redefine the importance of Benjamin Franklin's famed adage: "Early to bed and early to rise makes a man healthy, wealthy, and wise." Here are some of the scary problems that can develop from lack of sleep:

✔ **Increased cortisol levels:** University of Chicago researcher Eve Van Couter discovered that sleep deprivation left healthy volunteers with increased levels of cortisol, the stress hormone, as well as impaired glucose tolerance and insulin resistance, paving the road to diabetes. A rise in cortisol levels can also lead to hardening of the arteries and hypertension.

✔ **Obesity:** A lack of sleep, particularly in the young, inhibits the growth hormone, which speeds up the fat-gaining process. Some research shows a lack of sleep lowers production of the hormone testosterone. This can increase fat gaining as well as muscle loss.

✔ **Sweet cravings:** Increased carbohydrate cravings happen more frequently in the sleep deprived because a lack of sleep negatively affects the hormone leptin. This hormone tells the body that it's full after eating. However, when leptin is decreased, the body craves calories, particularly simple carbohydrates, even though its nutritional or blood sugar needs may have been met.

✔ **Breast cancer:** Research at the University of Connecticut indicates a direct connection between breast cancer and hormone cycles disrupted by late-night light. Melatonin, which is primarily secreted at night, triggers a reduction in the body's production of estrogen, which is a good thing because estrogen is known to promote the growth of breast cancer. However, light interferes with melatonin release, which allows estrogen levels to rise, leading to a likelihood of developing breast cancer.

✔ **Depression and irritability:** Research has shown that a lack of sleep causes depletion in the brain neurotransmitters that help regulate mood. As a result, sleep-deprived people have a shorter fuse and tend to get depressed more easily.

✔ **Weakened immunity:** Medical research shows that sleep deprivation negatively affects human white blood cell count, which can impair the body's ability to fight infection and disease.

Chronic emotional stress

Chronic stress has been shown to cause overproduction of different *neurochemicals* (chemicals of the nervous system) that can cause serious problems with our immune function. Additionally, the release of cortisol from the adrenal glands during emotional stress can depress immune function, resulting in conditions such as bacterial or viral disorders, hypertension, cardiovascular disease, asthma, diabetes, irritable bowel syndrome, ulcers, cancers, multiple sclerosis, arthritis, and a host of others.

The instant a person perceives something stressful is happening, the brain signals the nerves to release adrenaline and related chemicals, sending quick energy to the muscles. At the same time, a hormone called corticotrophin is released into the bloodstream and tells your adrenal glands to release *more* stress hormones called *glucocorticoids*.

Rethinking the search-and-destroy approach to healing

Research from a Johns Hopkins University study discovered that the normally larger molecules of milk proteins bond to some of our tissues, including the insulin-producing pancreatic cells. This causes the body's immune system to attack and destroy the milk proteins, as well as the insulin-producing cells of the pancreas. This research is convincing scientists that some people who are sensitive to animal meat and dairy foods, such as milk proteins, may be at risk for autoimmune disorders, as well as diabetes.

Until recently, the accepted method of dealing with immune-related diseases was chiefly to kill the invader, whether it was a bacteria, virus, or cancer cell. In the last 25 years, this approach has become less popular, and alternate strategies designed to support the body's immune system are now more popular and accepted. The new healing focus in alternative medicine is to find different ways to strengthen and bolster immune function, because this combats toxins and fights cancer's spread.

The health and vitality of your immune system is critical for healing. In fact, immunity is the foundation for healing. Strengthening immunity is more a matter of nutrition and lifestyle factors than simply "destroying invaders." Modern medicine has spent billions of dollars in the last 25 years for antibiotic, antiviral, and antifungal medicines to decreasing results. If this invader-killing approach were as effective as medical marketing would have us believe, there would be far fewer overall deaths from infections. However, statistics have shown just the opposite.

Acting as the Jekyll and Hyde of stress biology, these stress hormones direct the body to dump sugar into the bloodstream, providing quick energy for a sprint away from danger. However, in situations where there is repeated stress, the glucocorticoids overwhelm the body, and the beneficial effects of stress hormones are reversed. The result is a decrease in memory function, energy levels, and immunity, making you more susceptible to sickness. A wide range of stresses, from losing a spouse to facing a tough examination, can also deplete immune function, causing levels of immunity activity to dramatically decline, leading to sickness and eventual disease.

That ideal of no stress exists only in death. You need to make your stress manageable, and this is based on your perceptions. The way you evaluate a stressful event is the key to how you biochemically react to it. Take a lesson from Jeanne-Louise Calment, an unflappable French woman who lived to be 122, who said, "If you can't do anything about it, then don't worry about it."

Depression and negative attitudes

Our personality is usually defined by our attitudes, behaviors, and reactions to the everyday challenges of life. When faced with difficult situations, pessimists often perceive themselves as helpless and frequently surrender to circumstances they feel they can't change.

Optimism has been shown to have a positive effect on immune response and seems to be a key element for feeling in control and successfully coping with stressful situations. Optimists usually feel more in control of their situations than pessimists do. When a situation becomes challenging for an optimist, she usually creates an alternate approach or strategy, having faith that things can turn out positively in the long run.

Learned helplessness is another form of stress that is particularly harmful to immune function. Learned helplessness is thought to occur from constant exposure to "uncontrollable" stressors — specifically, finding yourself in a painful or uncomfortable situation from which there seems to be no hope of relief or escape.

People who are depressed have shown higher levels of the stress hormones cortisol, adrenaline, and noradrenalin, all of which negatively alter immune function.

Behaviors that stem from dark moods can influence immune health. Typically, depressed people get less sleep, consume more alcohol, exercise less, often smoke tobacco, and frequently use more drugs, either therapeutic or recreational. These behaviors strongly manipulate and eventually exhaust immunity activity.

Too much or too little exercise

Too much exercise may *decrease* immune function. Research has shown that more than 90 minutes of high-intensity endurance exercise can make athletes susceptible to illness for up to 72 hours after the activity. Stress hormones such as cortisol and adrenaline raise blood pressure and cholesterol levels while suppressing immune function. This has been linked to frequent infections that plague endurance athletes after extreme exercise, such as marathon running or Ironman triathlon training.

Regular moderate exercise has been linked to a positive immune system response and a temporary boost in the production of white blood cells, the cells that attack bacteria. Regular, consistent exercise can lead to substantial immune health benefits over the long term. Here are a few examples:

- Moderate exercise helps immune cells circulate at a quicker pace throughout the body, so they can detect illnesses earlier than normal. The increased rate of circulating blood may trigger the release of hormones that "warn" immune cells of intruding bacteria or viruses.

- Some research indicates that regular exercise helps flush bacteria out from the lungs, while increasing the output of wastes, such as urine and sweat.

- The temporary elevation of body temperature also inhibits bacterial growth, allowing the body to fight infection more capably, in the same way that the mechanism of fever works.

> ✔ Exercise slows the release of stress-related hormones, creating a reduced chance of immunity damage from these hormones.

Phytochemical deficiency

Traditional folk wisdom has always emphasized the importance of vegetable and fruit consumption, but only within the last 30 years have scientists understood why. Nutritional science has isolated compounds in plants and vegetables that have literally restored life. These are called *phytochemicals,* the *phyto* referring to "plant."

These phytochemicals help plants survive in varied environments and stimulate the production of self-repairing cells. Conveniently, they produce the same results in humans, reducing our susceptibility to disease. Phytochemicals that appear in vegetables have proved to be strong immune enhancers as well as antioxidants (for more about antioxidants, see the "Exposure to free radicals" section earlier in this chapter).

Although phytochemicals are important for health and immunity, it's equally important to consider how you're getting them. Generally, most antioxidants are more effective when you get them the old-fashioned way: as a part of the whole food you're consuming! Nutrients such as vitamins, minerals, and trace minerals work more effectively in their natural state. For maximum protection, you should eat at least five servings of assorted colored vegetables per day; this amounts to roughly 2½ cups of vegetables in various styles of preparation: steamed, lightly sautéed, in soup, and raw.

Excess of simple sugars

The quality of complex carbohydrates in whole grains, vegetables, beans, and fruits is good for you. The simple sugars found in candy, pop, icing, commercial cookies, and packaged treats can do harm, particularly when eaten to excess.

Excess sugar depresses immunity. Studies have shown that consuming 75 to 100 grams of a sugar solution (about 8 tablespoons of sugar — the amount contained in two 12-ounce sodas) suppresses the body's natural immune responses by a minimum of 40 percent. Simple sugars such as glucose, table sugar, fructose, maple syrup, and honey cause over a 50 percent decline in the ability of white blood cells to destroy bacteria. In the studies, the immune suppression was most noticeable two hours after ingestion, but the effect was still evident five hours later!

Conversely, ingesting a complex carbohydrate solution (starch) didn't lower the white blood cells' ability to engulf bacteria.

Nutritional deficiencies and mineral loss

Your immune system is compulsively busy: An adult body produces approximately 126 billion white blood cells daily. Normally, more than 25 billion are patrolling the blood, and another 2.5 trillion are headquartered in the bone marrow, while 10 trillion other immune cells are housed in lymph tissues.

The need to feed these hungry warriors good nutrition is crucial to maintaining optimum immunity. Nutritional deficiencies can decrease your natural capacity to resist infection and its aftermath, while decreasing the overall functioning of your immunity. No doubt, poor nutrition adversely affects *all* aspects of immunity.

Vitamins A, C, E, and B-complex, plus zinc, iron, copper, and selenium keep your immune system on its toes. The function of natural killer cells and other white blood cells is improved with as little as 30 milligrams of beta-carotene per day — approximately the amount in two large carrots.

Minerals can be considered the microscopic metals in your food; metallic fragments of the earth's crust (which are released through rivers, wind, and rain) get into the soil, where they're absorbed by the plants you eat. Healthful whole food sources of minerals include whole grains, beans, leafy greens, vegetable roots, sea plants, and fruit.

Although animal protein is another rich source of mineral content, it's also rich in fat and acids that can weaken immunity. In this regard, it is best as a supplemental rather than a daily food.

The mineral issue is simply not settled by adding supplemental minerals to your diet. You should also understand that some foods weaken mineral storages. Therefore, a healthy macrobiotic eating plan should not only provide minerals but also guard against mineral loss. The main mineral thieves are the acid residues from foods high in protein and simple sugars. Because acids threaten the blood's alkaline status, an instant adjustment is made by a buffer reaction where the blood instantly solicits minerals from bones and cellular fluids to neutralize this sudden increase of acid.

Excessive fat and food allergens

Fats can impair your immune response. Reducing fat from your diet can help to strengthen the immune defenses against cells that can potentially turn cancerous. Researchers in New York tested the effect of low-fat diets on immunity, placing healthy volunteers on a diet that limited fat content to 20 percent, reducing *all* fats and oils — not just saturated or unsaturated fats. After three months, the researchers took blood samples from the volunteers and examined their immune function. Immune cell activity was greatly improved.

Some foods, such as dairy or nuts, can cause an allergic reaction in which immune cells don't recognize a harmless substance and attack it, causing temporary inflammation. This reaction compromises immune function. With prolonged allergic reactions, the intestinal lining becomes damaged, which enables toxic substances to be absorbed into the blood stream and weaken digestion, absorption, and immunity. This condition is known as *leaky gut syndrome.*

Alcohol and recreational drugs

Excessive alcohol intake can harm the body's immune system in several ways. First, it produces a general nutritional deficiency that deprives the body of valuable immune-boosting nutrients. Second, alcohol, like sugar, consumed in excess reduces the ability of white blood cells to kill germs. Large amounts of alcohol suppress the ability of the white blood cells to multiply, inhibit the effectiveness of natural killer cells on cancer cells, and reduce the ability of white blood cells to attack tumors.

Three or more drinks (one drink is the equivalent of 12 ounces of beer, 5 ounces of wine, or 1 ounce of hard liquor) burden the immune system. Damage to the immune system increases in proportion to the quantity of alcohol consumed. Amounts of alcohol that are enough to cause intoxication are also enough to suppress immunity.

Marijuana is the most frequently used illegal drug in the world today, and its effects on immunity are well known to researchers. Marijuana depresses the immune system's ability to protect itself against invading bacteria, viruses, chemicals, foreign particles, parasites, fungal microorganisms, and infections. It also decreases the body's ability to prevent the growth of cancer cells. Some studies suggest that THC (the main psychoactive substance found in the Cannabis plant) has a general immuno-suppressive effect on a variety of immune cells, particularly those in the lungs.

Chapter 9

Healing Common Diseases and Conditions Macrobiotically

*E*very day, millions of people who have adult-onset diabetes, heart disease, bowel inflammation, early-stage arthritis, depression, and a host of other conditions reach for medications to alleviate pain or the annoying symptoms of body breakdown, be it an immune-related condition, inflammation, unstable blood sugar, or hormonal dysfunction. In most cases, they are told that their conditions require a lifetime of medications that, at best, may *slow* the development of their condition. Side effects are incidental and dependent on many factors, but they are real and potentially dangerous. The result for many on such medications can become a journey toward disease.

Of course, if their choices stand between being in pain and not being in pain, most people would opt for some kind of relief. Unfortunately, behind medications for symptomatic relief, the public remains ignorant of safe, non-invasive, less expensive, and natural means available for healing.

Most patients are *not* told that an alternative solution to their problems may lie in what and how they eat and exercise on a daily basis. It is known that food influences our blood quality and chemistry. This is a fact. Changing your nutrient balance can influence cancer growth, stabilize blood sugar levels, reduce inflammation, regulate hormonal levels, harmonize mood swings, and promote increased immune function. These are facts that have a scientific basis.

The United States has been rapidly expanding in girth and degenerative disease. The illnesses on the rise include allergies, arthritis, cancer, diabetes, digestive irregularity, heart and artery disease, and many more. Overwhelming research as well as the living testimony of many exceptional individuals has documented that the primary cause of this rise in illness has more to do with our daily nourishment of food and drink.

This chapter focuses on offering dietary suggestions for a number of conditions and diseases that are becoming increasingly common. I outline recommended foods, herbs, supplements, exercises, and lifestyle suggestions to show some of the more subtle distinctions in attempting to heal or halt further progression of each condition. Keep in mind that these suggestions don't qualify as specific recommendations because each individual differs in his makeup and sensitivity. Instead, I show general healing choices from a macrobiotic perspective that can make a positive difference.

General Macrobiotic Healing Strategies

Because we must eat to sustain life, food is the basis of life. Therefore, the first and essential steps on the macrobiotic path to health and harmony concern the selection, preparation, manner, and consumption of food. I outline the dietary templates you should follow in Chapter 6. Read that chapter, choose the template that fits your needs, and give it a shot.

So following the right diet is the first step to healing. The following sections present many more things you can do in your daily life.

Essential dietary healing strategies

The following health strategies are the first essential steps for healing:

- ✔ Reduce or eliminate all animal protein, refined sugars, and dairy foods from your diet.

- ✔ Reduce cravings for foods that don't support healing, making diet change less of an effort. Eating less volume more frequently can help reduce the urge to overeat or consume sweets. This makes your new health transition less of an effort and more results oriented.

During the first four to six weeks of dietary change, it's best to eliminate *all* saturated fats and try to keep dietary fat to a minimum. After this time, your personal experience becomes your barometer.

If you tend to have high cholesterol, my recommendation would be to have three blood tests: one prior, another after 6 weeks, and a final test after 4 weeks. Note your original cholesterol. Let's presume you have a 225 cholesterol level (this is now considered high). After six weeks with healthy dietary change, no sugar, low fat, no saturated fat, consistent exercise, and daily whole grains, vegetables, and beans, get your second test to compare with the original. Some clients have seen drops in this short time of up to 90 points! Note the difference. Then, at this point, if you decide that you would like to have some of these foods again, try small amounts, less frequently, for a period of four weeks. Then get a final test. You may see noticeable cholesterol elevation. At this point, knowing that you have the power to change, you make your own choice. This experiment can be very empowering because your experience creates new convictions about what works best for your good health.

Essential non-dietary healing strategies

While change of diet is critical, it's not the whole enchilada. You can accelerate your progress by actively engaging in some non-dietary healing strategies:

✔ Get moderate, consistent exercise for a minimum of half an hour a day; exercising for two half-hour periods (one in the morning and one in the evening) is ideal. Examples of good exercises include walking, biking, and swimming.

✔ Discover new ways to combat stress. Meditation, T'ai Chi, qigong (or ch'i kung), massage, deep breathing techniques, yoga, and similar techniques can go a long way toward distressing your body and restoring a steady calm.

✔ Spend some time in nature, if possible, away from the electromagnetic energy of computers, televisions, cellphones, and other electronic devices. Walk barefoot in the grass, walk along the shoreline in wet sand, expose your body to the elements, and breathe some quality air.

✔ Sleep! Rest is critical for recovery because it nourishes immunity (see Chapter 8 for more on your immune system). The old saying "One hour before 12 is worth two after 12" is a bit of traditional wisdom that science has verified. Your body releases healing chemicals (particularly melatonin) during the deep sleep hours after midnight. Make your room dark and keep it cool, if possible. Avoid watching the news before turning in for the night. Your mind needs to be peaceful just before going to sleep, and a fresh memory of traumatic television visuals parading around your brain doesn't help.

Essential dietary practices

The following dietary tips will enhance your general health:

✔ Consume a whole-grain source of fiber with at least two meals a day. These can include brown rice, a mixed-grain combo, or oatmeal.

✔ Consume 3 to 4 cups of vegetables prepared in a variety of styles: steamed, as soup, lightly sautéed in oil, water-fried, or raw. Include the sweet category of vegetables in your daily diet: onions, carrots, squash, parsnips, cabbage, corn, and so on. The category of sweet vegetables can sometimes avert sweet cravings and helps with overall satisfaction.

✔ Use approximately 1 to 2 teaspoons of vegetable oil daily. The best choices are sesame and olive oil. You can get this serving in salad dressing or in a stir-fry with grains, vegetables, or beans.

✔ Consume a concentrated protein source such as beans or bean products every day. Add freshly cooked or canned beans to a salad; blend them to make a vegetable dip; add beans to grains and vegetables in a tortilla wrap; or prepare a hearty bean-and-vegetable soup.

✔ Experiment with sea plants (commonly called seaweed) for their rich mineral content.

✔ Make sure to use the five flavors (discussed in Chapter 4) in your cooking and learn more about the various cooking styles described in Chapter 13. Having a number of cooking styles under your belt allows you more meal versatility and a variety of flavors that will make meals more satisfying.

✔ Do *not* avoid adding salt to your cooking. Purchase bright white *damp* sea salt (damp salt usually indicates the presence of some magnesium chloride, which attracts moisture from the air) and add pinch amounts to your cooking.

✔ Eat four to six meals daily. Some people may find it easier to eat more frequently in order to curb overeating and reduce sweet cravings. If this sounds like you, have 4 to 5 smaller meals throughout the day.

✔ Enjoy a cup of noncaffeinated tea (grain tea or herbal tea) after each meal to aid digestion (see Chapter 16 for tea recipes). Often this is an easy way to curb your appetite.

✔ Eat a small amount of fermented food to help digestion and improve intestinal bacteria. Some sauerkraut or several pieces of pickled vegetable aid grain digestion. Miso is a fermented soybean paste used like chicken bouillon; put 1 round teaspoon of the paste into a bowl, dilute it with several teaspoons of hot water, and then fill the bowl with hot vegetable soup and stir to mix in the paste mixture.

Food "no-nos"

I once had a client who left me a memorable telephone message: "I've been on your "no-no" diet for two weeks and not only do I feel great; I don't even want those foods! It's "yes-yes" all the way."

The "no-no" foods are not "never" foods but foods that can slow your progress toward feeling noticeably better, so it's best to avoid them for a while. Actually, many people find that after a brief period of eating balanced whole foods, they rarely even want those foods.

Here's the list of foods to avoid:

- ✔ Avoid *all* fruit juices because they contain concentrated sugar with little or no fiber. Enjoy fresh, whole, seasonal fruit instead.

- ✔ Eliminate all alcohol, canned, and packaged foods, refined and processed foods, dried fruits, sodas, and any food with artificial coloring or preservatives.

- ✔ Avoid red meats, gravies, pork, and dairy products. If you are craving fish, have it once or twice weekly, for now.

- ✔ Minimize salad dressings. The more finely cut your salad, the more you can stretch a small amount of dressing without sacrificing taste. The reason for this has to do with excess oil.

General supplement suggestions

In the ideal Shangri-La of clean air and water and bodies that haven't been abused for years by toxic elements, you may be able to extract all the nutrients you need from food. Because life is far from ideal, I cautiously recommend some form of supplemental support, but supplements clearly aren't for everyone.

It's also easy to become dependent on supplements, so if you want to experiment with supplements, a five-day-on, two-day-off plan works best.

If obtainable (ask at your local natural foods market), try a food-based supplement for the first two months of a macrobiotic diet, and then gradually reduce or eliminate them and go without for a while. You'll determine what works best over time. However, research shows that you absorb very little of the vitamins and minerals found in supplements — some estimates suggest 10 to 20 percent of what you take can only be absorbed.

The following supplement recommendations can help *if* you have poor nutrient absorption, *if* you're anemic or pre-anemic, *if* you eat out exclusively, or *if* the transition to a more natural diet simply proves difficult.

✔ **Vitamin B-complex (including B-12):** Take 50 milligrams five days a week. Vitamin B helps your body with carbohydrate metabolism, absorption, hydrochloric acid formation, and nervous system functions.

✔ **Multivitamin/mineral:** Take the standard milligram or microgram dosages five days a week. Nutrients such as magnesium, calcium, iron, zinc, selenium and vitamins A, C, D, and E can give you a nutritional boost while making a whole foods transition. It's as if you have a good car, but you left the lights on and now the battery is drained. You don't need a new car — just a jump-start. Sometimes during an initial change, a multisupplement makes this transition easier.

Looking at Low Blood Sugar

Low blood sugar, or *hypoglycemia*, is an increasingly common condition in which there is a low level of sugar (glucose) in the blood. *Reactive hypoglycemia* happens when the blood sugar drops to unusually low levels approximately 1¹/₂ to 4 hours after eating. The symptoms of hypoglycemia include hunger, fatigue, lightheadedness, insomnia, sweet cravings, headache, rapid heartbeat, and — more extremely — anxiety, nervousness, fainting spells, sweating, tremors, seizures, and loss of consciousness.

These symptoms happen when the level of blood sugar has become dangerously low. With high or low blood sugar you can end up in a coma, so in the case of low blood sugar, the body signals its need by the low blood sugar symptoms. This doesn't always mean that you actually need sugar, but that you need food! However, if you've allowed the blood sugar to get too low, then after a meal, you will have not sufficiently elevated the sugar level and you will then have those after-dinner sweet munchies.

Think about insulin as cellular keys that open the cells to provide nourishment. However, when the message is internally broadcast that insulin is required to shuttle sugar into your cells in order to keep the sugar levels in the blood from becoming too high, an unregulated about of insulin comes pouring out. Eventually, you end up with too much insulin. Sometimes, diabetics take too much insulin and they go into insulin shock. For this reason, many diabetics carry a small amount of candy or chocolate in case this may happen.

When blood sugar falls to a significant low, the body's stress hormones, cortisol and adrenaline, are released to prevent blood sugar from continuously falling.

The most common of the numerous types of hypoglycemia is *functional hypoglycemia,* which is likely the result of a faulty diet. The major players that instigate this condition are an excess of sugar, caffeine, tobacco, alcohol, pop, and sometimes waiting too long between meals.

Another kind of hypoglycemia, often called Adrenal Fatigue Hypoglycemia, has to do with poorly functioning adrenal glands. Normally, these glands produce *glucocorticoids* when the blood sugar is low to elevate blood sugar. If this function isn't working properly, hypoglycemia results. Strong stimulants, such as sugar, dietary acids, coffee, and tobacco, can weaken adrenal strength. Frequent low blood sugar can be an early sign of diabetes. Dietary changes can help determine the degree of this condition, so before leaping to the conclusion that your pancreas is betraying you, make immediate dietary changes and see whether they make a difference. Often, they can, and fairly quickly.

Some health books recommend lots of supplements for hypoglycemia, but simple dietary strategies often suffice. This condition is rarely a problem of nutrient deficiency. The problem is usually more about nutrient *balance*. Hypoglycemia is complicated by eating sugar, waiting long periods between meals, and not consuming enough whole-grain fiber.

Understanding blood sugar

Eating refined sugar and flour as well as stimulants like caffeine can create big swings in blood sugar (see the top of Figure 9-1), releasing excessive amounts of insulin and promoting inflammation, sweet cravings, and fatigue. These swings affect you not only physically but also emotionally, and you become prone to mood swings.

The swings are usually called a *blood sugar wave* because of their natural movement toward high and low points. If blood sugar is between the middle of both extremes, it is said to be *regular* or *even*. When sugar levels go up, it's because some form of simple or complex sugar has been introduced into the blood.

The more refined the sugar, the higher the upward swing. Spend a number of hours without food and as your muscles use all available sugar, the blood sugar level goes down. Additionally, when the blood sugar elevates, insulin is automatically released, which transports sugar into the cells. If for some reason this insulin cannot transport the sugars, they build up in the blood, resulting in high blood sugar. Essentially, this is a simplistic explanation of diabetes.

The complex-carbohydrate quality of whole grains, beans, and vegetables is composed of thousands of sugar molecules. Eventually, these complex sugar masses (think of a necklace) are broken apart into smaller units (think of beads), so they can be gradually absorbed into the blood. As you can see at the bottom of Figure 9-1, consuming complex carbohydrates results in a more regulated blood sugar wave. Think of complex carbohydrates as wood, burning with a consistent flame in a fireplace, and of simple sugar as newspaper that you toss in for a sudden big flame that soon extinguishes itself.

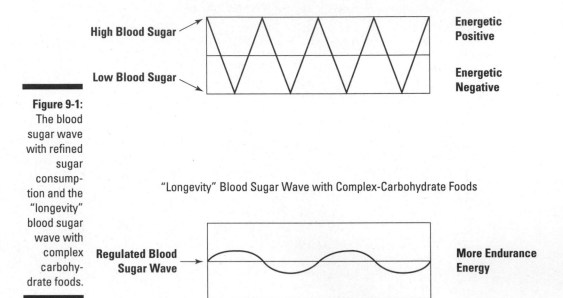

Figure 9-1:
The blood sugar wave with refined sugar consumption and the "longevity" blood sugar wave with complex carbohydrate foods.

The regulated blood sugar wave in Figure 9-1 is the wave of long-lived cultures. This wave produces greater endurance and vitality. Sugar waves that go through extreme rise and fall movements create short bursts of energy but little endurance. Eventually, with steady irregular blood sugar levels, either the pancreas or adrenal glands weaken, which can lead to numerous disease symptoms.

Additional dietary healing strategies for low blood sugar

In addition to the general strategies presented at the beginning of this chapter, you should also do the following:

- Understand how to regulate blood sugar by planning proper meals.
- Don't wait long periods between meals. This is often the reason that people end up eating late at night. Allowing your blood sugar to drop in this way can also trigger sweet cravings.

Additional non-dietary healing strategies for low blood sugar

In addition to the general strategies presented at the beginning of this chapter, you should also do the following:

✔ Remember that stress is always a chief player in hypoglycemia, because it directly affects blood sugar levels and adrenal function. So make sure you take the advice provided earlier in the chapter on reducing stress.

✔ Give your exhausted adrenal glands the benefit of strong circulation flush. External treatments such as plaster's fomentations and compresses were a standard part of folk medicine treatment. This hot circulatory stimulant is simple and economical. Use a hot water bottle (not too hot!) on the kidney area to stimulate toxin elimination and circulation throughout what is known in Chinese medicine as your Vitality Organs. Here's how to do it.

1. Fill $\frac{1}{3}$ of the bottle with hot water.

2. Push all the air out of the bag.

3. Cap the bottle tightly.

4. Place the hot water bottle on your back horizontally by the last rib (adrenal/kidney location).

5. Allow the gentle heat to remain for about 15 to 20 minutes.

6. Repeat several times weekly.

This treatment brings more circulation to the adrenals, stimulates lymph flow, and improves kidney filtering function.

Additional practical dietary suggestions for low blood sugar

For the most part, you can follow the percentages in the revised version of the Macrobiotic Standard Template (see Chapter 6) when treating hypoglycemia with a macrobiotic diet. Sometimes, though, you may need to increase the whole-grain percentage to 35 percent.

✔ For hypoglycemics who are at their target weight, slightly increasing the grain to 40 percent may work better.

✔ For hypoglycemics who need to lose weight, keeping the grain low — at 25 to 30 percent — is usually more effective and promotes quicker weight loss.

In addition, you'll find that the following dietary tips can help you keep your blood sugar levels regulated:

- ✔ Use approximately 1 to 2 teaspoons of oil daily. Your best choices are sesame and olive oils. They can be used in a salad dressing or in a light stir-fry with grain or vegetable or beans.

- ✔ Try sea plants. Also known as *seaweeds,* these highly mineralized vegetables can be nourishing and satisfying.

- ✔ Enjoy a moderate amount of barley malt, rice syrup, agave syrup, maple syrup, or molasses no more than twice weekly, until you develop more control over this condition.

Additional food "no-nos" for hypoglycemics

Follow all of the food no-nos at the beginning of the chapter. Also, don't wait long periods between meals. This is often the reason that people end up eating late at night. Allowing blood sugar to drop in this way can also trigger sweet cravings.

Diabetes: Trouble in Pancreas Land

Diabetes is a chronic disease caused by an inherited (usually type 1, or juvenile, diabetes) or acquired deficiency (type 2, or adult onset, diabetes) in the production of insulin by the pancreas, or by the ineffectiveness of its insulin secretion. This deficiency can cause increased concentrations of glucose in the blood, which can damage many of the body's systems, in particular, blood vessels and nerves.

Type 1 usually affects children, while type 2 typically develops as people gain weight.

- ✔ **Type 1:** In this form of diabetes, the body has insufficient insulin to meet its metabolic needs and requires insulin injections, usually made from animal sources, as a treatment.

- ✔ **Type 2:** This form of diabetes develops as people mature and gain weight. This type of diabetes is also known as *noninsulin-dependent diabetes* because insulin therapy is initially not needed as treatment. Unlike type 1 diabetes, type 2 is more treatable because damage to the pancreas is limited.

Diabetes affects more than 240 million people worldwide and contributes to more than 3 million deaths yearly. One out of three children born after 2000 will develop this disease. The incidence of diabetes is twice as high in the Latino population as it is among Caucasians. Native Americans, Asians, and African Americans also have high rates of the disease. The most frightening aspect of this disease is that one-third of the people with diabetes in America don't yet know that they have it.

The progression of diabetes can result in complications such as heart disease, stroke, high blood pressure, blindness, kidney disease, pregnancy complications, limb amputation, and increased susceptibility to other diseases.

The good news is that for many with type 2 diabetes, reversing this condition is possible with healthy diet and lifestyle changes.

How diabetes affects the body

Insulin is made in the pancreas, and its job is to regulate the volume of sugar circulating within our blood. Insulin escorts the sugar through cell membranes and into the cells' inner machinery. Think of insulin as the door key to the cell membrane. After the sugar is inside the cell, it's converted into chemicals that produce energy.

The word *insulin* is derived from the Latin *insula,* meaning "island." This refers to the islets of Langerhans, the tail end of the pancreas where insulin is produced.

However, if less insulin is produced, as happens with type 1 diabetes, or if the insulin is less effective, as in type 2 diabetes, the cells become starved for energy because sugar isn't accessible. Unable to enter the cell, sugar remains in the blood and elevates the blood sugar.

In the absence of sugar, the body switches to fats as an alternative fuel source. Normally, body fats are broken down into fatty acids that can easily pass through the cell membrane without needing help from insulin. These fatty acids can provide fuel for cells. The downside of using fats for energy is the resulting byproducts. When the body burns fats, the process produces byproducts that cause the body fluids and blood to become acidic temporarily. The result? Loss of cell fluids, inflammation, and mineral imbalances. Additionally, high levels of sugar pass through the kidneys and into the urine. The sugar then draws water out of the body, risking potential life-threatening dehydration. One of the early signs of advanced diabetes is frequency of urination and severe thirst — signs that the body is naturally attempting to replace its lost fluids.

However, as this way of eating can help lower or regulate blood sugar, your medication dosage, whether it's oral medication or insulin, may need immediate adjustment. For this reason, it's *critical* to make sure that you are being monitored by a knowledgeable physician who will adjust medication accordingly. Blood sugar readings, energy levels, mental clarity, and cravings are all important indicators when monitoring.

Additional diabetic dietary healing strategies

Take the following advice along with the essential healing strategies presented earlier in the chapter:

- ✔ Understand how you can regulate your blood sugar with proper meal planning and frequent eating.
- ✔ Reduce cravings for refined sugars, fats, and animal protein by a whole foods, macrobiotically oriented approach, eat more frequently, and eliminate sugar. (See Chapter 20 for sweet-craving reduction tips.)

Additional non-dietary healing strategies for diabetes

For folks with diabetes, along with the non-dietary healing strategies presented at the beginning of the chapter, it's also a good idea to try circulation rubs, such as massage and skin brushing. These techniques can be of enormous help in supporting good circulation. Vigorously rub your legs, arms, and trunk with a skin brush daily to promote lymph flow as well as blood circulation. Chapter 7 has more information on skin brushing.

Additional diabetic dietary suggestions

Transitioning to a macrobiotic diet benefits diabetics because of the reduction in saturated fat, the inclusion of foods that regulate rather than elevate or depress blood sugar, the strategy of eating smaller volumes more frequently, and the combination of a balanced whole foods diet and daily movement.

All of these elements conspire to help the diabetic transform their health. Sometimes, the grain percentage may need to be slightly higher than 30 percent. You frequently hear that carbohydrates are "the worst foods for diabetics," and this is true, but remember that this statement refers to simple sugars, refined flour, and refined grains, not whole grain.

✔ For diabetics who are at their target weight, slightly increasing the grain total to 40 percent may work better for healing.

✔ For those needing to lose weight, keep the grain percentage a bit lower — at 25 to 30 percent. This will be more effective and promotes quicker weight loss. Lowering the grain may make it necessary to add another small meal or two or make other adjustments to your diet.

- Increase the vegetable percentage.

- Eat some kind of protein twice daily.

- Include 1 to 3 teaspoons (1 tablespoon maximum) of oil in your food.

Follow the advice at the beginning of the chapter and do the following as well:

✔ When eating your vegetables, make sure to emphasize the onion and radish families. These vegetables help the body break down fat.

✔ If you're craving sweets, enjoy a moderate amount of barley malt, rice syrup, agave syrup, maple syrup, or molasses no more than two to three times a week until you develop more control over your diabetes.

Additional food "no-nos" for diabetics

Follow all of the food no-nos at the beginning of the chapter. Also, don't wait long periods between meals. This is often why people end up eating late at night. Allowing the blood sugar to drop in this way can also trigger sweet cravings.

Prompt and proven pancreatic punishment

Type 1 diabetes (also known as juvenile diabetes) has been associated with dairy food consumption. The milk protein bovine serum albumin (BSA) produces an autoimmune reaction targeted at the pancreas's insulin-producing glands. A *New England Journal of Medicine* article reported that in all of 142 diabetic children studied, abnormally high levels of BSA antibodies appeared.

Researchers concluded that a specific dairy protein (dairy products may contain up to 25 different proteins) sparked an autoimmune reaction believed to damage vital insulin-producing pancreatic cells.

Despite what conventional nutrition suggests, dairy foods are not a healthy food group for children, especially diabetics or those with immune concerns. Dairy is considered by many credible nutritional authorities to be the number one cause of food-based allergies.

Diabetic supplement suggestions

Over the years, a number of diabetic supplements have been advertised as "best for glucose control" or "helpful for lowering blood sugar." However, conflicting information would surface, and everyone would scratch their heads, wondering what to do until the next miracle supplement appeared.

Fish oils, cinnamon, fructose, red yeast extract, chromium picolinate, fenugreek, selenium, magnesium, spirulina, and a host of others have been reputed to have negative effects on blood sugar, despite advertisements that recommend these supplements to diabetics.

My down-to-earth advice is to first experiment with changes to your diet. As your dietary sensitivity increases and you regain control of your health, you can experiment with supplements because you'll be more sensitive to their effects and able to gauge their effectiveness. I recommend that you simply follow the supplement suggestions presented at the beginning of the chapter.

Arthritis: Pain That Immobilizes

Arthritis is a degenerative condition in which the joints become inflamed. More than 100 forms of arthritis have been identified. The most common are

- **Rheumatoid arthritis:** This is a chronic inflammatory disorder of the autoimmune system that predominantly affects woman and young girls.
- **Osteoarthritis:** This degenerative disease typically occurs in adults in their mid-40s and involves deterioration of *cartilage* (the material that protects the ends of the bones). Most often, osteoarthritis is the result of wear and tear over the years, but diet and lifestyle can influence this type of arthritis.

Less common forms, such as gout, lupus, infectious arthritis, scleroderma, fibromyalgia syndrome, and ankylosing spondylitis, have increased steadily.

Arthritis affects 1 in 5 adults, bringing the approximate total of Americans with doctor-diagnosed arthritis to more than 24 million women and 17 million men. Additionally, as many as 300,000 children in the United States are affected by arthritis.

People afflicted with arthritis usually experience stiffness and pain, particularly in the morning or after exercise. Arthritis can limit the range of motion, cause swelling, and eventually lead to deformity.

Reversing diabetes?

Reversing type 1 diabetes isn't possible, because you never get over the insulin deficiency. However, a 2001 decade-long National Institute of Health study of type 1 diabetes found that diabetics who kept their blood sugar levels near normal dramatically reduced their risk of eye, kidney, and nerve damage up to 70 percent! Uncontrolled sugar levels increased the risk of blindness, stroke, heart disease, nerve damage, kidney failure, skin problems, and more. This important clinical trial Diabetes Prevention Program demonstrated conclusively that diet with the addition of exercise severely cut the risk of Type 2 diabetes by up to 58 percent.

A group of scientists at the Los Angeles Pritikin Center achieved equally spectacular results by recommending a low-fat, plant-based diet of whole grains, vegetables, beans, fruit, and limited amounts of animal proteins along with daily exercise. Of 40 patients on medications at the beginning of the program, 34 were able to discontinue all medication after 26 days. The research group also illustrated that the benefits of a whole foods, plant-based diet can last for years if that way of eating is followed consistently.

The traditional macrobiotic understanding of arthritis points the finger primarily at the modern diet of excessive acid-forming foods — specifically, a diet high in animal proteins, simple carbohydrates, and fat. Foods that foster cartilage inflammation often press against nerves in the joint, which results in pain.

According to Herman Aihara, a well-known Japanese macrobiotic teacher, too much acid-forming food, especially when coupled with a low- or no-salt diet, causes the fluid between the cartilage in the joints to become overly acidic. If the body lacks alkaline-forming elements (such as calcium, sodium, potassium, and magnesium), calcium is then dissolved from bones to neutralize the joint fluid. This results in a calcium deposit. With sharp protruding edges, the deposit can cause pain with joint movement. Eventually, these calcium deposits can deform the joint.

Additional dietary suggestions for arthritis

When dealing with arthritis, the most important dietary adjustments are the following:

- You want to greatly reduce your dietary acid — foods such as sugar, nightshade vegetables, and excessive protein that may contribute to inflammation.

✔ You want to reduce and eventually eliminate these foods, which contribute to immune weakening: sugar, gluten-containing foods, possibly corn and corn products, excess saturated fat, and dairy products.

✔ You need to reverse these lifestyle factors: inactivity, staying up late, stress, and waiting too long between meals.

When you transition from your current diet to a macrobiotic diet to treat arthritis, you can follow the percentages in the revised version of the Macrobiotic Standard Template (see Chapter 6). However, you may need to increase the whole-grain percentage.

✔ For those with arthritis who are at their target weight, increasing the grain total to 40 percent may work better for healing.

✔ For those needing to lose weight, keeping the grain percentage low — at 25 to 30 percent — is more effective and promotes quicker weight loss. Lowering the grain may make it necessary to add another small meal or two or make other adjustments to your diet.

  • Increase the vegetable percentage.

  • Eat some kind of protein twice daily.

  • Include 1 to 3 teaspoons (1 tablespoon maximum) of oil in your food.

Follow the advice at the beginning of the chapter and do the following as well:

✔ Avoid the gluten grains (wheat, barley, rye, and sometimes, oats) for the first two or three weeks. Then begin to add them back to your diet and see if you notice a difference within a two- or three-week period.

✔ When choosing which vegetables to consume, avoid corn and corn products initially. Make sure to have two servings of daily greens. These can be steamed, lightly water-fried, and sometimes raw. The best cooking greens with abundant minerals are dark leafy greens, such as collard greens, kale, bok choy, Napa cabbage, mustard greens, tops of various vegetables, and mega-nutritious broccoli.

✔ Minimize fruit and concentrated natural sweeteners for at least two to three weeks during your initial dietary experiment. When you experience strong cravings for sweets, have the minimum amount that satisfies your sweet tooth.

Additional arthritis food "no-nos"

Follow the guidelines at the beginning of the chapter and also do the following:

- ✔ Avoid soy and soy products, particularly mock soy meats, soy cheeses, and soy milks. A small amount of tofu or a tempeh soybean burger once or twice a week is permitted.

- ✔ Initially, avoid nightshade vegetables: tomatoes, potatoes, eggplant, and all peppers. After a time, you can try eating these foods again to see if avoiding these foods makes any difference in your joint sensitivity. (See Chapter 8 for more on nightshade veggies.)

Here's an interesting reminder on the front and back aspect of Mother Nature: Although eating peppers (a member of the nightshade family) can trigger joint inflammation in some people, a topical ointment made from an ingredient in chili peppers, called *capsicum,* applied externally can *soothe* inflammation. Capsicum is responsible for the pungent and irritating effects of cayenne pepper. However, some capsicum preparations halt the transmission of pain impulses from the nerves to the spinal cord. As a result, even though the condition causing the pain may continue, no perception of that pain reaches the brain.

Arthritis supplement recommendations

A number of arthritis supplements have been advertised as "best for bone building," "helps cartilage regenerate," or "replaces mineral loss." However, some conflicting information indicates otherwise.

People suffering from arthritis should avoid iron or multivitamins containing iron, because iron is thought to contribute to pain and swelling. You can take a multivitamin as suggested at the beginning of the chapter, but choose one without iron.

Digestive Disorders: When the Breakdown System Breaks Down

When you eat, your body breaks down food to a form it can use to build and nourish cells and provide energy. This process is called *digestion* and occurs in a series of hollow organs joined in a long, twisting tube of various widths and lengths. This tube runs from your mouth to your anus and includes the esophagus, stomach, and small and large intestines. Your liver, gallbladder, and pancreas also contribute to the process by producing secretions to help digest food matter. There are many types of digestive disorders, and symptoms can vary widely depending on the problem.

According to the American College of Gastroenterology, more than 100 million Americans suffer from some form of digestive disorder. That's almost half of the U.S. population. Digestive problems are the number-one problem in North America and include conditions from hemorrhoids to colon cancer. These disorders also seem to be occurring with greater frequency — while many of them were uncommon during our grandparents' time, they are on the rise at earlier ages more than ever before.

"Digestive disease" is a broad umbrella that can include a number of common conditions directly affecting digestive organs. The most common conditions are the following:

- **Acid reflux (also known as heartburn):** The symptoms of heartburn are difficult to ignore. You've just eaten a big dinner and now lean back to settle into your favorite chair. As you begin to relax, your chest begins to hurt so much that it feels like it's on fire. Welcome to heartburn. This condition — a burning sensation in the food pipe (esophagus), just below the breastbone — is actually a *symptom* of acid reflux. Frequent burning is a common symptom of gastroesophageal reflux disease (GERD), a condition in which stomach acid, or even bile, occasionally flows back up into the esophagus. Some 60 million Americans are thought to suffer from heartburn.

  One of the structural problems to blame for this condition is a swollen *esophageal sphincter,* which acts like a lid on stomach contents, keeping food out of the food pipe. This allows acid fluids and vapors to escape. They rise and create the burning sensation in heartburn and a host of other conditions. In 2005, a pharmaceutical giant that manufactures acid reflux medication grossed more than $12 billion from acid reflux medication sales.

  Some troublesome foods for this condition are sugar, caffeine, spices, carbonated beverages, peppers, tomatoes, chocolate, alcohol, fried foods, citrus, and fruit juices. Overeating and eating prior to bed can contribute to the problem as well.

- **Irritable bowel syndrome (IBS):** Irritable bowel syndrome is a common complaint: Nearly 50 million Americans experience the diverse symptoms this syndrome causes. IBS is known by several names, including *spastic colon, colitis,* and *functional bowel disease.* IBS is a collection of symptoms that can appear in any number of combinations. These symptoms include bloating, gas, diarrhea, constipation, abdominal pain and spasms, and nausea.

  Most health practitioners agree that food allergies, high sugar consumption, medication, stress, hormone changes, low-fiber diets, infection, parasites, lactose intolerance, laxatives, and antibiotic abuse could all be involved. Just about anything that upsets the intestinal bacterial balance — the ratio of good bacteria to bad bacteria — can have a part in causing IBS. IBS is not life-threatening; however, it makes for a very uncomfortable life, and progressive IBS can often evolve into inflammatory bowel disease.

✔ **Inflammatory bowel disease (IBD):** Inflammatory bowel disease is the name given to a group of disorders that cause the intestines to become inflamed (red and swollen). The inflammation can last for long periods and, after normalizing, can return repeatedly. Each year, more than 600,000 Americans experience some kind of inflammatory bowel disease symptoms. If you have inflammatory bowel disease, you may have abdominal cramps and pain, diarrhea, weight loss, and bleeding from your intestines. Two kinds of inflammatory bowel disease are Crohn's disease and ulcerative colitis. While these conditions have different characteristics, they share many IBS symptoms.

- **Ulcerative colitis:** This is the continuous inflammation of the mucosal lining of the colon and/or rectum and can be fairly mild or extremely severe. The most common symptoms are diarrhea and bleeding.

- **Crohn's disease:** This condition also results in inflammation, but it can occur anywhere from the mouth to the rectum. Frequently, it occurs in the colon near the *ileocecal valve,* which separates the contents of the small intestine and colon in the right lower part of the abdomen. The inflammation in Crohn's disease is more severe than ulcerative colitis and can develop into abscesses and *fistulas* (an abnormal, narrow passage formed by disease between a hollow organ and the body surface).

A whole foods cooked diet with the avoidance of sugar and minimal well-cooked fiber, or in some cases *no* fiber, can be critical in combating both of these conditions.

✔ **Ulcers:** Essentially, an ulcer is a type of sore, which means it's an open, painful wound. Some ulcers (peptic ulcers) are formed in the stomach or the duodenum, the upper part of the small intestine. Peptic ulcers are fairly common, and it's estimated that almost 1 in every 10 Americans will get an ulcer at some point in their lives. For the longest time, stress, spicy foods, and alcohol were thought to have caused most ulcers. In the early 1980s it was discovered that a particular bacterial infection in the stomach and upper intestine was the cause of most peptic ulcers. The medical term for this bacterium is *Helicobacter pylori* (or *H. pylori,* for short). A very high percentage of Americans have *H. pylori* infections. Nearly 2 out of every 10 people below 40 have this bacterium in their digestive systems. While the bacterium may be ruled as an aggravating factor, it is probable that a weakened immune condition, faulty diet, and the physiological effects of stress play a big part in the development of ulcers.

Digestive disorder dietary healing strategies

Take the advice provided at the beginning of the chapter and also make an effort to control food volume by eating less at each meal.

Additional non-dietary healing strategies for digestive disorders

Follow the healing strategies at the beginning of the chapter. In addition, to assist bowel movements, rest your feet on a small stool or several thick telephone books to elevate your knees when you have to empty your bowels. This natural bend simulates the "squat" posture and facilitates in an easier and much quicker bowel release. Simple intestinal massage (applying pressure and kneading sections of the ascending transverse and descending colon) can help make bowels more regular.

Additional dietary suggestions for digestive disorders

A week of a balanced menu of whole grains and vegetables will show you how quickly your intestinal condition can improve. Digestive sensitivity, gas, bloating, constipation, loose bowel, and so on can all be remedied fairly quickly with moderate volumes of whole foods such as grains, vegetables, and beans (well chewed, of course). This high percentage of whole fiber and complex carbohydrate has a very soothing effect on digestion and regulation.

When you transition from your current diet to a macrobiotic diet to treat a digestive disorder, you can follow the percentages in the revised version of the Macrobiotic Standard Template (see Chapter 6). However, you may need to increase the whole-grain percentage.

- ✔ If you have a digestive disorder and you're at your target weight, increasing the grain total to 40 percent may work better for healing.
- ✔ If you need to lose weight, keeping the grain percentage low — at 25 to 30 percent — is more effective and promotes quicker weight loss.

Lowering the grain may make it necessary to add another small meal or two or make other adjustments to your diet.

- Increase the vegetable percentage.

- Eat some kind of protein twice daily.

- Include 1 to 3 teaspoons (1 tablespoon maximum) of oil in your food.

✔ Avoid gluten grains (wheat, barley, rye, and sometimes, oats) for the first two or three weeks of eating macrobiotically. Then slowly reintroduce them to your diet and see if there is a difference as you add them back.

✔ For digestive regularity, have a serving of whole grain, such as oatmeal, or soft rice at breakfast. The transit time of bowel passage in a healthy intestine ranges from 17 to 24 hours. Eating whole grain at breakfast will usually ensure a bowel movement for the following day.

✔ When choosing vegetable, make sure to include at least one serving of greens every day. These can be steamed, lightly water-fried, or sometimes raw, according to your taste, digestibility, and preference. The best cooking greens with abundant minerals are dark leafy greens, such as collard greens, kale, bok choy, Napa cabbage, mustard greens, tops of various vegetables, and mega-nutritious broccoli.

Additional food "no-no's" when you have a digestive disorder

All of the no-nos at the beginning of the chapter apply. Adhere to these restrictions as well:

✔ Avoid soy and soy products, particularly mock soy meats, soy cheeses, and soy milks. A small amount of tofu or tempeh soybean burger once or twice weekly is recommended.

✔ Reduce nuts and seeds as snacks. Instead, use them as food condiments for flavoring and to add a small healthy dose of fat to the meal.

✔ I would suggest that you resist the temptation to spice your food if you have digestive weakness, as most spices, despite any nutritional benefits, can contribute to inflammation of the intestinal lining. Later, as you become familiar with the foods and comfortable with this way of eating, you can add some back into your meals.

TECHNICAL STUFF

Bacteria wars: Good versus bad

Annually, Americans spend more than $100 billion on drugs and antacids attempting to fight digestive disorders. It's estimated that more than 400 different types of bacteria live in the gastrointestinal system. Some are good, some are bad. Naturally, you want a larger population of good, because the body depends on the colon being able to get the maximum nutrients from your food.

The colon's beneficial bacteria manufacture B vitamins, which includes biotin, niacin, folic acid, and pyridoxine. These microorganisms produce antibacterial substances that kill disease-causing devils such as *salmonella* and some types of *E. coli*. These bacteria keep your digestive system in top shape. Two important beneficial bacteria are *acidophilus bacteria* and *bifid bacterium*. Having a slightly acidic pH in the colon helps support these beneficial

bacteria and helps keep bad organisms from spreading, because most of the bad organisms don't like an acidic environment. Unfortunately, the colon's pH can be altered by many conditions, which causes the beneficial bacteria to be reduced. This throws off the delicate balance among the different microorganisms.

Factors that interfere with the colon's pH are high-meat and high-fat diets, alcohol, stress, and antibiotics. *Probiotics,* dietary supplements made of beneficial microorganisms, can renew the good bacteria in your intestines. Many people are familiar with yogurt, which contains acidophilus, but you can also get probiotics in supplement form. If you suffer from digestive problems or just want to keep your digestive system functioning at optimum efficiency, consider a probiotic supplement.

Digestive disorder supplement recommendations

Here are some standard recommendations for folks with digestion disorders:

✔ Take probiotic supplements. Follow the label recommendations (usually five days a week). These supplements help restore beneficial intestinal bacteria and aid in vitamin absorption.

✔ Choose a multivitamin/mineral without iron. Take the standard milligram/microgram dosages five days a week.

Heart Disease: When Your Ticker Takes a Licking

Heart disease includes a number of abnormal conditions that directly affect the heart and the blood vessels within the heart. The types of heart disease include:

✔ **Coronary artery disease (CAD):** This is the most common type of heart disease and is the leading cause of heart attacks. Artery disease, also known as *arteriosclerosis,* occurs when deposits of hardened fat and cholesterol build up along the arteries' inner walls and obstruct the flow of blood transporting oxygen and nutrients to the brain, kidneys, heart, and lower limbs. When blood flow is inhibited, it has a hard time getting to the heart, so the heart doesn't get all the blood it needs. CAD can lead to

- **Angina:** Angina is the name for chest pain or discomfort that happens when the heart can't get enough blood. It feels like a pressing or squeezing pain and often occurs in the chest, but sometimes people feel it in the shoulders, arms, neck, jaw, or back. It can also be mistaken for indigestion.

  Angina is *not* a heart attack, but having angina means you are *more likely* to have a heart attack.

- **Heart attack:** A heart attack occurs when an artery is severely or completely blocked, and the heart can't get the blood it needs for more than 20 minutes.

✔ **Heart failure:** Heart failure happens when the heart can't efficiently pump blood through the body. As a result, other organs can't get enough blood. It does *not* mean that the heart stops. Signs of heart failure include:

- Shortness of breath (you feel you can't get enough air)

- Extreme fatigue

- Swelling in feet, ankles, and legs

✔ **Heart arrhythmias:** These are changes in the beating pattern of the heart. At one time or another, many people have felt dizzy, faint, or out of breath or experienced chest pains. These changes in the heartbeat are, for most people, nothing to worry about. However, as you age, arrhythmias become more common. If you have a few flutters or if your heart races once in a while, it may not be a concern.

However, if you have flutters *and* other symptoms, such as dizziness or shortness of breath, then a visit to the ER (or calling 911) may be a lifesaver.

The role of nourishment on heart health

From a macrobiotic perspective, heart health depends on how you nourish yourself in body, mind, and spirit, with balance being the key factor. Your daily diet may be composed of foods that alter your physical structure as they digest and become part of your chemistry. Some foods produce the reaction of *expansion,* either by loosening, swelling, and enlargement. Other foods produce symptoms of constriction, narrowing, and tightening, generally referred to as *contraction*. With consistency, both extremes can evolve into disease symptoms. Table 9-1 sums up the types of foods that cause these reactions in your body.

Table 9-1	The Expansion/Contraction Chart
Foods That Expand	*Foods That Contract*
Sugar, alcohol	Animal meats
Coffee and tea acids	Caffeine, Sodium
Most chemical preservatives and additives	Salted cheeses, eggs

In Table 9-1, although meats are in the contracting column, it is the salt within the tissue of the meat and its effect on male hormones that keeps it in this column. Ultimately, meat, which is a protein, breaks down into various acids and exerts a more acid (or expansive) influence. This supports the principle that says nothing is solely of one essence but composed of layers. The same can also be seen in coffee. While caffeine exerts an alkaline effect in our bodies, coffee has over 40 different acids that do not contribute to good health. Always look for the predominance in these factors.

Foods such as sugar and liquid sugar (sodas, fruit juices, and so on), alcohol, and stimulants like caffeine can cause inflammation when consumed to excess on a regular basis. This can result in different conditions of artery inflammation (as in aneurysm), as well as enlargement of the heart muscle.

At the other end of the scale, excessive salt use and a diet heavy in saturated fats and cholesterol can cause hardening and narrowing of the arteries. Foods that contribute to this condition are from meat, eggs, and other dairy sources. The potential result of this excess is a loss of arterial elasticity, blocked arteries, and fat accumulations around the heart. Because these foods are usually eaten in combination, heart disease symptoms can be uniquely varied.

There is some nutritional controversy today about what really constitutes heart-healthy foods. At the extremes, some research suggests a heart-healthy diet should avoid saturated fats, emphasizing a predominantly vegetarian path. At the other extreme, some recent research suggests that it is permissible (and even healthy) to eat high-quality, natural saturated fats such as olive oil, walnuts, flax seeds, and fish oil (optional), as long as they have not gone through standard high-heat food processing.

Considering that the majority of 20th-century Americans were brought up with an assortment of meats as a principle food, abundant simple sugars, plentiful amounts of milk, butter, cheese and eggs, and processed nut and "vegetable" oils, as well as enough trans fats for each of us to fill a municipal swimming pool, the dietary suggestions for handling heart disease that follow favor limiting, or even eliminating, these extreme foods to establish a baseline of sensitivity.

Although there may be negligible risk in consuming a limited number of saturated fats from natural sources, it may be best to consider a semi-vegetarian or full vegetarian approach as a starting point. A number of documented studies have shown that a whole foods vegetarian diet, along with practical lifestyle changes, such as exercise and meditation, can reverse arterial plaques that were previously thought irreversible.

Additional dietary suggestions for a healthy heart

Our blood is constantly nourishing our heart. Good heart health has two components: diet and consistent exercise. Excessive animal proteins and sugar are two of the worst extremes for this system. Fibrous complex-carbohydrate foods are best for regulating blood sugar (this is important for good cardio health) and better arterial pathways where blood can flow without impediment.

When you transition from your current diet to a macrobiotic diet to treat a heart condition, you can follow the percentages in the revised version of the Macrobiotic Standard Template (see Figure 9-1). However, you may need to increase the whole-grain percentage.

✔ For those with heart disease who are at their target weight, slightly increasing the grain total to 40 percent may work better for healing.

✔ For those needing to lose weight, keeping the grain percentage low — at 25 to 30 percent — is more effective and promotes quicker weight loss. Lowering the grain may make it necessary to add another small meal or two or make other adjustments to your diet.

- Increase the vegetable percentage.

- Eat some kind of protein twice daily.

- Include 1 to 3 teaspoons (1 tablespoon maximum) of oil in your food.

Follow the advice at the beginning of the chapter and do the following as well:

✔ Include in your diet a daily complex carbohydrate whole grain source, such as brown rice, barley, oats, millet, and so on. In some individuals, grain products, such as muffins, pasta, flour, and so on, can create blood sugar swings. These swings may lead to cardiac stress. These foods do not qualify as whole grains. They are *particle foods,* and because the grains have been refined, they often get absorbed quickly and can elevate blood sugar.

✔ Consume a low-fat diet in which the fat percentage remains below 20 percent of total calories. For more advanced cardiac problems, restrict your fat intake even further; no more than 10 to 15 percent of your calories should come from fat.

✔ The omission of simple sugar and alcohol is critical. Omitting these foods, or at least keeping them to the minimum, allows you to better control your blood sugar. Blood sugar can aggravate arrhythmias and foster cravings for sweets or overeating, so consuming foods that create a mild blood sugar wave (see the earlier section on low blood sugar for more about this) are essential for cardiac health.

✔ As mentioned earlier in the chapter, do *not* avoid adding salt to your cooking, but use it *very sparingly.* Purchase bright white damp sea salt and add it to your cooking in pinch amounts. Use a very small amount with grains ($^1/_{10}$ teaspoon per cup of grain) and perhaps 1 teaspoon (maximum) of natural soy sauce in vegetables for its valuable fermentation and enzymes

Heart health supplement recommendations

In addition to the suggestions I give at the beginning of this chapter, I also recommend these supplements:

✔ Take Co-Q10 after meals. Take a 100 to 200 milligram supplement five days a week. Co-Q10 is more effective when taken with dietary fat. This supplement helps to restore cell functioning, strengthen the heart, and helping gum tissue for those with early stage periodontal disease.

✔ Drink dandelion root tea. This is a wonderful, slightly bitter herb that, according to herbal texts, strengthens the walls of the heart. You can drink this as often as you like. It's especially nice with several drops of lemon juice.

Chapter 10

The Ultimate Recipe for Self-Healing

As a health counselor for many years, I wondered what the essential elements of healing were. Was it diet? Emotional work? Physical labor and exercise? Spiritual practice? Human will? After spending many years counseling, the only pattern I could see among people who were happiest and healthiest, or those who had recovered their health, was that these people had achieved their health and happiness through these factors. Most focused their efforts on the factor (or factors) that they believed needed more attention.

The ultimate recipe for self-healing is a combination of what I call ten directives for self-healing.

You know the word *choice,* but many people misunderstand the role of choice in healing. Your life revolves around the many choices you make on a daily basis. Choice determines the quality of your life, through its opportunity to empower or enslave, create safety or challenge, invite love or keep it distant. Because you're always engaged in making choices, seeing the *possibilities of choice* is the first step toward creating a happier and healthier life. By choosing to pay attention to each directive, you can uncover primary and powerful tools for self-healing.

This chapter details critical macrobiotic factors that make up a self-healing individual and explains how these ten essential directives can help you live a healthy, happy, and passionate life.

Strive for a Meaningful Life

Is your will to live motivated by a sense of meaning for your life? Beyond the accumulation of material goods and status, what significance does this life hold for you? Whatever deep meaning you have defined for your life often feeds inspiration and hope. In times when it's needed most, a committed sense of meaning can rally the will to support the deepest levels of healing.

Self-healing individuals often are energetic, responsive, and have a great appetite for learning. They seem to embody the literal meaning of the word *enthusiasm* — from the Greek *enthuousiasmos,* which means "to be inspired, or possessed, by a God." People who have survived terminal diagnoses and gone on to have thriving, healthy lives have demonstrated a strong passion for living. Their passion is fueled by having a purpose for their lives — something that provides vital meaning to daily life and gets them out of bed in the morning to start the day with enthusiasm.

The work of creating a meaningful life begins with first understanding the importance of meaning and then finding time to pursue our passions —things that resonate with personal importance for us.

Personal belief and the quest for meaning

Finding meaning in life usually means discovering meaning in your personal life. However, for a deeper quality of happiness, this may be a limited concept. Famed author and therapist Viktor Frankl, who wrote extensively on finding meaning, suggested that true meaning arises from two beliefs that represent a personal as well as universal perspective:

 ✔ Belief that your life has significant meaning

 ✔ Belief that life itself has meaning

I discuss each of these beliefs in the following sections.

Belief that your life has significant meaning

You can find meaning in your life through relationships, work, and in believing in a cause.

 ✔ **Relationships:** Relationships offer individual growth, education, and meaning to your life. In family relationships, you receive satisfaction from loving, being loved, having a sense of belonging, and feeling that others need us.

You also find personal meaning through your relationships with friends who act as mirrors to help you better understand yourself and provide support in times of need. One of the most disappointing features of senior life, I've been told, is the loss of primary friendships, either through death or the inevitable alienation that fragility and sickness bring.

✔ **Work:** If your daily work is something you feel passionate about, dedicated to, and challenges your personal growth, it adds great meaning to your life. On the other hand, if you are indifferent and work exclusively for money without any real redeeming value, you get less meaning from this large commitment of time.

For many, work isn't a source of joy and self-challenge. People who dread their work can relate to the popular quotation that says, "No one on their deathbed claims, 'I really should have spent more time at the office.'" Being forced to choose between income and meaning in the work you do often creates an internal conflict that inevitably breeds resentment and potential sickness.

✔ **Cause:** Commitment to a cause can also create a profound sense of meaning to life as long as it doesn't place your work and relationships at risk. This is the back and front of the benefit from having a cause.

Although causes bring a rich sense of meaning to life, the most satisfying sense of meaning usually comes from the personal relationships in which you allow yourself to love and be loved.

Belief that life itself has meaning

For many people, finding meaning in their personal lives isn't enough. To find a deeper sense of meaning and happiness, you must also believe that life itself is meaningful.

The belief that life has meaning is essential to all religions. A religious or spiritual perception of life in which we acknowledge a God, higher being, or some guiding force makes for a more purposeful universe — a grander sense of meaning than one that is simply personalized.

Work, relationships, and other causes provide a sense of meaning (see the preceding section for details of these), but without the understanding that life itself has meaning, independent of human achievement, these things become less meaningful. They have an artificial air to them, as if we've created these meanings because we needed purpose. To believe that life itself has no meaning may be a sign of deep spiritual conflict. A larger view of a meaningful universe reminds us that personal meaning and life's daily comforts are insufficient to satisfy the human need to live in a meaningful universe.

Your statement of purpose

The word *purpose* is often confused with the word *goal,* but the distinction between these words is critical. Purpose is not a goal; it is focused action and movement. It's not something to be accomplished and checked off as you would on a to-do list. A *purpose* is something you continuously accomplish, whereas goals can be considered stopovers in the journey of life.

What's *your* statement of purpose? Without purpose, your life motivation diminishes. A sense of purpose allows you to be discriminating in the life choices you make by asking, "Is this compatible with my purpose?" In making choices that further your purpose, you live a healthier and more passionate life.

You will only want to take care of your life when you value the life that you're living.

People who have triumphed over cancer usually have a deep purpose for living. They "don't have time" to get sick, and they're "not ready" to let go of this body for another world. Their passion for living is their elixir for healing.

Author Richard Kinnier and his colleagues at Arizona State University studied the quotations and thoughts from hundreds of eminent people on the meaning of life. The following ten themes emerged, many of which can be seen as a statement of purpose:

- ✔ Life is to be enjoyed.
- ✔ We are here to help others.
- ✔ The meaning of life is a mystery.
- ✔ Life is meaningless.
- ✔ We are here to serve God.
- ✔ Life is a struggle.
- ✔ We are here to contribute to society.
- ✔ We are here to seek wisdom and self-actualization.
- ✔ We must create meaning for ourselves.
- ✔ Life is absurd.

Choose one (or several) and find meaning in it!

Improve Your Attitude: Establishing a Personal Philosophy

Your attitude toward life is strongly influenced and fortified by a personal philosophy, which is one of the most important features of the self-healing individual. A personal philosophy evolves as a result of self-reflection and life study. Bound by a moral credo and developing value system, a philosophy of life reflects your beliefs and reveals itself in your daily attitude. A healthy personal philosophy enables you to see things from a flexible perspective that minimizes stress, bolsters faith, and inspires motivation.

Self-knowledge, core values, and our deeply held convictions define your personal philosophy. The way you experience so many things — triumph, loss, happiness, grief, love, death, success, ambition, devotion to a cause, worship, friendship, and risk taking, as well as physical, emotional, intellectual, and spiritual growth — depends on the kind of personal philosophy you create.

Creating a personal philosophy means to question yourself about your feelings and values in core areas of your life. *Values* are best described as ethics, beliefs, guiding principles, virtues, ideals, and a specific moral compass that you live by. These values help you achieve happiness, confidence, clarity in decision making, satisfying relationships, and more awareness and balance in daily life. These core values also exist in other facets of daily life, from social concerns, politics, and religion to health management. They assist you in making positive decisions, establishing goals, and determining a sense of purpose.

Confronting the following issues and redefining your opinions and feelings allows you to re-create yourself to support your *new* existence:

- What are your spiritual beliefs?
- What do you feel deeply about?
- What kind of goals do you have in the areas of health, emotions, finances, creativity, work, and relationships?
- What are your opinions on hardship, compassion, forgiveness, patience, humility, commitment, responsibility, discipline, trust, fear, faith, self-respect, expectation, humor, love, sickness, will, and passion?
- What are you willing to take responsibility for?
- How would you like to spend your time?

Your attitude about life and the way you approach its challenges stem from a personal philosophy that is constantly changing, expanding, and growing. A philosophy motivated by love and guided by gratitude can help you maintain a sense of inner control that is sustained by the certainty that you can influence the experiences of your life. You can develop the ability to see these experiences as purposeful and necessary, and this can lead to an abundance of profound, joyful meaning.

Consume Balanced Nourishment

Balancing your daily nourishment, as this book emphasizes, is the essential key to transforming your health. By way of absorption, food influences the health and chemical balance of your blood, eventually nourishing tissues and regulating blood sugar, cellular functions, and the distribution of nutrients.

Diet has been estimated to contribute up to 60 percent of all cancer-related deaths. Although there is no definitive dietary formula for healing, in general, specific foods, food group percentages, and a growing field of *specific supplements* can bolster immunity, diminish tumor growth, and support overall fitness and good health.

The simple factors that support good absorption of nutrients from the foods you eat include the following:

- ✔ Thorough chewing to initiate digestion in the mouth.
- ✔ Eating in a relaxed manner.
- ✔ Consuming a variety of foods at each meal for optimum nutrition.
- ✔ Controlling the amount of food you eat.
- ✔ Consuming a low-fat, high complex carbohydrate whole food diet with minimal natural sugars, reduced caffeine intake, and moderate alcohol use.
- ✔ Not drinking with meals. Well-chewed, balanced food choices replace the need to "wash" anything down.

Following a healthy diet and lifestyle plan can bring benefits to every area of your life. It can improve stamina, sharpen senses, regulate mood, deepen sleep quality, lower susceptibility to stress, increase appetite for healthier foods, strengthen immunity, and promote mental clarity, flexibility, and inner peace. When your body is responsive and sensitive, you feel a greater sense of control over your health. This control gives you the opportunity to realize your goals.

Live a Healthy Lifestyle

Lifestyle is about how you design your life to realize and support your goals, good health, creativity, and peace of mind. Your daily schedule, the balance between work and play, sleeping habits, sexual expression, creative work, and physical exercise can strengthen immunity and improve the odds of halting, or even reversing, disease. The lifestyle you choose can enhance other self-healing factors or work against the healing process.

The following sections take a look at how you schedule your time to balance responsibilities, priorities, and self-care; where you spend your time; and how you express yourself creatively.

Making the most of your time

Living a healthy or self-healing lifestyle means making a conscious effort to balance your time. One effective way to do this is by listing everything you need to do and would like to do within your day.

Ask yourself

- What is the *most* important?

- What gives me the *most* pleasure? What is the most rewarding?

- What *must* I do to avert future stress by advance planning or incremental work?

- What obligations and responsibilities can I *delegate* so I can have more time?

- What *advance* planning can be done the day prior to ease the stress of becoming overwhelmed?

Figuring how to manage time for the things that enhance your health is the first step in creating a self-healing lifestyle. This list should include meal planning, cooking, eating, exercising, inspirational study, family time, work, partner time, personal creative time, mediation, visualization time, sleep time, and so on. But the question remains: How do you handle all the options? With flexibility and moderation! If you can recognize its importance, you'll find a way.

If you fail to make time for the things that are an integral part of the healing process, you'll feel stressed, overwhelmed, and victimized by time constraints. Then, we complain: "Gee, there aren't enough hours in the day." For those who have many passions or long workdays, this may be true. However, understanding the value of time means making sure to enjoy what you do and being grateful to at least have it included in your day in whatever amount of time you can comfortably allot.

On the other hand, excessive scheduling can be a recipe for insanity; it's inevitable you'll soon feel controlled by your regimen. Days packed with long agendas seem to have a staccato feel and lack spontaneity. Your furious inner rebel may even leap out and take you on a bender of self-destructive behavior because you feel so controlled and pressured to complete everything on your list. However, doing nothing is just as self-punishing.

The key is to seek a balance point. Your days should strike a balance between handling normal responsibilities and doing some of the things that nurture you, give you pleasure, or inspirationally challenge your abilities.

Improving your life with healthy environments

Your lifestyle is influenced by the environment around you through its sense of order, quality, comfort, and style.

It makes little sense to attempt to detoxify your body if you surround yourself with toxicity.

Unfortunately, it's virtually impossible to avoid pollution today — it's everywhere: pesticides, food additives, gasoline fumes, industrial chemicals, artificial home furnishings, toxic household cleaners, chemicalized hygiene products, toxic packaging materials, and municipal water with added chemicals. In virtually every realm of living, chemicals have infiltrated our lives.

You may not be able to completely avoid chemical hazards in daily life, but you can minimize them by using quality eco-friendly products and naturally fortifying your health. Your home should feel like a toxic retreat from the carcinogens you face outside — a protective fortress offering comfort, a sense of renewal, and an environment that contributes to your health. Does this sound like your home?

Fostering creativity — a healthy lifestyle's essential element

Whether you paint portraits, paint walls, fashion auto mounts with junk parts, or fit pipe, the need for daily creative play is an indispensable part of a healthy lifestyle. Performers such as actress Katharine Hepburn, pianist Vladimir Horowitz, and cellist Pablo Casals, all of whom remained successful and active late in their lives, continually radiated that *joie de vivre* that was such a part of their appeal. Joy, fulfillment, and creative playfulness are prime factors of the self-healing character.

Much evidence suggests that curiosity, stimulation, and exploration are essential ingredients in the self-healing soup, because we are focused on things outside ourselves. They represent challenges that have some degree of stress, albeit a positive type of stress. The same can be said for competitive sports, exotic travel, or those intricate 1,000-piece puzzles that can make you want to pull your hair out. Such agreeable challenges are considered "good stress." Therefore, stress can have a healthy side.

Do you have to be an artist to be creative? Of course not! Creative play is any activity where you can freely and spontaneously challenge your intuitive, artistic, logical, impulsive, or imaginative skills to tap into the universe's inspiration and create something that keeps you completely absorbed in the present moment.

Being absorbed in a creative moment puts you into a *timeless present*. You have little awareness of real time, and nothing seems to distract you. In such moments you are full of life, savoring your task with alert focus and passion. Timeless moments are periods that repair, inspire, and heal.

Reduce Stress

Finding new ways to reduce daily pressures, worries, overwork, and fear-based behaviors can't be overemphasized. Stress-related hormones influence disease progression, moods, and immunity weakness. Stress reduction begins by reevaluating what's important in your life and extends to letting go of perfection patterns and the extra things you're driven to do for approval or to create a feeling of being needed. The key to reducing stress begins with questioning behaviors that don't support health.

How stress is harmful

Stress and negative emotions play a featured role in the disease equation. Cancer is frequently diagnosed in people who have experienced the loss of a loved one or traumatic events within a two-year period. A number of studies have linked high levels of stress with an elevated risk of breast and prostate cancer.

Stress encourages the production and circulation of adrenal hormones, which inhibit the immune response by lowering levels of important, disease-fighting white blood cells. This adrenal response is commonly referred to as the *fight-or-flight mechanism*.

Genetically embedded in animals and humans, this mechanism prepares your body to respond to an attack and is part of your survival instinct. These days, however, this attack mechanism isn't in response to large roaming animals looking for a human snack but to the onslaught of job pressures, noise, environmental toxicity, emotional conflict, and myriad other 21st-century fears. In the flight-or-flight mode, our bodies overproduce chemical and electrical messages that disrupt immunity, digestion, respiration, and mental stability. Suddenly, our hormonal functions are in continuous emergency mode.

Stress can play havoc by depressing existing immunity within the digestive tract, a major entry route for *carcinogens* (cancer-causing agents) into the body. Considering that three-quarters of our immune cells are housed in the digestive tract, this is of critical consequence. Prolonged stress lowers a defense substance called *secretory immunoglobulin A* (sIgA), making the digestive system more vulnerable to carcinogens. This may explain why the risk of colon cancer becomes greater after a period of high stress.

Stress is primarily harmful when it's continuous. Experiencing long-term stress at threshold levels has reportedly affected the way cells develop and mature, causing premature cell death. If this happens in significant numbers, the pathway to disease or a shortened lifespan becomes probable.

Relieving stress

You can choose from a great number of effective and proven therapies to combat stress, including rest, hypnotherapy, visualization, hatha yoga, T'ai Chi, qi chong, meditation, chanting, biofeedback, exercise, being in nature, creative expression, and avoiding high-stress stimulating foods and substances. Psychological counseling can help challenge stress patterns that you unconsciously engineer or uncover the reasons you find stressful behavior, in some cases, addictive.

It's up to you to become aware of how you engage in stress and discover the specific steps necessary to reduce it. Those steps are a primary part of the body, mind, and spirit self-healing paradigm.

Self-healing requires managing stress as well as reducing it. The state of no stress doesn't exist among conscious, living people. "No stress" actually describes the death state. Nonthreatening stress is manageable and doesn't compromise your health or mental stability.

Develop a Sense of Humor

Defined as the ability to laugh with others, laugh at ourselves, and discover humor in everyday life, a sense of humor is essential as an emotional coping tool. Humor provides a greater capacity to forge through the most adverse of situations. Its psychological value immediately transports you in the present moment as its physical benefits work their magic; immunity is stimulated, oxygen in your tissues increases, and stress evaporates in the simple exhalation of a laugh. Consider humor the "Vitamin H" of a healing regime.

In challenging times it's easy to forget about the healing power of humor. For someone facing a degenerative disease, the idea of developing a sense of humor or seeing the humorous side of things may seem frivolous and irrelevant to the serious business of healing. However, nothing can be further from the truth.

Here's a sample of some of the most provocative experimental findings over the last 20 years in humor research:

- Science has found that laughter showed a lowering of our stress hormones and an increase in our immune cell activity.

- After subjects viewed a humorous video, they increased their production of salivary immunoglobin A (IgA), which is believed to protect against some viruses.

- Laughter initially causes an increase in the heart and respiratory rate, raises blood pressure, increases oxygen consumption, gives the face and stomach muscles a workout, and relaxes the muscles not involved in laughing. Shortly following laughter, however, these cardiovascular indicators fall to levels below previous resting values.

- The experience of positive emotions, such as happiness, during exercise appears to produce beneficial cardiovascular effects.

- Individuals who said they turned to humor as a way of coping with difficult life situations had the highest initial concentrations of salivary IgA.

> ✔ Tears in response to laughter and pain have a different composition than do those induced artificially by cutting onions. Emotional tears have a higher concentration of proteins and toxins, suggesting that they may help the body rid itself of injurious substances.

Many events occur in your life that you have no control over. This sense of powerlessness can lead to depression and frustration. In developing a humorous perspective, you minimize these situations to your advantage. And while humor isn't a cure-all, a sense of humor helps you navigate through life's daily disappointments and upsets. Keeping a humorous perspective eases your suffering by giving you a refreshed power in what appears to be a powerless situation.

Make Friends and Find Love

Volumes of documented research have been published on the importance of being loved and loving in regard to health and sickness. Social connectedness is basic and vital to your health. The quality and depth of these relationships directly affect your blood pressure, the potential for heart disease, immune function, and even your will to live. Indisputable evidence shows that people with close, loving relationships have greater resistance to stress and disease while having more to live for.

How love keeps you healthy

The link between personal relationships and immune function is one of the most robust findings in the arena of the study known as *psychoneuroimmunology*. Having quality relationships that we value has even shown to improve our immune function, something of vital importance that helps us fight disease and normalize body functions.

According to a Journal of the American Medical Association, "married persons live longer, with lower mortality for almost every major cause of death, in comparison with single, separated, widowed, or divorced persons." Many of these studies conclude that the more a person is isolated from the social whole, the less healthy she is likely to be.

Love is intimately connected to your health. In one survey of 10,000 men with heart disease, researchers, over a five-year period, found a 50 percent reduction in frequency of chest pain (angina) among men who perceived their wives as supportive and loving.

Our immune system is also influenced by relationships that are non-nurturing and act as a subtle but consistent source of stress. By choice, you can redefine personal boundaries and choose relationships that encourage and support your health or healing path.

How buddies make us stronger

A positive element of joining organizations and groups is the *buddy factor.* Most often used in groups that cater to overcoming addictions, such as alcohol, smoking, overeating, or drug use, is the selection of a sponsor, or buddy, who has or is facing similar challenges and agrees to work with another member to develop mutual support. When you extend a helping hand for the benefit of others, you strengthen your own commitment and fortify discipline. As a result, by elevating your self-esteem, you often lessen the need for practices or substances that don't promote good health.

The buddy system gives you a mirror that reflects your own challenges, provides encouragement from someone who you feel understands you, and creates an extended family that aids your recovery and accepts you for who you really are.

Seek Emotional Equilibrium

We all feel emotion. However, what differs from person to person is an emotional awareness — our individual inhibitions, unexamined fears of emotional expression, and an ability to communicate those emotions when necessary. Research proves that emotional expression contributes to good health and healing. You surrender part of this healing power when you devalue your innermost feelings and resist voicing important feelings and opinions.

In our everyday lives, you diminish your personal sense of power when you devalue your feelings. Many people make conscious choices not to express how they feel for fear of "rocking the boat." They walk through their lives with unresolved feelings that often burst out at the wrong time or toward the wrong person. In psychology this is known as *emotional displacement.*

Continually suppressing feelings can result in feeling overwhelmed. Often, people also lack the awareness of how they feel and don't know how to articulate those feelings. When you're overwhelmed and frustrated, sometimes you find it easier to numb these suppressed feelings with food, extreme substances, alcohol, or other styles of compulsive behavior.

Does the need to express emotion mean you have to walk around constantly broadcasting every feeling? This would amount to a lot of effort due to the fleeting nature of emotions — and this is the greatest fear most people have about doing "emotional work."

You need to express the emotions that affect the way you feel: feelings that take your body or mind away from the present moment; and feelings that inspire sadness, fear, love, happiness, or sudden separation from someone close.

Presume, for a moment, that you're having a conversation with your mate and she says something critical or offensive, such as, "Marie says her husband never lifts a finger around the house, and I said you never do, either." Although your mate continues to speak, that critical comparison, specifically the word "never," causes your attention to falter as you feel the sting of her subtle criticism. If you, then and there, make it a point to tell her that it was an unfair comparison or that it hurt and that "never" may be an exaggeration, you can begin to disperse this tension buildup. But, to sit there and *not* say anything, hiding or devaluing those disconnected feelings, only hurts you (and others!) in the long run.

Expressing your emotions is only necessary to do with people whom you have some kind of relationship with (mate, family, friend, or business associate), but it's imperative to share how you feel when this sense of separation occurs. Then your future conversation and dealings can lack tension or suspicion.

Emotional expression is one of the most challenging demons of a self-healing protocol. It requires emotional courage to risk saying what is important to you and to take a position that people may judge you by. It is, for many, an atrophied muscle, and, like muscles that have not been used with frequency, expressing emotions may initially feel awkward and stiff. But as you feel more confident and articulate, you can self-monitor yourself more easily and rapidly. When you express how you feel, you move through the stagnation of pooling emotions to experience greater emotional strength and resiliency.

Take Part in Physical Exercise

Exercise is the opportunity to breathe life into your cells. If food helps to nourish the blood, exercise is the catalyst to stimulate its movement. This movement circulates valuable nutrients, helps remove waste products, and brings life-sustaining oxygen to hungry cells. Part of the resistance toward exercise is not only emotional and intellectual but also physical as well.

As a former long distance runner, despite my love for running, there was not a day that I ran (which was nearly daily) that I didn't hate the first 15 minutes. Why? My body had to wake up! When my circulation was finally zooming through my arteries and when the chemical endorphins in my body finally began to circulate and give me that "runner's high," the memory of loving what I was doing was refreshed. But to that point, it was misery and discomfort, questioning my sanity and thinking of all the other things I could be doing. Often, this is the stage when people quit. They never allow themselves to get past this point, so the need for patience and a minimum of 20 minutes of brisk walking, biking, or swimming is what's required for any real benefits to kick in and generate positivity.

You can unravel your emotional and physical blocks to exercising by beginning a smart and consistent exercise program tailored for your lifestyle and condition. This will demonstrate the power of movement in healing within days.

Exercise is a required element of a self-healing lifestyle. If you can influence the quality of your blood with nutrition, exercise is the catalyst for getting that blood to effectively circulate through the system, generate lymph flow, aid blood sugar regulation, enhance immune function, and even improve brain function.

Studies have shown that a consistent exercise program produces numerous benefits, including a longer life and reduced chance of developing major diseases. You feel better with regular exercise because it offers an optimum outlet for stress release, control of your body weight, and the stimulation of circulation and greater energy release.

For all the valuable information available about exercise, an often overlooked point is *that the time we put aside for exercise should be pleasurable*; something we look forward to and something that moderately challenges us. Of course, those first 10 to 15 minutes are always the most difficult; however, after our muscles warm and our stride is reached, it should become a moving mediation. Focusing on your body, breathing, and bodily sensations with movement that is repetitive can help to invoke the body's natural relaxation responses.

Have Faith

The consistency of a spiritual practice, such as prayer, worship, energetic therapies (T'ai Chi, yoga, and so on) and mediation, adds a potent dynamic to healing. Spiritual practices, for all their unseen value, support and reinforce the self-conviction that you can, and will, recover.

Faith is a word of profound significance to both secular and religious worlds. To the religious mind, faith has moved mountains, walked across water, healed the sick, and communed with the Almighty. Faith can either be a badge of glory worn by those with divine connections or a hopeful rationale lamented whenever efforts result in failure: "Your faith is not strong enough," you're told. Such a comment judges our efforts as mediocre. However, failure can also be a humbling motivator, allowing us to believe that with more faith, more love, more surrender, all things are possible. To the secular world, faith implies loyalty, trust, sincerity, and belief. "Keep the faith" reads a popular bumper sticker, a catchy phrase managing to straddle both worlds with equalized appeal.

Faith brings you into focus, making you a willing participant in the act of your own healing while allowing you to experience a more fulfilling and greater sense of value for living. "While we cannot count on miracles to save us," writes Rabbi David Wolpe in *Making Loss Matter,* "we can be miraculous. We can ourselves do things that change the world and reshape our own souls. Faith teaches us not that life will be easy, but that the difficulties of life yield beauty."

For anyone trying to heal herself, the question of faith becomes a more focused one. You either seek solace in your beliefs and trust that the healing process will strengthen your faith, or you begin to redefine the meaning of your beliefs as a preliminary path toward building faith. Its broadest meaning might be best explained in Antoine de Saint-Exupery's *The Little Prince,* where the fox shares his secret with the Little Prince: "It is only with the heart that one can see rightly; what is essential is invisible to the eye."

Honoring the spiritual realm has been the foundation for many remarkable recoveries from so-called terminal diseases. Such a spiritual dimension in healing is untouched by the mental, emotional, and physical realms. It inspires and reconfirms that you are greater than your sum total appearance and connected eternally to unseen forces beyond the physical realm. For some, this may mean conventional religious observation; for others, the word *spiritual* can be a substitute for the invisible world of energy — "what is essential is invisible to the eye." The wisdom of the fox may be invaluable for redefining spirituality.

Establishing reverence for energy and for opening your body to this energy is foundational for true healing. How does this relate to healing disease states? You limit the scope of your healing potential by remaining isolated, separate from others, and detached from the infinite source of energy itself, if you're not cultivating it. In such a limiting ego-driven mind-set, you reduce your essence to being dependent on the laws of nature, physics, and biology. You exist as oblivious, defiant, or fearful that a larger source of energy exists and can be accessed.

Medical research has confirmed the value of prayer; having faith in a higher power can be good medicine, regardless of the type of religion practiced or your style of worship. Whether you're on an evangelistic path or hold your convictions privately, religious activity and its supportive fellowship encourage healing on numerous levels. These activities include group and private prayer, socializing, volunteer activities, well-known rituals, and heartfelt music that reaffirms faith.

In the shelter of faith you are free to suspend your fear, extend your trust, and find peace. A life navigated by faith is enriched by unseen influence and marked by gratitude, hope, and reverence.

Part III
Planning and Preparing Your Macrobiotic Adventure

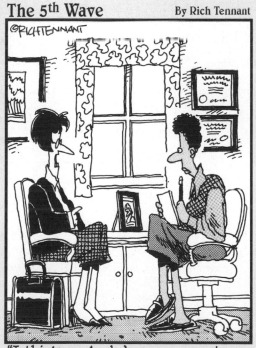

The 5th Wave   By Rich Tennant

"I think my body's energy centers ARE well balanced. I keep my pager on my belt, my cell phone in my right pocket, and my palmtop computer in my inside left breast pocket."

In this part . . .

Planning and preparing is half the work and when you can do it in an organized and efficient way, it makes everything easier and more inspirational. This section explains how you can make healthier lifestyle changes to support a new way of eating and great tips on creating a macro-friendly kitchen.

Chapter 11

Transforming Your Current Lifestyle into a Macrobiotic One

A healthy lifestyle has a powerful influence in your daily life. Just as you nourish your body with food, you gain support and nourishment from your home and its environment, its sense of order, and health qualities.

In this chapter, I explore the important points of a healthy lifestyle, which includes the different ways we can care for our health from the outside, such as our home environment, our physical activity, the products we can surround ourselves with, and the toxins we want to avoid. These factors all influence our health and are part of a macro approach that looks at the larger picture.

Revamping Your Space with an Eye toward Macrobiotics

Transitioning to a macrobiotic lifestyle is simple, yet it can bring many profound benefits. Although changing the food you nourish your body with brings you more vitality and better health, making changes to the way you live in your home also can enhance your health and sense of well-being.

In the following sections, I explain why it's important to think about the materials you surround yourself with and what you should look for when you're ready to give your home and furnishings a macrobiotic makeover.

Making healthy home changes that matter

Macrobiotics isn't just about healthy eating — it's about the complete picture of what constitutes healthy living. That doesn't mean you have to go nuts and toss out everything in your home. It just means being more thoughtful about the quality of what you use or bring into your home. No matter how well you eat, the pollutants and toxins in your immediate environment can still have a dramatically adverse effect on your health.

Many of the modern materials in home construction and interior décor, including flooring and furniture, use chemical compounds known to be toxic. These chemicals release into the air you breathe toxins that can be detrimental to your health. This means you need to minimize your exposure to industrial and household pollutants. A healthy, toxin-free home environment is critical to protecting your immune function and promoting good health.

Toxins are not only found in the building and decorating materials of your home. They're also found in many items commonly used in the kitchen, such as plastic cooking utensils, plastic storage containers, aluminum foil, plastic wrap, and aluminum or nonstick pots and pans. Some varieties of stainless steel cookware give off metal toxins that are absorbed by food during cooking; nonstick coatings, such as Teflon, have been known to chip or peel during cooking; plastic wrap contains carcinogenic byproducts; and not only does aluminum foil leave aluminum particles behind in food, but most varieties aren't biodegradable, meaning every piece you use will be on Earth indefinitely.

So what are your options? Safer choices would be wood utensils, enamel-lined cast iron pans as well as 3-ply stainless steel pans, and glass or ceramic for food storage. For wrapping food, you can use cellulose, wax, or brown paper. Choosing better quality, nontoxic products for cooking and storing food, as well as for cleaning up afterward, will take you on a healthier home path. I cover cookware and food storage in much more depth in Chapter 12.

Choosing nontoxic products for you and your home

Whenever possible, choose natural products that are healthier for your body as well as the environment. For instance, paint, one of the most popular wall coverings, emits *volatile organic compounds (VOCs),* which are organic chemical compounds that exert extremely high vapor pressures under normal conditions. These VOCs seep into the air not just when the paint is applied to walls but long after it has dried. Paint's harmful VOCs irritate the lungs and respiratory tissues, no matter how sound or balanced your whole food diet is. The simple solution? Choose one of the many VOC-free or low-VOC paints on the market. They cost just a few dollars more yet take you one step closer to creating a low-toxin environment.

Building materials and furnishings

In the last few years, many household fabrics, floor coverings, building materials, and furniture have become available in sustainable and eco-friendly forms. Here are just some of your choices:

- VOC-free carpets
- Furniture made from sustainably harvested or managed forests, Bamboo wood or from recycled timber
- Upholstery fabrics and bed and bath linens made from organically grown plants, such as organic cotton, hemp, and bamboo, and colored with low-impact dyes.

Don't forget to focus on your sleeping space. Good sleep is essential to strong immunity and sustained health. You can increase the quality of your sleep and its rejuvenating benefits very simply. Just remove, or unplug, electronic items in the bedroom, such as TVs, clocks, electric blankets, waterbed warmers, and so on. These "conveniences" usually emit what can amount to disturbing electromagnetic frequencies (EMFs) that have a depleting effect on the body's natural energy field.

Television can project EMFs 10 feet or more, even when the TV is switched to standby. You can replace electric clocks with battery-operated ones and place them far from your where your head rests, which promotes a more restful and healthier sleep.

You can soothe allergies by choosing hyper-allergenic bedding, including pillows, mattresses, mattress pads, and eco-friendly bedding materials.

Cleaning products (for yourself and your stuff)

Take a look beneath your kitchen sink at the cleaning products you currently use. Read the ingredients label. Can you even pronounce some of them? Lose 'em! Just keep those harmful chemicals far away from your home. Most commercial cleaning products are loaded with a virtual parade of toxic chemicals.

While these products may do a respectable job of cleaning, they're harmful not only to you and your family but also to your pets. Rover or Kitty, being low to the ground and frequently resting his snout barely an inch from those surfaces, inevitably breathes the chemical aroma or petroleum derivatives.

Fortunately, many eco-friendly, biodegradable products are available that enable you to replace dish soap, washing powder, and other cleaning products with natural and safe alternatives. In a pinch, you can revert to more traditional methods that use time-tested results, such as baking soda, vinegar — and even a little bit of old-fashioned elbow grease!

What we put *on* our bodies is just as important as what we put *in* our bodies. Consider your skin; with more than two million pores that travel down to blood capillaries, they are a direct link to your blood. Therefore, what you put on your skin is soaked up like a sponge, and what doesn't evaporate goes into your blood.

Like cleaning products, many body lotions, soaps, shampoos, deodorants, and creams usually contain a plethora of chemicals that can be harmful. Although some chemical compounds need to be added to stabilize products to prevent bacterial growth when opened (or to maintain shelf life), a wide range of natural-based toiletries on the market aim to keep such chemicals to a minimum.

The availability and range of quality goods grows by the day. Now you can find eco-friendly products in nonspecialty stores as well as from online retailers.

Performing a personal space makeover

Clutter is a seven-letter word that can spread its subtle havoc into every area of your life. When your living space is full of clutter, or just consistently disorganized, it makes the energy around you stagnant and inert. Clutter arrives in many forms: from too many clothes, books, and collectables to just plain piles of . . . stuff! Energetically, it can make you feel weighed down and inhibit you from moving forward with your life. When you make the conscious decision to switch to a macrobiotic lifestyle, part of that choice is cleaning up your environment to free you up energetically.

Living with clutter can be exhausting. It can make you feel out of sync with your home and your life. If you're finding parts of your life too challenging and not working in the way that you want, chances are it's usually reflected somewhere in your home. Living in a clean, open environment offers you the freedom to move with ease and grace, to focus more effectively, and to attract greater possibilities. Removing clutter creates a healthier environment that's clean, peaceful, and full of energy. It's what a home should be: your oasis of sanity where you restore and recharge your essence.

The kitchen

A great place to begin your purge is the kitchen — the hub of macro-living. There are two good reasons for lightening the load in your kitchen:

- ✔ You won't be tempted to smother ketchup on your *tempeh*.
- ✔ You'll need the space for the new and healthier additions to your grocery repertoire.

Keeping your countertops clear also provides the space and inspiration to feel more comfortable in the kitchen, so you may be more motivated to experiment with new recipes and snacks.

First, thoroughly clean your pantry, drawers, and cupboards. Remove everything from these spaces, sort through all your food products, dishes, and utensils. Only return those that will be used in food preparation. Place any unopened dry goods and unwanted dishes in a box and donate them. Now do the same with your fridge contents.

The bathroom

Go through your bathroom and linen closet and do some heavy-guns cleaning. Replace old junk products with quality, earth-friendly versions. Let go of products that you bought but never used and that are still taking up valuable space (while you keep promising that you're going to use them soon). They are likely to have passed their sell-by date anyway and are no longer useful. Removing chemical-laden products is a major step toward giving your home a healthy makeover.

The rest of the house

You can organize other areas of your home by sorting through your piles (no matter what they contain) and your closet spaces. Create separate piles for the items you want to keep, those you want to donate, and those that no longer work or are useful. By paring down and streamlining your closets and collections, you'll feel more settled and calm and be able to relax in your own space. You will have room to move and grow, to expand and embrace your new lifestyle.

Strengthening the Body You Live In

Western culture is driven by external appearances. However, many problems that appear to be "cosmetic" often indicate deeper internal imbalances.

As an example, I've seen clients with skin conditions who had made appointment after appointment with skin specialists for years, taking one medication after another and paying through the nose for specially formulated chemical soaps, lotions, and external treatments, all to no avail. Typically, when external treatments failed, the doctor would suggest psychological counseling as a last resort. But rarely did doctors ever suggest a dietary change, beyond the trite adage of "Be sure to eat a healthy diet."

Although what you eat can strengthen your body's natural discharge systems, continually challenging your body is equally important. Stretching your muscles, increasing your respiration, lowering your heartbeat through sustained aerobic activity, and succeeding at goals to challenge yourself creates a state of well-being. Fortunately, this doesn't need to be documented with long-term studies or peer-reviewed reports, because it's good common sense and almost always feels intuitively right.

Putting one foot in front of the other

Regular exercise is a key component to healthy macrobiotic living. It strengthens circulation, respiration, digestion, and will. Regular aerobic movement (20 minutes of steady, repetitive movement) and stretching exercises are important at every age to burn fat, build muscle, promote flexibility, and retain bone density. If you're a gym fanatic or a yoga diehard, you're right up there on the macro health-ometer. However, if you struggle to find the time or motivation to exercise, now is the time to make a personal vow to set yourself up with a manageable exercise plan that will complement your new macro lifestyle.

Exercise helps increase your energy, and the endorphins your body generates through exercise automatically help relieve stress and tension. Your mind will find a welcome peace and calmness as you take time to nurture yourself this way.

If walking is the only exercise you can do every day, do as much as you can! Brisk walking not only keeps you fit but increases your heart rate (so during later resting periods your heart actually slows), gets your blood and lymph fluid systemically pumping, and can be done literally anywhere, anytime for free!

Plan an exercise routine that's realistic and manageable. A weekly game of tennis, golf, or other sport is a fun way to bring exercise into your lifestyle.

Additionally, grab 10 minutes a day to do some basic stretching exercises. This does wonders for increasing your body's flexibility. Stretching helps ease tight areas in the body, relieves joint and muscle pain, and opens you up to a more flexible attitude in the process.

Energizing acupuncture meridians with exercise

Hundreds of years ago, the acupuncture system of energy pathways, called *meridians*, were mapped out on the human form. People began experimenting with point and energy channel stimulation using needles *(acupuncture)*, finger pressing or body part pressure *(acupressure/shiatsu/do-in)*, hot herbs that were ignited to heat acu-points on the skin *(moxa)*, or general massage techniques that follow energy pathways.

Much like a battery that has a current running through it to keep it active and charged, some theorize that the human form also has a series of energy pathways that run through the body and connect with different organs and systems, feeding it energy and giving it energetic support.

In a form of self-acupuncture called *do-in* (pronounced doe-*een*), practitioners rub, pound, massage, and pressure different acupuncture points. Actually, people do this almost intuitively; you rub your eyes when tired or awakening (acu-points around the eye stimulate the liver and help with fatigue), or you may rub your intestines when you're hungry.

Although physical forms of activity can help you improve your health, exercise has an energetic aspect to it that people miss entirely because we're always looking at physical matter. We deny the energetic because we can't see it, but we do perceive it. The testimony of that is in our everyday language with common words such as:

"I got a really good *vibe* from those people . . . ."

"I *knew* it; I just had a feeling . . . ."

"I don't like that home. It just *felt creepy* to me . . . ."

Exercise, while having profound physical effects, also stimulates our energy body. The fascinating thing is that any motion creating muscle movement, such as stretching or a yoga pose, has an energy-promoting effect on a specific, or group of, energy line and the points along that particular pathway. Although this form of energy is subtle, its consequence eventually makes its way to an organ.

Be aware of your body. It speaks to you. As you become acquainted with some general acupuncture points, you'll note your increasing sensitivity to their effectiveness when those points are massaged or stretched. Pain in these areas can give you a read on the low energy areas of your body that need more attention and are related to these organ named pathways throughout the human form.

Here are a couple examples to demonstrate this point.

Doing yoga to stimulate acupuncture points

In the yoga camel pose (see Figure 11-1), you kneel on the floor, stretch your arms behind you, and grasp your ankles. This pose places emphasis on the area of the front shoulder just at the corner of the collarbone. In acupuncture charts, this is the beginning of the lung meridian. Stretching this area also stimulates the lungs. Tarzan must have instinctively known this when he beat those points on both sides as he yodeled that jungle scream.

In the plough pose (also in Figure 11-1), you lie on the ground, place your arms on the ground next to your sides for support, and stretch your legs back over your head so your feet touch the ground behind your head. This pose focuses on stretching the lower back and neck area. Many of these points relate to digestion, as well as the mid-organ area (liver, kidneys, pancreas, stomach, spleen, gall bladder), so this pose also energizes each organ.

These are basic yoga exercises and can be easily learned from a DVD or class. Also, *Yoga For Dummies* is probably the best place to start for an easy introduction, Dummies style.

Figure 11-1:
The camel pose and the plough pose.

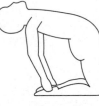
Camel Pose

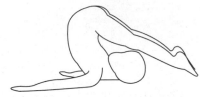
Plow Pose

Go with the flow: T'ai Chi

When I first saw a young man doing T'ai Chi in a park, I thought he was delusional and probably had lost his medication. However, those gentle dance poses that look like anything but exercise actually are designed to stretch various muscles in a way that also uniquely stimulates acupuncture points.

After I had moved into a macrobiotic community and was making dietary changes, I took a T'ai Chi class. I don't remember being particularly impressed; it felt like a lame sort of dance that I didn't find very challenging. About 20 years later I took another T'ai Chi class and was amazed at the result. I felt highly energized and profoundly calm and left with a strong, centered feeling. I can only attribute a growing energetic sensitivity to this positive experience of the later T'ai Chi class.

I think that learning energy-related therapies such as yoga, meditation, and T'ai Chi can be vital tools for keeping a foot in the spiritual world — the world of energy, what we can perceive, but not see.

I would encourage readers to learn the Basic 82, a T'ai Chi routine. You can do it anywhere, anytime, and your sense of awareness will increase. There's also some partner work you can do, such as "push hands" movements that are both bonding and challenging, not to mention fun. Most local schools that offer night courses have T'ai Chi classes.

Relearning how to breathe

You gotta learn this — because it's powerful! Breath work can actually help discharge systemic acids through the breath, promote lymph flow, and improve respiration while centering and calming the mind. Breath work is an important part of any meditation practice and becomes a stabilizing focus for concentration, intuitive work, or to induce deeper sleep.

Three-part breathing — that is, a full inhalation using the abdomen, the chest, and the upper chest — allows more air to enter your lungs and thus more acids to be discharged during your exhale. In yoga, this is known as the *full breath*. In three-part breathing, the breath path is divided into three cavities: the lower digestive cavity, the chest cavity, and the upper lung and shoulder area.

Before I offer a brief three-step outline, first consider *how* you currently breathe. Most of us (except for babies and animals) constrict our mid-section as we inhale. We should actually be doing the reverse: expanding our stomach as if it is filling with the air we are taking in.

This three-part breathing exercise is the basic deep-breathing exercise that you can use to re-create immediate calm, ease your temper, and get clear as you flush your body with life-giving oxygen and wake up sleepy cells. It is broken in three parts, or thirds, to illustrate each part of the technique but should be woven into one long breath.

1. **Inhalation:** Breathe in and expand only your abdomen. Think about when we were kids trying to imitate having, in kid lingo, a "fat stomach." Now hold that pose.

2. **Continued inhalation:** When you've taken as much breath as possible (and you now look pregnant), expand only your chest as you breathe in as if you are filling the middle of your chest with air. It's a "look proud" visual. Now, hold that pose.

3. **Concluding inhalation:** As you've expanded your chest to its limit, breathe in deeper while slightly raising your shoulders. Filling the last third of your upper chest allows more air into the top of the lungs, thereby giving you the distinct feeling that you have taken a very deep and fulfilling breath.

   Your exhalation ideally should take twice as long to completely exhale.

Practice this technique. When I was a long distance runner, I did this breath in rhythm to my steps, taking one breath section at every stride (three strides, or large steps, to every full breath) and it enabled me to increase my endurance and speed. Learn to do it naturally, when sitting, waiting, when cold, when you need to focus, or when tired.

Try taking 5 to 10 deep full breaths right before you drift off to sleep at night. It'll be only a minute or two before you find yourself floating on a cloud into a peaceful slumber.

Chapter 12

Setting up and Stocking Your Macro-Friendly Kitchen

Y ou're more likely to stick to a macrobiotic diet if you enjoy being in the kitchen and have the right cookware and foods to support your lifestyle. In this chapter, I show you how to create a healthy, working kitchen, which should result in more orderly and efficient food preparation. I include tips on food storage, which kitchen tools you need, and how to organize shopping lists.

In addition, I offer some advice for healthy shopping, which requires identifying undesirable label ingredients and spotting the health saboteurs.

Organizing Your Kitchen

It's time to get your kitchen ready for its macro-transformation. With the right tools and organized space, your kitchen can become an inspiring environment that you'll relish cooking in as it regains its rightful place as the heart of your home.

Properly setting up your kitchen allows your cooking time to be less stressful and more pleasurable. The most efficient kitchen allows you to easily find the equipment and ingredients you need. Begin by finding the best home for all key ingredients and cookware. Here are some tips:

✔ Store frequently used items, such as brown rice, grains, and beans, together in the pantry or on the countertop. On the wide countertop that leads to my stove, I have different grains stored in large Mason jars that give me easy access to ingredients I use often. (The jars also give the space a unique look.)

✔ Organize your dried herbs and spices so you can quickly identify those you need for cooking.

✔ Place cooking utensils close to the preparation area with easy access to mixing bowls, pots, and pans.

✔ An efficient kitchen has a triangle of floor space located between the sink, refrigerator, and stove.

✔ Avoid placing furniture where you can bump into it as you maneuver throughout the kitchen.

✔ Create a conversation area with bar stools at the countertop so friends and family can join you as you cook or play TV chef and add pinches of salt or herbs with a stylized flourish. Of course, you'll need a white chef's hat for this!

Storing whole grains, vegetables, and condiments

Whole grains and dried beans are usually considered *dry goods*. Dry goods keep best in dry environments (hence, their name), so be sure to use airtight containers like glass or ceramic jars.

If stored properly, dry goods can last up to six months. You can store most fresh vegetables in plastic or cotton bags and place them in the crisper drawer of your refrigerator. If you store your vegetables in plastic bags, you can keep them fresh and longer lasting by squeezing all the air out of the bag.

You can purchase green plastic storage bags in many natural food stores that use this method to seal in vegetable freshness for longer periods of time. This bag-squeezing technique also ensures that your vegetables can be kept in a cool, dry pantry.

Figuring out the utensils and small appliances you need

Macrobiotic cooking doesn't require any magical mystery appliances or utensils. You probably have the basics — pots, pans, a cutting board, knives, a blender, a stainless steel or bamboo vegetable steamer, and an array of cooking utensils. If you don't, this is a great time to begin building your kitchen toolbox.

However, one thing that no kitchen can be without is a good sharp knife! Sharp knives make food preparation easier and safer. A good vegetable knife and sharpening tool are essential when you're eating large quantities of fruits and veggies. If you're consuming small amounts of animal protein, sharp fish and meat knives are also handy.

No kitchen is complete without a large chopping board. Boards come in all kinds of shapes, sizes, and materials. Bamboo is becoming a favorite because it's durable, sustainably harvested, harder than maple, and naturally anti-microbial — one of its biggest advantages.

A pressure cooker can also be a useful asset to any whole foods kitchen. One of the chief advantages of pressure cooking whole grain is that the force of consistent heat penetrates the outer covering of the grain, making it easier to digest and preserving more nutrients. Pressure cooking also brings out the naturally sweet and nutty flavor within the grain. Of course, it also saves time, and that's a big plus for many folks.

Minding the materials and methods of your cooking tools

When you cook, your goal is to take a large volume of food and, by using heat, concentrate its nutritional goodness and weaken the cellular walls where the nutrition is stored so your body can absorb it. Ideally, you want to cook, not overcook, in a variety of ways that allow you to get the most from what you choose as nourishment.

The cookware you use to prepare your foods can affect your health. Some materials don't interact with the foods you cook or store in them, so no worries there. Other materials give off particles that the foods absorb, and then you consume those particles. Yuck! You also have to be cautious about the methods you use to cook food, microwaving in particular.

My personal choice for the best cookware is hands down cast iron enamel coated cookware (CIECC). The common complaint about CIECC is that it's heavy to lift, and it is, but it's worth it if you've got the arm strength. Another alternative is the lightweight, ceramic-coated Nano-Glaze cookware that cooks with a far-infrared heating process and contains no lead, cadmium, copper, aluminum iron, chromium, or nickel. These products are fairly new on the market, contain natural coatings, and are far less expensive than enamel coated cast iron. I also recommend cast iron, earthenware, and quality stainless steel 3-ply pots and pans.

Say no to Teflon and aluminum

I recommend replacing aluminum or nonstick pots pans with those made from stainless steel, stoneware, or porcelain-covered cast iron. Buying these pots and pans is one of the most sensible and health-rewarding investments you'll ever make. If you take care of them properly, they will last a lifetime.

You may be thinking, "What's wrong with my nonstick pans?" Perhaps you love the fact that you avoid burning the pan and cleanup is a snap. However, every back has a front, as the principle goes, and that applies to cookware.

Certain materials such as nonstick coatings and aluminum pans eventually leech toxic particles into food during the cooking process. Aluminum is a reactive metal and has been suspected to be a potential factor in Alzheimer's disease.

When you're following a macrobiotic diet, the last thing you want to add to your meal is a fine coating of toxic Teflon.

Teflon-coated aluminum contains perfluorooctanoic acid (PFOA). This synthetic chemical creates a soap-like slipperiness and nonstick finish. When heated, Teflon and other nonstick pans quickly reach temperatures that force toxic fumes into the air — also known as your breathing space. The coating begins to break down and discharge its toxins at 446 degrees. PFOA has become a very controversial issue because of its reputed dangers connected with human absorption. PFOA has already been associated with a potential for instigating cancer in the pancreas, liver, testicles, and mammary glands. Miscarriages, thyroid problems, weakened immune systems, and low organ weights have also been connected with PFOA excess.

For the sake of your long-term health, try the healthier options of 3-ply stainless steel, cast iron, ceramic coated cookware, enamel coated cast iron, or earthenware. Most waffle makers, baking trays, and even a number of rice cookers are typically made of aluminum or are Teflon coated.

Some years ago, I realized that I missed having a waffle maker. I thought to myself, "So what if it's Teflon or some newer chemical coating. It's not going to kill me." I bought one at a cooking supply store. I enjoyed using it until I realized that the strange odor permeating my kitchen was the heated coating. The toxic fragrance diffused into my living room, dining room, and anywhere else it could linger. I tossed it and happily went back to a family pancake recipe when the craving struck.

Avoid the microwave

Not only are Teflon and aluminum not your friends, but the microwave is also problematic. This issue is close to many hearts, because currently about 50 percent of U.S. homes have a microwave. However, many years of scientific testing has shown that microwave cooking lessens the nutritional content of food. Microwaving, though very convenient, destroys the very nutrients you need to maintain your health. And not only do you eat less nutritionally valuable food, but you also ingest microwaves!

Research published in the British medical journal *The Lancet* suggests that microwave cooking can cause structural, functional, and immunological changes in your body by converting the amino acid L-proline into toxins detrimental to the nervous system, kidneys, and liver. Other studies show that eating foods cooked in a microwave can reduce muscle strength; cause a free-radical, highly carcinogenic effect in fats; and limit the amount of vital vitamins and minerals available for your body to absorb.

Microwave cooking also takes away the joy, love, and nurturing you would otherwise put into cooking. Through its convenience, you're tempted to buy processed, ready-made, nuke-in-a-bag food. And then you miss out on some loving home cooking!

Saying adios to plastics

Sometimes as I walk through a supermarket or pass a toy store in a mall, I look at the products and can't help recalling the words of a well-meaning friend of Mrs. Robinson in *The Graduate*, who turns to Benjamin and gives him some very succinct advice: "One word: Plastics! It's the future!"

And sure enough, we're now swimming in it. Although the plastics industry has made some convenient and useful products in recent years, the downside poses great threat to human well-being as well as planetary health. We now consume more nonbiodegradable plastic bags and water bottles than the earth can handle, and they're not magically going away — at least not in the next 300 years!

When it comes to using plastic in relation to food or drink, plastics' real threat is in its ability to give off toxins into whatever it holds.

A simple solution is to avoid plastic as much as possible in your kitchen. Glass and ceramic containers are terrific for food storage and are available at most department or specialty stores. Storage jars and glass bowls with resealable lids allow you to store food without using plastic wrap. Stainless steel utensils can replace plastic ones for just a few dollars. Even wood utensils, particularly bamboo, work well.

Ideally, you want to avoid making bottled water a regular habit because of the plastic component. For more on this topic, see the section "Choosing a healthy water source" later in this chapter.

Stocking Your Kitchen

No matter how big or small your kitchen, having a good supply of essential macrobiotic ingredients ensures you can always prepare a delicious meal or snack. Dry goods are easy to store and can last ages, allowing you to just purchase fresh delicious vegetables to complete any recipe.

Choosing bulk foods: Buy lots; save money

Many natural food stores sell dry goods in bulk. Buying bulk goods has many advantages: First, you save money because you don't have to pay for packaging and marketing. It also saves on resources because the goods aren't shipped off to food manufacturers for additional packaging, and therefore less energy is consumed.

All sorts of foods can be bought in bulk (check out the list later in this section). When choosing bulk foods, buy larger quantities of those goods that you'll use more frequently, such as short-grain brown rice, rolled oats, and lentils. It also helps to keep a stock of dried legumes, like chickpeas, split peas, and black beans, or other grain products on hand, so you always have ingredients for favorite recipes.

Check out the many bulk goods at your local health food store or natural foods market. Even many commercial markets have begun to carry some of these foods. Here's a list of food items you can typically by in bulk:

- Almonds
- Amaranth
- Barley
- Buckwheat
- Bulgur wheat
- Chickpeas
- Corn grits
- Couscous
- Cracked wheat berries
- Dried beans
- Dried fruit
- Kamut

- Lentils
- Millet
- Mixes (falafel, pancake, broth, burger, and so on)
- Muesli and cereals
- Oils
- Pumpkin seeds
- Quinoa
- Rice (various types)
- Sesame seeds
- Spelt
- Split peas

- ✔ Tea
- ✔ Teff
- ✔ Walnuts

- ✔ Wheat or non-wheat flour
- ✔ Whole or rolled oats

Selecting condiments, oils, herbs, and spices

You can find many of the seasonings and condiments used in macrobiotic kitchens in most health or natural food markets and even some regular grocery stores. Begin with the basics, such as fine-quality cooking oil like sesame seed oil for sautéing foods and extra virgin olive oil for salads and dressings.

Some basic spices, such as chili powder, ground coriander, cumin, curry powder, tumeric, cinnamon, and nutmeg and herbs such as oregano, bay leaf, basil, garlic powder, rosemary, sage, thyme, and onion powder, can all be wonderful and inspiring additions to your culinary creativity.

The key to healthy and flavorful cooking is in purchasing the best-quality ingredients available, and this equally applies to herbs, spices, and condiments. Good-quality sea salt and oil enhance the flavor, nutrition, and digestibility of your food. The crème de la crème of sea salt is called *Fleur de Sel* (from France) or *Flor de Sal* (from Portugal) — it's a hand-harvested sea salt. And insisting on organic quality also ensures that your food is pesticide free.

Condiments are not just options for flavoring. They have specific functions. Some offer a jolt of alkalinity — like the Japanese salt plums called *umeboshi*, which calm upset stomachs. You can use umeboshi in vegetarian sushi and salad dressings or as a condiment. Sometimes a third of a teaspoon of umeboshi on a plate can help with whole-grain digestion, in the same way sauerkraut does. Each condiment lends a different quality and most important, allows you to customize your own needs from your very own kitchen. Table 12-1 lists condiments that I recommend, organized by whether the condiment contains salt.

Table 12-1	Macrobiotic Condiments
Without Salt	*Containing Salt*
Sesame oil and olive oil (extra virgin)	Sesame salt
Nuts (almonds, walnuts, so on)	Sauerkraut
Almond butter	Pickles

(continued)

Table 12-1 *(continued)*

Without Salt	Containing Salt
Seeds (pumpkin, sesame, so on)	Miso paste
Seed butter (pumpkin, tahini, so on)	Sea salt
Rice wine vinegar	Natural soy sauce (*tamari* or *shoyu*)
Quality herbs and spices	Salt plums or paste *(umeboshi)*
Lemon juice	Sea vegetable flakes or sheets
Mirin (sweet rice wine)	
Herbs (bay leaves, basil, garlic powder, and so on)	
Spices (chili powder, curry powder, and nutmeg)	

When choosing natural soy sauce (fermented enzymes of soybean and rice) look for labels that say "traditionally brewed," which indicates that the soy sauce has been fermented according to Japanese traditions and is free from artificial ingredients. Avoid commercial "soy sauce" at all costs. It tends to be highly processed, is often made from genetically modified soybeans, and is high in salt.

Look for the Japanese words "tamari" or "shoyu" on the label; these are commonly used as a quality marker. Though such products are indeed Japanese, they are medicinal preparations that are common to many cultures. Essentially, they are fermented brews of grain, beans, water, and sea salt, but blended with a cultural technology that is thousands of years old. Their fermented alkaline quality adds a rich ingredient to most meals and is known to have a slight blood sugar lowering effect.

Choosing a healthy water source

Switching from bottled water to home water filtration is one of the most ecological, economical, and practical steps you can take to secure a better water source.

What's wrong with bottled water? Most bottled water is nothing other than tap water sitting in a toxically infiltrated plastic bottle. The U.S. Federal Drug Administration (FDA) regulations that govern bottled water quality are only applicable if a product is transported across state lines. The guidelines also require bottled water to be "as good as tap water." Frankly, this isn't saying much. Nearly 70 percent of bottled water companies produce and sell their elixir in their home states to get around the federal purity standards. And disposing of all those plastic bottles creates environmental headaches.

The environmental impact of bottled water

On a daily basis, more than 60 million disposable plastic water bottles go into U.S. landfills. Beyond the impact on landfills, bottled water pollutes the environment in numerous other ways. Each year, 17 billion barrels of oil are used to produce the discarded bottles, which creates more than 2.5 billion tons of carbon dioxide pollution. It requires three times the amount of water to produce the bottle as it does to fill it.

The annual energy resources used to transport bottled water are estimated at more than 49 million barrels of oil, the equivalent of running 3 million cars for an entire year.

Municipal drinking water doesn't fare much better; it contains hundreds of contaminants, including lead, copper, arsenic, iron, manganese, and microscopic parasites. The sources of these contaminants range from sanitary waste to acid rain.

Although several types of water filters are available, carbon filters are the most economical, effective, and available choice.

Carbon is the most powerful absorbent known, and its use in water filtering is highly effective. One pound of carbon contains a surface area of approximately 125 acres, and it can absorb thousands of chemicals. Activated carbon has a minor electro-positive charge added to it, which makes it a better bonding agent for impurities and chemicals. A typical countertop filter contains 12 to 24 ounces of activated carbon. You can also buy models that go under your counter.

Other forms of water filtration are available, but one thing is certain: Having some kind of filtration is important.

Gearing Up for Macro Shopping

Grocery shopping can be overwhelming. If I'm not prepared, two things happen — either I'm so hungry that I overstuff my cart with goodies that I have to devour the minute I've paid for them (or more likely, I'm consuming them while I shop), or I have no plan and if I'm tired or not in the mood to shop, I wander aimlessly, for what seems like ages, and leave the store with only a fraction of what I need.

The secret is to be armed with a plan before you leave home. If you give yourself a few minutes to plan your shopping experience, you'll find that you end up making fewer trips to the store for forgotten ingredients, making your entire shopping experience less daunting, maybe even fun. In the following sections I give you some hints to help you make the most of your shopping trips.

Eat before you shop. Make an effort to avoid shopping on an empty stomach. It can often lead you down that never-ending path of distracting indulgence. On the other hand, shopping with a full stomach can be just as unsettling. The thought of buying more food when you just stuffed yourself easily inspires impatience and "shopping-aisle fatigue." So you want to be not too hungry but not too full either!

Organizing meal plans

When you plan your meals before you head to the store, shopping becomes a breeze. Think about what you'd like to cook and eat over the next couple of days or week (depending on how frequently you like to shop). Choose recipes for breakfast, lunch, and dinner. It's a good idea to include dessert and some snacks as well, because they can be convenient when food isn't prepared or your blood sugar drops.

Although variety is key to a healthy diet, you may want to prepare an extra portion or two of certain dishes so you can enjoy them as leftovers the next day. Don't forget to allow for a few extra ingredients so you can spice up your leftovers.

Seasonal cooking is an excellent way to enjoy the best and freshest ingredients. When in season, vegetables are available in abundance, and prices tend to be lower as well. When possible, support your local farmers and buy organic. Make it a point to purchase the freshest ingredients, because these will last longer.

Composing your shopping list

When you have some meals planned, check to see what ingredients you already have in your kitchen and what you need to complete the dishes you plan to make. Add any bulk items or condiments that you may be running low on to the shopping list. Voilà! You now have a list that will keep you focused when you set foot in the store.

Get to know the aisles of your local market. If you're a really savvy shopper, you can organize your list based on the order you find the items in the grocery store. (Okay, that may be asking a little too much.) But truthfully, knowing where items are located not only speeds up the shopping process because you'll know exactly where to find your goods, but you'll also know which aisles to avoid before temptation strikes. (Yep, the middle aisle where the potato chips lurk is a good one to avoid; ditto for the cookie aisle, the ice cream fridge, and the soda aisle!) Becoming familiar with your market's floor plan means you'll be in and out before you can say "fair-trade chocolate."

Detecting Harmful Ingredients on Labels

Sometimes I spend more time reading food labels than I do novels. This is because manufacturers and marketers have a deceptive way of telling us one thing on the front of the label such as "sugar free," and yet, hidden on the back of the label, in minuscule type, loom the words "evaporated cane juice." Right there on the pretty label, they're testing your intelligence.

Reading labels and knowing what to look for helps you avoid foods with additives and chemicals with names you can't possibly pronounce. If you can't pronounce it, how can something be edible? I used to joke in seminars that this was one scientist's way of talking to another.

The following food additives are frequent ingredients in many processed and packaged food. If you care about your health or the health of your loved ones, they are best avoided.

- **Acesulfame-K:** This fairly new artificial sweetener is put into baked goods, chewing gum, and even gelatin desserts. Testing on this product has been lacking, with some studies indicating that this additive may cause cancer in rats.

- **Aspartame:** Generally known by brand names such as Equal and Nutrasweet, aspartame is a concentrated chemical sweetener found in nearly every diet food — low-calorie desserts, gelatins, drink mixes, and soft drinks, to name a few. It may cause cancer or neurological problems, such as dizziness or hallucinations. *Note:* Other popular sugar substitutes, such as Splenda, high fructose corn syrup (HFCS), or Sorbitol, all have numerous complaints. But in the end, your best and most trusted barometer is to avoid these and try them after you've had three or four weeks of whole foods with natural sweeteners such as fruits. Your taste buds will tell you everything you need to know about them — the artificiality will be nothing other than distasteful, chemical tasting, and grossly sweet. You'll wonder why you never noticed it before.

- **BHA and BHT:** Butylated hydroxyanisole (BHA) and butylated hydrozyttoluene (BHT) are used to preserve many household foods.

Found in cereals, chewing gum, potato chips, and vegetable oils, they are classified as oxidants and have been linked with cancers.

✔ **Food colorings:** Blue 1 and 2, red 3, green 3, and yellow 6 are five toxic food colorings that have clearly been linked with cancer in animal testing but continue to be used in food production. Blue 1 and 2, found in beverages, candy, baked goods, and pet food, have been linked to cancer in mice. Red 3, used to dye cherries, fruit cocktail, candy, and baked goods, has been shown to cause thyroid tumors in rats. Green 3, added to candy and beverages, has been linked to bladder cancer. The frequent use of yellow 6, which is added to beverages, sausage, gelatin, baked goods, and candy, has been linked to tumors of the adrenal gland and kidney.

✔ **Monosodium glutamate (MSG):** MSG is an amino acid used as a flavor enhancer in soups, salad dressings, chips, frozen entrees, and restaurant food. It can cause headaches and nausea, and animal studies link it to damaged nerve cells in the brains of infant mice.

✔ **Olestra:** Olestra, a bad-news synthetic fat found in some potato chip brands, can cause severe diarrhea, abdominal cramps, bloating, and gas. Olestra also inhibits healthy vitamin absorption from fat-soluble carotenoids, which can be found in fruits and vegetables.

✔ **Potassium bromate:** This is used most frequently as a bread additive to increase flour volume. Like many other chemical additives, it's known to cause cancer in animals. Even small amounts in bread pose a risk to humans.

✔ **Propyl gallate (PG):** A food preservative aimed at preventing oxidation, PG is often used with BHA and BHT. It's found in meat products, chicken soup base, and chewing gum. Animal studies link this substance to cancer development

✔ **Sodium chloride:** A dash of sodium chloride, more commonly known as table salt, may add flavor to your meal, but in significant amounts, it creates cardiac and kidney problems.

✔ **Sodium nitrate (also called sodium nitrite):** Sodium nitrate can take the form of a preservative, coloring, or flavoring and is frequently added to bacon, ham, hot dogs, luncheon meats, smoked fish, and corned beef. Numerous studies have associated eating it with a variety of cancers.

✔ **Trans fats/hydrogenated oils:** Trans fats contribute to heart disease and are now banned by many restaurants and in future food policies. Restaurants, particularly fast-food chains, often feature foods that contain trans fats.

✔ **White sugar:** It's everywhere — baked goods, cereals, crackers, sauces, beverages, and so on. White sugar doesn't belong in a healthy daily diet.

Chapter 13

Cooking Tips for Macrobiotic Newbies

In This Chapter

▶ Turning favorite recipes into healthier ones

▶ Making meals more satisfying and diversified

▶ Conquering veggie phobia

▶ Exploring different cooking methods

. . . .

The more familiar you are with your kitchen and how to produce simple yet satisfying meals, the greater sense of joy and accomplishment you'll feel about taking better care of your health.

In this chapter, I help you take your first culinary steps into a multicultural macrobiotic world. I show you how to re-create familiar foods with healthier ingredients, offer strategies for introducing the family to a new way of eating, provide creative suggestions for preparing lunches and repurposing left-overs, and review various cooking methods.

Easing into Macrobiotic Cooking

Most people are very protective and passionate about their food. Often, a change of diet may not be a logical or even pleasing sensory choice. I've met individuals who just could not wrap their head around how food can taste good or be satisfying without meat, sugar, or dairy.

When you begin eating a macrobiotic diet, you quickly discover that none of the perceived flavor is lost in macrobiotic cooking. Your pallet grows more sensitive to discovering new flavors and textures in macrobiotic foods. And chewing food slowly enables you to taste and savor the unique and subtle flavors of whole foods (see Chapter 6 for more on chewing).

Transition takes time and patience, and it may take a while to engage those around you. In the following sections, I give you some tips to help your family and friends see a macrobiotic lifestyle as a sensible choice.

Re-creating familiar foods in healthy, macrobiotic ways

At a first glance, macrobiotic foods can seem very unfamiliar because of the number of multicultural ingredients, such as tempeh (Indonesia) and tofu (China), tamari (Japan) and tahini (Middle East). So many T's and yet so little knowledge of them! But many foods used in macrobiotic recommendations are familiar. They include ingredients such as rice, beans and vegetables — simple ingredients used by many cultures. Macrobiotic cooking uses different varieties of these foods, prepared in different styles and methods of cooking.

 When beginning your journey with macrobiotic cooking, a great first step is to get yourself a reliable cookbook that you'll enjoy referring to for menu planning and inspiration. I include macrobiotic recipes in Chapters 14, 15, and 16.

Take some of your favorite recipes and see how well they translate into more balanced macrobiotic meals. For instance, if you love rice and stir-fry vegetables, try using short-grain brown rice instead of long-grain white. Add some new ingredients to your stir-fry, such as kale or sea vegetables, and season with a sprinkle of natural soy sauce *(tamari)* instead of your usual spices. You'll find it to be just as delicious and really not such a drastic change.

Table 13-1 presents everyday items that are easily replaced by healthier alternatives that fit into a multicultural macrobiotic diet. Note that many cookbooks abbreviate "whole-wheat" *WW*.

Table 13-1	Ingredients for a Healthy Transition to Macrobiotics
Ingredient	*Macrobiotic Alternative*
Baked goods	Sugar- and dairy-free cookies, muffins, and cakes
Black tea	Herbal teas, dandelion, twig tea, rooibos (see Chapter 16 for tea recipes)
Canned beans	Dried beans and legumes, or canned natural varieties
Cheese	Mochi (sweet brown rice), finely grated and roasted, can be used as a "cheese topping" for many dishes
Common white bread	Sourdough, unleavened, or leavened varieties

Ingredient	Macrobiotic Alternative
Cornstarch	Kuzu powder or arrowroot powder
Iodized salt	Solar-Evaporated Sea salt
Meat	Seitan (wheat meat) and tempeh can be used in dishes to replace meat (for example, prepare a tempeh Ruben), or use small volumes of quality meats less frequently
Meat stock	Miso, dulse, or vegetable stock
Milk	Rice, oat, or almond milk
Pasta dishes	Whole wheat, rice pasta, or soba noodles
Scrambled eggs	Tofu (soft or firm — both scramble well)
Soy sauce	Natural soy sauce (tamari or shoyu)
Sugar	Brown rice syrup, barley malt, or maple syrup, honey
White flour	Whole-wheat flour, whole-wheat pastry flour, or Kamut flour
White rice	Short-, medium-, or long-grain brown rice

Introducing whole foods to the family diet

Getting every member of the family to eat and enjoy the same foods can be a difficult task, so when introducing whole foods to your family, begin with subtle changes until everyone becomes familiar with the new tastes and styles.

Start with simple changes, such as substituting brown rice for white rice or mixing the two together, and introduce some new vegetables, such as kale and collard greens. Initially, greens are best when they're finely chopped because this makes them easier to chew. You can also add greens to soups and stews, or hide them in a vegetarian sushi roll, without making your spouse or kids feel like you're trying to turn them into Popeye.

Make sure you continue to serve some familiar foods so everyone remains comfortable through the transition process. Gradually phase out processed foods completely, or replace them with a whole-foods version. As your family becomes more familiar with new ingredients and tastes, you can become more adventurous and experimental with your meal planning.

Involve your family in the shopping and cooking so they gain familiarity with the new ingredients and have a deeper value for what goes into a meal, instead of just meeting the food as it arrives on the table. Have your children help you bake cookies and macro desserts so they not only have fun cooking but look forward to eating as well.

Putting macrobiotics in the lunchbox

If you're feeding your family healthy foods at home, the last thing you want is for your kids to go off to school and eat the unhealthy foods of a typical school lunch. So I encourage you to pack your kids' lunches. Here are ten lunch box tips:

- ✔ Flexibility is the key. Kids will get exposed to conventional foods at school, birthday parties, and friends' houses. Don't even try to insulate them. Think about all the junk you had growing up and be grateful that they have a better and more conscious start. You can control what you give your children when you prepare the food yourself and teach them how to make wise choices when someone else does the cooking. Let them taste different foods and show them, by example, that everything is okay in moderation.

- ✔ When you first introduce whole foods, begin with small, tasty changes. Don't force tempeh and brown rice on them from day one! Gradually introduce foods such as brown rice (kids love it lightly fried), bulgur, or quinoa salads into their lunchbox.

- ✔ Include fresh carrot sticks or crispy celery spread with almond butter.

- ✔ Use homemade sourdough or whole-grain bread instead of store-bought varieties.

- ✔ If your kids love peanut butter–and–jelly sandwiches, choose almond butter and a good-quality, sugar-free jelly.

- ✔ Instead of potato chips, serve baked organic corn chips.

- ✔ Give them fresh fruit, a small fruit salad, or sugar-free cookies as a snack.

- ✔ Make lunch fun! Prepare foods your kids will enjoy and find delicious.

- ✔ Involve your kids in the process. Let them have a say in what they'd like for lunch; that way they're more likely to eat it.

- ✔ Don't force anything. Remember, happy kids make happy parents!

Finding Fun and Healthy Ways to Cook and Eat Vegetables

You can cook vegetables in lots of fun ways that can appeal to all tastes. No matter what method you choose, avoid overcooking your veggies — they should be slightly crunchy and still retain their full color. Table 13-2 offers some cooking options for various vegetable types.

Table 13-2	Options for Cooking Vegetables
Vegetable Type	**Cooking Styles**
Asparagus, beets, bell peppers, carrots, cauliflower, celery, corn, leeks, lettuce, mushrooms, onions, plantains, pumpkin, squash, zucchini	Boiled, blanched, broiled/grilled, curried, glazed, juiced, marinated/pickled, pressed, pressure cooked, raw, steamed, stir-fried, sautéed
Daikon, parsnips, rutabagas, turnips	Boiled, broiled/roasted, steamed, stir-fried
Bok choy, broccoli, Brussels sprouts, cabbage, chard, collard greens, kale, mustard greens, spinach, watercress	Curried, juiced, sautéed, steamed, stir-fried

Your diet always has room for more vegetables. Breakfast, lunch, dinner, and snacks should ideally contain vegetables, when possible. Aim for 3 to 5 cups (cooked measurement) each day for optimum health. Packed full of fiber, vitamins, and minerals, vegetables can be eaten in abundance, especially leafy greens. The nutrients you receive from vegetables are far superior and easier for the body to absorb than those from the animal kingdom.

Variety is key to any meal plan, and most veggies mix and match pretty well. Buying and eating seasonal vegetables ensures that your vegetables are ripe and at their peak. Whenever possible, choose organic or locally farmed produce, but supplement where you need to with conventionally grown vegetables to ensure you always have variety in your diet.

There are a couple of caveats, though. An overindulgence of *nightshades* (potatoes, tomatoes, eggplant, and peppers) may aggravate some arthritic conditions. Greens, such as chard, contain ample amounts of oxalic acid, which can hinder the body's ability to absorb minerals such as calcium. A simple solution is to eat these delicious greens with other vegetables to neutralize their effect.

Creating Meals that Sing with Variety

You can eat the same thing for just so long. Sooner or later, you're bound to freak out and crave the kitchen sink. This tendency toward extremism happens more often than you think. You behave in such uninspiring, seemingly unchanging, and mechanical ways for several reasons: you're bored; you don't know how to prepare foods differently; you have negative associations with the kitchen; you don't value the possibilities of what you can create or how you can benefit.

Make a commitment to try one new recipe each week. That's all, just one little ole recipe. In three months, you'll have 12 different recipes in your mental recipe bank. Then the fun begins. After you have some mix-'n'-match knowledge, improvising becomes much easier because your confidence level is higher and you have some background to lean on.

Eventually, you begin to develop more positive associations with food preparation. You figure out some shortcuts, so you can have something cooking while you're doing other things. Your sense of planning develops.

That's the real work: planning. Being organized enough to plan makes everything easier. And when you feel healthier, have more energy, look better, sleep deeper, have bowel regularity, and feel more present in your own body, the act of taking nourishment becomes more sacred and powerful. Not with every meal. Sometimes the last place I want to be is the kitchen. But when I remember that I can prep things quickly and duplicate favorite dishes and create new ones, I become more creative and inspired in the kitchen. Of course, I'm not crazy about washing dishes . . . but that's another story.

Variety makes your meals more diversified and more nourishing. You can add variety through cooking styles, tastes, textures, combinations, colors, and fragrances. We miss out on a whole realm of senses because we're too busy trying to cut corners and boil water in the microwave. Be present in your kitchen. It's where you sustain and enhance life.

Using different cooking methods to prevent boredom

You have a unique assortment of cooking methods available to you, courtesy of many cultures with varied culinary styles. There is little excuse for claiming cooking boredom. All you need is a simple stove, a little energy, a dash of imagination — and you're on your way. Each method creates a precise flavor and texture. You can find recipes using many of these methods in Chapters 14, 15, and 16.

Here are some simple and tasteful ways to cook your food:

Steaming, boiling, and blanching

To steam, blanch, or boil food, you need a pot with a fitted lid and some water.

- **Steaming** uses a small amount of water and relies on the hot steam to penetrate and cook the vegetables. This method can be super quick and retains all the vegetable's nutrients. Simply place the vegetables in a stainless steel or bamboo steamer basket. Bring the water to a boil in a pot, add the steamer basket, and cover with the lid. Depending on how you slice the vegetables (thinner cuts cook faster), steaming usually requires a short cooking time. Steaming is also a handy way to reheat leftovers.

✔ **Boiling** requires more water and a longer cooking time than steaming does. Some nutrients are lost in the water; however, the liquid can be used for gravy, sauces, or stock.

✔ **Blanching** is a quicker version of boiling, where thinly sliced vegetables are quickly cooked in boiling water. This helps retain their crispness and color and, for some, makes them easier to digest than raw vegetables.

Pressure cooking

Pressure cooking slowly cooks food in a small amount of water under high pressure. This method is a good way to cook grains, beans, and grain or rice soups. The high pressure helps soften the outer coating of the grain, making it sweeter and easier to digest.

To use a pressure cooker, add your ingredients with the correct amount of water or stock, and then clamp or twist the lid into place and bring the contents to a boil. You know the liquid is boiling when you hear the unmistakable sound of jutting steam or a vibrating top-piece. That sound signals that the contents are under pressure, so you need to turn the heat down low to simmer for the remainder of the cooking time. Cook the contents for the required time and soon you'll have hearty-cooked grains, beans, or soup.

Stir-frying, sautéing, and water-frying

Stir-frying and sautéing rely on the use of oil or a small amount of water. Both methods use high heat to quickly cook vegetables. *Water-frying* (stir-frying or sautéing with water instead of oil) is an excellent way to cook leafy green vegetables.

The type of oil used to sauté or stir-fry food can enhance the food's flavor, and because the oil cooks quickly, it retains its chemical nature.

If your oil is smoking while you're cooking, you've altered its chemistry, and it's toxic to consume. Toss it.

To sauté or stir-fry with oil, first heat the pan. Then add a small amount of oil — generally less than a tablespoon. After the oil is heated, add your vegetables and move them around the pan (I use wooden implements like a rice paddle or cooking chopsticks). As you stir the vegetables, they'll get covered with a thin coat of oil, which seals in their flavor. Add a pinch of salt to bring out more moisture from the vegetables, thus avoiding burning, and cover. Return every so often to stir the veggies and test when they're ready.

To minimize the amount of oil I use, I often use a cook's brush. I dip it into a small amount of oil and brush the pan with a thin layer. (Do this quickly; otherwise you'll melt the brush!) This allows you to use the minimum of what you need.

For water-frying you use water instead of oil to sauté your ingredients. Add ¹/₃ to ¹/₂ cup of water to the pan (don't drown the veggies) and cook them, stirring frequently.

In the Chinese version of water-frying, you add a small amount of oil toward the end of the cooking process and allow the ingredients to cook for several minutes longer. The oil makes the meal feel bulkier and more satisfying and helps some nutrients absorb more efficiently; the water-frying technique keeps you from cooking the oil and adding free radicals.

Roasting or baking

The slower methods of roasting and baking use the oven. Roasting is great for vegetables such as squash, sweet potatoes, parsnips, asparagus, and potatoes. It brings out their natural sweet flavors. Baking is the preferred cooking method for cakes, breads, pastries, and cookies. To roast or bake foods, just follow the times and temperatures given in the recipe you're using.

Here's a sample baked onion recipe that can't be any easier. Preheat your oven to 350 degrees Fahrenheit and then simply place three or four onions, still in their brown wrapper skins, on a cookie sheet and place in the heated oven. Allow to bake for two hours! You don't have to stand there and watch them. When the time is up, remove from the oven, allow to cool for a few minutes, pull the skins off, quarter, and serve.

Making soup

Soup is one of the easiest and most delicious ways to prepare foods. A good bean soup is hearty in the winter, while a cold gazpacho soup can be refreshing in summer.

You can put anything in a soup. After you've made your stock (or you can just use water), play around with all kinds of combinations of rice, beans, noodles, barley, lentils, vegetables, herbs, and condiments. You'll usually end up with a delicious soup. A spoonful of miso added at the end of cooking increases the nutrients and enzymes and helps with digestion. You can also add leftovers with a bit of diluted miso to make a quick one-pot meal.

Broiling and grilling

Broiling and grilling are great for vegetables and give them a unique savory flavor, especially when you cook on a grill. For broiling, set your oven to broil, and as soon as heat is maximized between the upper and lower grill, place your food on the rack. Grill over an open grill, such as an outdoor grill or the stove grill that sometimes comes on large six-burner stoves.

You can grill or broil vegetables with a light coating of oil, with fresh herbs, or with a simple marinade for delicious taste sensations.

Pickling

One of my favorite condiments is fermented vegetables. Not only does the tart pickled flavor add punch to a meal; the fermentation aids digestion. Over centuries, most cultures have served fermented vegetables with meals from Japan (pickled ginger) and Korea (kimchi) to Germany (sauerkraut) and America (the good old pickle).

You can make fermented vegetables by using a combination of sea salt and herbs or marinade and hearty vegetables such as cabbage, carrots, onions, and cucumber. The concoction is either left to marinate in an airtight jar or pressed using a special pickle press. During the pickling process, the vegetables not only absorb the marinade but they become easier to digest. Because the pickling instructions can be overwhelming, here are some easy ways to get fermentation without having to pickle:

- Put miso in your soups and sauces.
- Look for places to add sauerkraut to your recipes. It's great as a wrap ingredient.
- Add umeboshi to various dishes

"Raw" cooking

Raw food is not exactly raw, but the word generally is used for foods cooked to a temperature lower than 106 degrees. This low temperature allows them to retain their natural enzymes, which assist in the digestion and absorption of the vegetables. Raw foods can be prepared in many different styles, such as raw whole vegetables, vegetable broth or shakes, salads, vegetable wraps, and so on. Many nutrition bars available in natural food stores are made from raw ingredients.

Additional preparations

Here are several categories of recipes you can consider to add variety to your macrobiotic repertoire:

- **Curries and chili:** If you like your food with a little spice, this recipe is perfect for you. Curries and chili can be made in many varieties. Beans, grains, and vegetables are staples for these dishes.
- **Glazes and sauces:** Glazes are a simple way to add extra flavor to your dishes — simply mix some chunks of white kuzu starch powder with water, add it to your dish, and you'll have a delicious thick glaze. Glazes

can be flavored with tamari or other condiments and herbs. Sauces come in many varieties, from tomato-based to creamier. Many sauces can be made from diluted seed and nut butters that thicken and add their own flavor to the sauce.

✔ **Juicing:** Juicing allows you to enjoy your fruit and vegetables in a fun, cool, and refreshing way — especially when the weather is hot. With a good blender and, if you like, a few ice cubes, you can experiment with different combinations of fruits and vegetables to create delicious and healthy shakes.

Juicing increases the sugar content because you're combining many fruits, minus the fiber. So fruit juices are, ideally, a refreshing treat food.

✔ *Nishime:* This Japanese style of cooking is great for cooking large root vegetables. Nishime cooking uses a little bit of water and the naturally occurring juices of the vegetables to create soft, juicy, sweet vegetables. Nishime cooking is generally done over low heat until the vegetables are tender.

✔ **Nori sushi and summer rolls:** These are my favorites for a fast lunch or snack.

Using sticky rice and nori, you can roll any ingredients into your sushi mat, so have fun not only making them but in choosing the ingredients you use too. My favorite is avocado, cilantro, carrots, tahini, and finely chopped almonds. Summer rolls are also light and refreshing, using Vietnamese rice paper rolls and a plethora of fresh ingredients and herbs.

✔ **Pasta and noodles:** Who doesn't love twisting spaghetti around their fork or slurping soba noodles? In Japan, slurping is practically a custom; it pays a compliment to the cook. Not only do pasta and noodles come in many different varieties and flavors, but you can also create an amazing array of dishes with them. From soups to stir-fried noodles, from hot and cold pasta dishes to mock lasagna, you'll never run out of ideas with these stringy guys.

✔ **Patties, burgers, and croquettes:** Not sure what to have for lunch today? Whip up a quick croquette or veggie burger. These are simple to make using combinations of grain (millet works well), finely chopped vegetables, and seasoning. They can be baked, lightly fried, or grilled and served with other grains, vegetables, salads, or soups.

✔ **Salads:** In this category, you've got your raw salads — those made up of fresh vegetables such as lettuce, tomatoes, onions, carrots, and many other veggies — and served cold. And you've got your *boiled salads,* which are generally served cold and are made from par-boiled vegetables so they retain their color and still pack a crunch.

You can create many varieties of boiled salads. Grains such as bulgur wheat and couscous make delicious combination salads when prepared with vegetables and nuts. Small cubes of tofu add protein to any salad.

Salads can be dressed with oil-based or creamy dressings made from diluted tahini or served with a squeeze of fresh lemon juice or balsamic or rice vinegar.

✓ **Sandwiches and wraps:** Sandwiches can be served cold or toasted or grilled on many types of bread with an endless variety of ingredients. You can place whatever you find appealing between two slices of bread — or make an open sandwich with just one slice. It doesn't take much to create a delicious and satisfying meal.

✓ **Stews:** Stewing is a slow method of cooking that allows the flavors of the ingredients to culminate in the stock to create a delicious gravy. Who doesn't love a hearty stew? It's so warming in cool temperatures, and, like soups, stews can be made from seasonal vegetables in many combinations. I prefer to use what I have in the fridge that day and play around with seasonings, so my stews always have interesting flavors.

Cooking with the five tastes

When considering variety in your meal planning, it's good to think about how you can incorporate the five tastes:

✓ **Bitter:** Foods featuring this taste include collard greens, kale, mustard greens, arugula, endives, radicchio, burdock root, dandelion leaves, sesame seeds, cereal grain, coffee substitutes, and parsley leaves.

✓ **Salty:** You find this taste mostly in condiments but occasionally in other foods, including sea salt, tamari, soy sauce, miso, umeboshi plums, pickles, sea vegetables, and sesame salt.

✓ **Sweet:** The secret here is to find foods that are naturally sweet. Some possibilities include whole grains, carrots, squash, pumpkin, parsnips, sweet potatoes, yams, fruits, corn, and cooked cabbage.

✓ **Sour:** Foods with this taste include pickles, umeboshi salt plums, lemons, limes, sauerkraut, fermented vegetables, sourdough bread, and vinegar.

✓ **Pungent:** Foods in this category have a strong flavor. Consider: garlic, ginger, raw onions, turnips, peppers, wasabi, scallions, daikon radish, horse radish, spices, and chili peppers.

When possible, every meal should have some degree of the five tastes, although they don't have to be in equal quantities. This not only stimulates all of your taste buds, but it also helps curb cravings by making the meal more satisfying. An example of a five-taste balanced meal would be brown rice (sweet) stir-fried with kale (bitter), sea vegetables (salty), carrots, onions, and cabbage (all sweet), ginger (pungent), and served with several slices of a pickle (sour). Including sour or pungent flavors when frying with oil also helps your body break down fat and digest the oil much easier.

Playing with textures

Texture plays a huge and often little-acknowledged role in the creation of a balanced meal. The following are the textures we typically associate with food: crunchy, chewy, creamy, soft, moist, and dry.

A combination of textures makes meals more satisfying and stimulating. A bowl of creamy oatmeal is complemented with a piece of crunchy toast or the addition of chopped nuts. Crunchy rice cakes are a great addition to soft foods, such as rice or other grains, and some chewy foods, such as wheat meat (tempeh), are delicious when served with a soft grain like millet or a creamy side dish such as soup. You can combine textures in one dish (for instance, take a soft dish like rice and cook it with chopped nuts for added crunch), or when making dishes with multiple ingredients, such as noodles and vegetables, use lots of different textured vegetables in contrast to the soft noodles.

Here are some examples of texture combinations:

- Chinese restaurants often give you some dry, crunchy noodles to eat with your gooey chop suey.
- A traditional dish of the American South is cornbread and bean soup.
- Salads are often complemented with crunchy croutons.
- Pasta is often served with hard sourdough bread that allows you to soak up remaining sauce.
- The traditional *knish* (cooked and pureed potatoes) or soft-cooked *kasha* (toasted buckwheat) is wrapped within a crusty covering.

Becoming texture-savvy makes meals more satisfying and can reduce your cravings. Sometimes when you're hanging on the refrigerator door and wondering what you want to eat, you may be looking for just the right texture.

Part IV

Morning to Evening Recipes: Your Dietary Path to Wellness

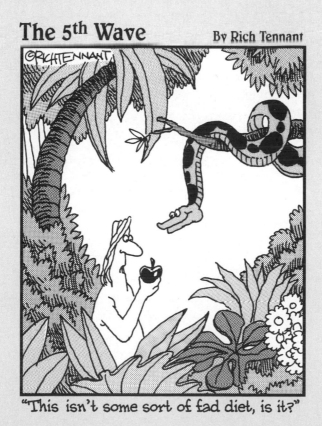

The 5th Wave   By Rich Tennant

"This isn't some sort of fad diet, is it?"

In this part . . .

Of course, you have to eat, and having a guide to creating delicious meals makes it less of an effort and more exciting as an adventure. This section offers delicious and easy-to-follow recipes that will have you leaping around your kitchen like the galloping gourmet you really are — or want to be. It's just a matter of practice! Some helpful advice for handling social situations and making healthy restaurant choices makes this adventure one that you can share and not feel restricted from socializing.

Chapter 14

Best Breakfasts and Lip-Smacking Lunches

In This Chapter

▶ Redefining the breakfast meal

▶ Whipping up breakfast foods

▶ Taking another look at lunch

▶ Preparing soups, salads, and sushi for lunch

Breakfast poses a problem for most people. They're typically short on time and low on inspiration when choosing foods that offer maximized energy, taste, and efficiency.

This chapter addresses the need for creating substantial breakfasts as a way to ensure you maintain your energy throughout the day. When you understand the importance of this foundational meal, you'll be inspired to find the time and creativity to make breakfast. I present several recipes you can use to experiment with and discover new tastes. I hope these dishes provide you with a vital sense of renewal.

In the second part of this chapter, I outline some interesting recipes for lunch that can keep your body powered throughout your busy afternoons.

Jump-Starting Your Day with Breakfast

Hands down, breakfast is the most important meal of the day. Not only do we hear this opinion echoed by nutritionists and researchers; artifacts indicate that traditional cultures regarded breakfast with great reverence, embodying the old European adage that you should eat like royalty for breakfast, a commoner for lunch, and a pauper for dinner.

The English term *breakfast* comes from a Middle English word that means "breaking the fast." It's the meal that ends or breaks the overnight fast that occurs while we sleep. Whenever I meet people who say, "I'm not the breakfast type," that usually indicates to me that they tend to eat late at night or overeat with the last meal of the day. As a result of digesting late into the night, they rarely awaken with an appetite. Often, someone who does this will grab what I call a *stimulant breakfast* of coffee and a muffin and head out the door. This practice creates an even greater need for stimulants and increases later appetites. On the other hand, a good macrobiotic breakfast helps you perform far better mentally and stay far more alert because you're not contending with low blood sugar or hunger pangs.

Eating Well to Start Your Day

As the pace of life today seems more instant, our choices have become increasingly irresponsible. The invigorating traditional morning meal has fallen by the wayside in favor of the morning "energy bar" — a foil-wrapped package containing refined sugar, bits of fruit, and odd chemicals that we swallow in two gulps in the car on the way to work, wash it down with highly caffeinated coffee, and then consider breakfast a done deal.

John Kellogg probably had something to do with this. In 1898, he introduced the first ready-made cereal he called granola. In 1902, John and his brother Will developed corn flakes — and the rest is ready-made cereal history. Breakfast foods have become a convenience of nutritional absurdity that manufacturers unceasingly promote with their "whole-grain goodness" messages, and unassuming consumers fall for these misleading claims.

In replacing nourishing, traditional complex carbohydrates with refined foods, juices, and simple-sugar pastries, we have, in essence, exchanged diamonds for pebbles.

The morning meal recipes I offer here include a variety of choices based on restoring complex carbohydrates as a central component of breakfast. Put some morning goodness in your bowl and chew to your heart's content! Bon appétit! Salud! Itadakimasu! L'chaim! To your health!

Winter Warming Oatmeal with Roasted Almonds, Raisins, and Cinnamon

Oatmeal, a staple grain for cultures around the world, provides a warm, satisfying breakfast that gives you the endurance you need until lunchtime. Raisins add a slight sweetness, while almonds provide some protein and oil content and extra texture. These mix-ins are best added two-thirds of the way into the cooking, allowing them to flavor the oatmeal. The key is to add a small amount of raisins to the oatmeal, as opposed to adding a little bit of oatmeal to a large amount of raisins! ***Note:*** For a one-person serving, use a total of $1/4$ cup of grain with $1/2$ cup of water (ratio 1:2).

Preparation time: *5 minutes*

Cooking time: *20 to 25 minutes*

Yield: *3 to 4 servings*

4 cups of water	*Handful of chopped roasted almonds*
1$1/2$ cups rolled oats	*2 tablespoons organic raisins*
$1/8$ to $1/4$ teaspoon sea salt	*Pinch of cinnamon to taste*

1 Add the water to a medium saucepan with the sea salt, cover, and bring to a rolling boil.

2 Gently stir in the oats as you lower the heat to a simmer. Cover the pot about four-fifths to allow the steam to escape. Cook the oats for 10 to 15 minutes.

3 Check occasionally to make sure the water hasn't evaporated. If the oats look dry, gently stir in $1/3$ to $1/2$ cup of water. You may have to repeat this step if the heat is too high or if you want a creamier texture.

4 Add the almonds and raisins.

5 Cook for another 10 minutes. Stir in the cinnamon and serve.

Tip: *To get a creamy consistency, cook the oats longer while continuously adding small amounts of water until you reach the desired consistency.*

Tip: *Almonds are usually available already toasted at natural food stores. For a nuttier flavor you can chop and dry roast the nuts in a skillet over medium-low heat for approximately 15 minutes, or until they turn slightly brown, and then add them to the oatmeal.*

Vary It!: *Mixing in ingredients like roasted seeds or nuts, a pinch of salt, or whatever else suits your fancy adds variety to this standard breakfast.*

Per serving: Calories 481 (From Fat 247); Fat 27g (Saturated 2g); Cholesterol 0mg; Sodium 113mg; Carbohydrate 47g; Dietary Fiber 10g; Protein 18g.

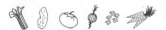

Southern-Style Corn Grits with Roasted Walnuts and Maple Syrup

Start your day with a delicious bowl of Southern-style corn grits topped with roasted walnuts for crunch and sweetened with a hint of maple syrup. It's quick and satisfying!

Preparation time: *8 minutes*

Cooking time: *9 minutes*

Yield: *4 servings*

1 cup corn grits

3 cups water, divided

¼ teaspoon sea salt

1 cup chopped walnuts

Maple syrup to taste

1 Whisk together the corn grits with 1½ cups of water in a small bowl and let it stand for 3 minutes.

2 Bring the remaining 1½ cups of water to a boil in a medium saucepan.

3 Pour the grits into the boiling water. Add the salt.

4 Reduce the heat to low, and stir the grits vigorously until they become thick and creamy.

5 Dry roast the walnuts in a skillet over medium-low heat for 3 to 4 minutes.

6 Stir the walnuts into the grits. Divide into 4 bowls and drizzle with maple syrup before serving.

Per serving: *Calories 367 (From Fat 181); Fat 20g (Saturated 2g); Cholesterol 0mg; Sodium 147mg; Carbohydrate 42g; Dietary Fiber 3g; Protein 8g.*

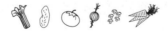

Spiced Mexican Tofu Scramble with Tortilla Chips

Send your taste buds on an adventure with a taste of Mexico! This delicious tofu scramble is the perfect healthy substitute for traditional scrambled eggs. You can add a finely chopped avocado at the end of the cooking for even more flavor.

Preparation time: *5 minutes*

Cooking time: *10 minutes*

Yield: *Approximately 4 servings*

1 tablespoon of sesame oil	*¼ teaspoon sea salt*
1 red onion, finely chopped	*¼ teaspoon Cayenne pepper*
1 cup sliced mushrooms	*1 pound tofu*
1 cup finely sliced red pepper	*¼ cup chopped fresh cilantro*
1 celery stalk, chopped into small pieces	*1 small package organic tortilla chips*
1 cup cooked yellow corn kernels (about 2 ears of corn)	

1 In a large skillet, heat the oil over medium heat and sauté the onion, mushrooms, and red pepper until they're slightly soft (about 3 to 4 minutes). Drain off any excess liquid.

2 Add the celery, corn, salt, and pepper, and sauté for another minute.

3 Crumble the tofu and stir it into the vegetables.

4 Cover the skillet and steam the tofu for 3 to 4 minutes, stirring once or twice.

5 Add the cilantro and serve with the tortilla chips.

Per serving: Calories 220 (From Fat 86); Fat 10g (Saturated 1g); Cholesterol 0mg; Sodium 205mg; Carbohydrate 25g; Dietary Fiber 4g; Protein 13g.

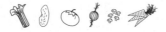

Banana Pecan Buckwheat Pancakes

Perfect for a lazy weekend breakfast or brunch with friends, pancakes are everyone's favorites. Pair the sweet pancakes with the tempeh bacon and you've got a mouth-watering delight. (You can find the recipe for tempeh bacon elsewhere in this chapter.)

Preparation time: *30 minutes*

Cooking time: *20 minutes*

Yield: *Approximately 10 to 12 pancakes*

¾ cup of sparkling or still water

1 cup soy or rice milk

½ teaspoon sea salt

4 tablespoons cold-pressed walnut or sesame oil, divided

1¾ cups whole wheat pastry flour

¼ cup buckwheat flour

1 tablespoon baking powder

½ cup chopped pecans

3 medium bananas, sliced

Maple syrup to taste

1 Mix the water, milk, salt, and 3 tablespoons of the oil together in a medium mixing bowl.

2 Sift the flours and baking powder together in a large mixing bowl.

3 Pour the wet ingredients into the dry ingredients and mix lightly with a whisk to a thick creamy consistency. Add a little more water if the batter is too thick.

4 Chill the batter for 20 minutes until it's cold.

5 Dry roast the pecans in a skillet over medium heat for 5 to 7 minutes.

6 Pour a small amount of oil into a heavy skillet that's been heated over a high heat.

7 Spoon ¼ cup of the batter into the skillet, add a few pieces of banana and some pecans, and cook until bubbles form on the top of the pancake.

8 Flip the pancake and cook until it's lightly brown on both sides. Remove the pancake from the skillet, and repeat Steps 7 and 8 until you've used all the batter.

9 Drizzle the pancakes with maple syrup before serving.

Per serving: *Calories 163 (From Fat 59); Fat 7g (Saturated 1g); Cholesterol 0mg; Sodium 234mg; Carbohydrate 25g; Dietary Fiber 4g; Protein 4g.*

Tempeh Bacon

Tempeh is a high-protein food made of soybeans and used as a meat substitute. If you're missing that familiar taste of bacon, try this as a delicious and healthy alternative — far fewer calories, fat, and cholesterol, and it's especially pig-friendly!

Preparation time: *15 minutes*

Cooking time: *30 to 40 minutes*

Yield: *4 servings*

½ cup water	2 bay leaves
2 tablespoons sweet miso paste	¼ teaspoon white pepper
3 garlic cloves, thinly sliced	½ pound tempeh cut into 8 to 10 thin strips
1 tablespoon mustard	Sesame, walnut, or canola oil

1 Boil the water in a medium saucepan and stir in the miso until it is diluted. Add the garlic, mustard, bay leaves, and pepper.

2 Add the tempeh strips, cover the pan, and simmer for 20 minutes.

3 Preheat the broiler.

4 Remove the tempeh strips and place them on a lightly oiled baking sheet.

5 Broil the strips for 5 to 8 minutes until they're crisp and golden brown on one side.

6 Turn the strips over and cook for another 5 minutes before serving.

Per serving: *Calories 137 (From Fat 63); Fat 7g (Saturated 2g); Cholesterol 0mg; Sodium 338mg; Carbohydrate 10g; Dietary Fiber 0g; Protein 11g.*

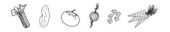

Hearty Miso Rice Porridge

Rice porridge is an excellent way to use last night's leftover rice to make a delicious breakfast. And it's so simple that you leave it to simmer on the stove while you take a shower and prepare for your day! It's a great dish that leaves you satisfied and energized. Add a slice or two of whole wheat toast with tamari-tahini topping (you can find the recipe elsewhere in this chapter), and you're good to go until lunch!

Preparation time: *10 minutes*

Cooking time: *35 minutes*

Yield: *4 servings*

2½ cups of brown rice	1 small piece of kombu
1 tablespoon sesame oil	5 cups water
1 leek, thinly sliced	1 tablespoon barley or light-colored miso
1 cup tofu cut into small cubes (optional)	1 teaspoon tamari or shoyu
1 cup dried shiitake mushrooms	Fresh parsley for garnish (optional)

1 Cook the rice as directed on the package or use leftover rice.

2 Add the oil to a small skillet and gently stir-fry the leeks over medium heat until tender. Add the tofu (if desired) and cook for 3 to 5 minutes

3 Cook the mushrooms, kombu, and water in a large saucepan and cook over medium heat until the mushrooms are soft, approximately 5 to 8 minutes. This creates a mushroom broth for the porridge.

4 Remove the kombu pieces and pour the mushrooms and broth over the rice. Bring the broth to a boil.

5 Stir the miso and tamari and most of the leek into the rice and simmer over low heat for about 30 minutes.

6 Spoon the rice into serving dishes and garnish with a small amount of cooked leek, parsley, or mushrooms.

Per serving: *Calories 699 (From Fat 99); Fat 11g (Saturated 2g); Cholesterol 0mg; Sodium 1,002mg; Carbohydrate 125g; Dietary Fiber 14g; Protein 27g.*

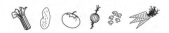

Whole Wheat Toast with Tamari-Tahini Topping

This crunchy toast is delicious on its own or paired with miso porridge (see the recipe elsewhere in this chapter). The toast provides a satisfying texture and savory flavor that complements the miso porridge nicely. Try toasting some of the non-yeast breads, which are a little chewier but definitely more substantial. You can also try the Asian method of briefly steaming bread. Sounds strange, no doubt, but it's very delicious.

Preparation time: *5 minutes*

Cooking time: *2 to 3 minutes*

Yield: *1 to 2 slices per person*

1 tablespoon tahini	*1 to 2 slices whole-wheat bread, toasted or steamed*
1 teaspoon tamari	

1 Mix the tahini with the tamari until it is blended well and creates a thick paste. If the mixture is too dry, add a teaspoon or two of water until you get a thick spreading consistency.

2 Spread the paste evenly over toasted (or steamed) bread and serve.

Vary It!: *To steam bread, bring ¹/₂ inch of water to a boil. Layer slices of bread into a steamer basket and place into boiling water. Cover with lid and steam for about 30 seconds. Remove bread from steamer and enjoy!*

Per serving: *Calories 161 (From Fat 82); Fat 9g (Saturated 1g); Cholesterol 0mg; Sodium 460mg; Carbohydrate 16g; Dietary Fiber 3g; Protein 6g.*

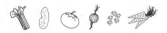

Mouth-Watering Breakfast Muffins

These yummy breakfast muffins are perfect for those mornings when you're on the go. You can also serve these muffins for afternoon tea with some almond crème (almond butter diluted with a bit of water) for the perfect topping!

Preparation time: *15 minutes*

Cooking time: *30 minutes*

Yield: *12 servings*

2½ cups unbleached flour

½ cup whole wheat flour

½ teaspoon sea salt

2 tablespoons baking powder

½ teaspoon cinnamon

½ to 1 cup dried fruit and/or nuts

1½ cup soy milk

½ cup maple or rice syrup

½ cup corn or cold-pressed canola oil

1 apple, peeled and cut into small pieces

1 Preheat the oven to 350 degrees Fahrenheit. Line a muffin pan with paper liners or lightly grease the pan.

2 Combine the flours, salt, baking powder, cinnamon, and fruit or nuts in a large mixing bowl.

3 Stir together the milk, syrup, oil, and apple in a medium mixing bowl.

4 Slowly add the wet mixture to the dry ingredients, stirring gently using a wooden spoon until thoroughly mixed.

5 Spoon the mixture into the prepared muffin pan.

6 Bake for 30 minutes at 350 degrees Fahrenheit until the muffins are lightly browned on top. Do not open the oven door during the first 20 minutes of baking or the muffins may sink in the middle.

7 Remove the muffins from the oven and let them cool on a wire rack, or serve while they're still slightly warm.

Vary It!: *You can substitute blueberries for the apple, adding them to the wet mixture after it's been blended.*

Per serving: Calories 257 (From Fat 91); Fat 10g (Saturated 1g); Cholesterol 0mg; Sodium 293mg; Carbohydrate 38g; Dietary Fiber 3g; Protein 4g.

No-Time-to-Eat Nondairy Green Smoothie

Green smoothies are an excellent way to pack in lots of essential nutrients, vitamins, and minerals at breakfast time. Think of your smoothie as a cool summer soup. You can whip it up with different combinations of vegetables, although leafy greens such as spinach, kale, chard, cabbage, and lettuce make the best smoothies. Here are a few of my favorite combinations, guaranteed to kick-start your day!

Preparation time: *10 minutes*

Cooking time: *None*

Yield: *1 serving*

1 cup water plus any of the following combinations:

2 cups cut raw broccoli

½ cup cut raw green cabbage

1 stick of celery, chopped

1 apple, peeled and cut into pieces

Or

4 apples, peeled and cut into pieces

Juice from ½ lemon

4 to 5 leaves of kale, roughly chopped

Or

2 ripe pears, cored and cut into pieces

4 to 5 leaves of kale, roughly chopped

2 tablespoon freshly chopped mint

Or

8 leaves of romaine lettuce, chopped

2 to 3 sticks of celery, chopped

2 small to medium carrots, chopped

Or

1 large apple, peeled and cut into pieces

Half cucumber, chopped

2 sticks of celery, chopped

½ fennel, chopped

Handful of spinach roughly chopped

Handful of parsley

Juice of half a grapefruit (optional)

1 Make sure all the vegetables are thoroughly washed, dried, and peeled if necessary.

2 Chop into small chunks that can be easily blended.

3 Place all the ingredients in a blender and add just enough water to create a smoothie-like consistency.

4 Blend, serve, and enjoy!

Vary It!: *You can also add a tablespoon of green food powder that contains chlorella, blue green algae, or spirulina for extra punch.*

Per serving: *Calories 132 (From Fat 9); Fat 1g (Saturated 0g); Cholesterol 0mg; Sodium 95mg; Carbohydrate 31g; Dietary Fiber 8g; Protein 5g.*

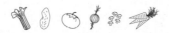

Boston Baked Beans with Sourdough Toast

Navy beans make the perfect baked beans. This delicious recipe works great with some crunchy toast. You can also try this hearty bean dish with tempeh bacon (see the recipe elsewhere in this chapter), fried bread, and a few mushrooms for a memorable breakfast.

Preparation time: *15 minutes*

Cooking time: *40 minutes*

Yield: *4 servings*

1 onion, cut into large slices	1/2 teaspoon sea salt
1 sweet potato, peeled and diced	1 tablespoon shoyu (natural soy sauce)
1 carrot, washed and diced	1 tablespoon tomato paste
One 15-ounce can navy beans	1 1/2 tablespoons balsamic vinegar

1 Preheat the oven to 450 degrees Fahrenheit.

2 Layer the onion, sweet potato, carrot, and navy beans in a large saucepan. Add enough water to just cover the beans.

3 Cover the pan and bring the contents to a boil over high heat. Reduce the heat to low and simmer for about 15 minutes.

4 Add the salt, shoyu, and tomato paste, and cook over medium heat for 2 to 3 minutes.

5 Add the balsamic vinegar and mix gently.

6 Place the beans and vegetables in a 2-quart baking dish and bake at 450 degrees Fahrenheit for 15 minutes.

7 Remove the dish from the oven and serve with thick slices of toasted sourdough or whole wheat bread.

Per serving: Calories 142 (From Fat 4); Fat 0g (Saturated 0g); Cholesterol 0mg; Sodium 856mg; Carbohydrate 28g; Dietary Fiber 6g; Protein 7g. Does not include bread.

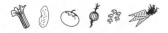

Fast Morning Muesli with Soy or Rice Milk

If you can't give up your familiar breakfast cereal, you'll love this delicious and simple way to make muesli. Your leftover muesli can be refrigerated in an airtight container for up to two days.

Preparation time: 20 minutes (overnight optional)

Cooking time: None

Yield: 4 servings

1 cup rolled oats	1 cup chopped almonds
¼ cup dates or raisins	½ cup chopped walnuts
3 cups soy or rice milk	½ cup sunflower seeds
1 teaspoon vanilla extract (optional)	

1 Place the oats and dates or raisins in a large mixing bowl.

2 Cover the oats with milk. Stir in the vanilla extract, if desired.

3 Leave the oats to soak for 15 to 20 minutes or overnight.

4 When ready to serve, stir in the almonds, walnuts, and sunflower seeds.

Vary It!: Soak the oats overnight in apple cider instead of milk.

Per serving: *Calories 417 (From Fat 238); Fat 27g (Saturated 3g); Cholesterol 0mg; Sodium 24mg; Carbohydrate 34g; Dietary Fiber 10g; Protein 17g.*

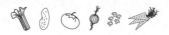

Keeping Your Fire Fueled With Lunch

The abbreviation *lunch*, in use from 1823, is taken from the more formal German word, *lunchentach*. Some reports show this word in use from 1580, as a word for a meal that was inserted between "more substantial meals."

But to me, as a grade school student suffering through the tedium of a morning history class, dreadful mathematical equations messing with my brain, Eddie Wisbeck's spitballs ricocheting off the back of my head, and that biology quiz Mrs. Sobel surprised us with, it was all made tolerable by knowing that as the noon hour approached, my favorite period of the day would finally arrive: *lunch!* — educational reprieve. I'd watch the classroom clock as if trying to move its hands with sheer mental power.

Opening the brown lunch bag prepared by my mother was a ritual of surprise and response: tuna sandwich, chips, an apple, and a thermos of juice, which made me happy, or an egg salad sandwich with celery sticks and milk, which made me nauseated. Still, it was lunch and the occasion most school kids eagerly awaited the entire morning.

Lunch is the energetic anchor between early day and early evening. If you have an ample breakfast and hearty lunch, you won't find yourself feeling deprived with a light dinner. As a result, you'll sleep more deeply, require less sleep, and usually awaken with more energy the following morning.

What follows are a dozen recipes for lip-smacking lunches. Feast well!

Vegetable Miso Soup with Spelt Noodles

Try the likes of a hearty bowl of miso soup for lunch. Noodles add another dimension of flavor, texture, and variety to this simple and strengthening meal.

Preparation time: *10 minutes*

Cooking time: *30 minutes*

Yield: *4 servings*

4 cups water	1/4 cup well-packed seasonal green (kale, bok choy, collard greens, napa cabbage, or watercress
1 round tablespoon of ready-to-eat wakame sea vegetable	
1/4 cup onion, leek, or green onion	1/2-inch slice tofu, cubed
1/4 cup carrot or other root vegetable	One 12-ounce package of Udon noodles
1/4 cup daikon	3 tablespoons miso
	Spring onions, chopped

1 Bring the water to boil in a large saucepan and add the wakame.

2 Let the wakame simmer while you cut the vegetables, excluding the spring onions, to similar sizes and shapes.

3 Add the vegetables and the tofu to the pan.

4 Cook over medium- heat until the vegetables are cooked but still crunchy, about 10 to 15 minutes.

5 In a medium saucepan, cook the noodles according to the instructions on the package, usually 6 to 8 minutes.

6 When the noodles are cooked, drain and rinse them under cool water.

7 Spoon a little bit of soup broth into a small bowl and dilute the miso. Add the miso and some of the spring onions to the large pan during the last three minutes of simmering.

8 Divide the noodles into 4 soup bowls. Ladle the soup and vegetables over the noodles. Garnish with the rest of the spring onions.

Per serving: Calories 223 (From Fat 29); Fat 3g (Saturated 0g); Cholesterol 0mg; Sodium 860mg; Carbohydrate 39g; Dietary Fiber 1g; Protein 9g.

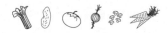

Veggie Nut Bulgur Salad

Bulgur wheat is made from cracked wheat berries, so it's quick to cook. You can use bulgur as a basis for many different salads, and it can also be served warm. Try bulgur salad with a side of kale for a super-nutritious meal.

Preparation time: *15 minutes*

Cooking time: *25 minutes*

Yield: *4 servings*

1 to 1¼ cups water	⅛ cup celery	Tamari
½ cup bulgur	¼ cup kale	¼ cup sauerkraut with a little juice
Pinch sea salt	¼ cup walnuts	1 teaspoon parsley
¼ onion	¼ cup pine nuts	
¼ carrot	1 teaspoon sesame seeds	

1 Bring the water to a boil. Place the bulgur in a medium saucepan and pour the boiling water over it. Bring the water to a boil again.

2 Add the salt, cover the pan, and reduce the heat to low. Simmer for about 15 minutes until the bulgur is soft and fluffy.

3 Remove the pan from the heat and place the bulgur in a large mixing bowl. Stir the bulgur to cool it off.

4 Dice the carrots and celery into small pieces.

5 Boil ½ inch of water in a shallow pan and cook the kale for 2 to 3 minutes until it's tender.

6 When the kale is cool, chop it finely.

7 Chop the walnuts into small pieces.

8 Toast the pine nuts in a small pan over medium-low heat for 5 to 7 minutes until they're golden brown.

9 Toast the sesame seeds in a small pan over medium-low heat for 3 to 5 minutes until they start to pop. Add a few drops of tamari after 3 minutes and stir.

10 When the bulgur is cool, add the vegetables, nuts, seeds, parsley, sauerkraut, and juice, and mix thoroughly.

Vary It!: *For a sauerkraut substitute, use dill pickle relish, lemon juice, or umeboshi vinegar.*

Per serving: *Calories 163 (From Fat 81); Fat 9g (Saturated 1g); Cholesterol 0mg; Sodium 108mg; Carbohydrate 18g; Dietary Fiber 5g; Protein 6g.*

Spring Quinoa Salad with Zesty Lemon Dressing

Quinoa is a delicious nutty grain that makes a wonderful salad. What's more, it's full of protein and can be mixed with many vegetables to create nutritious warm or chilled dishes.

Preparation time: *20 minutes*

Cooking time: *1 hour*

Yield: *4 servings*

1 cup quinoa	*1 apple, peeled and chopped*
2 cups water	*¼ cup chopped mint leaves*
Sea salt	*2 tablespoons fresh cilantro, chopped*
1 cup corn kernels	*2 tablespoons fresh mint, chopped*
½ cup chopped scallions	*2 tablespoon fresh parsley, chopped*
1 cup chopped walnuts	*½ cup pitted black or green olives*
1 cup chopped cucumber	

1 Wash the quinoa and drain.

2 Bring the water and a pinch of salt to a boil in a large saucepan.

3 Add the quinoa and bring the water back to a boil. Cover the pan and reduce the heat to low so that the contents simmer until all the liquid has been absorbed. This usually takes 25 to 30 minutes.

4 Remove the pan from the heat and allow the quinoa to cool.

5 In a small saucepan, bring about ½ inch of water to boil. Add the corn and cook for 2 to 3 minutes until it's tender. Allow the corn to cool.

6 Transfer the quinoa to a large mixing bowl and add the remaining ingredients. Stir.

7 Drizzle the lemon dressing over the salad and stir it in. Season the salad with a pinch of sea salt.

8 Allow to the salad to sit for 20 to 30 minutes to allow the flavors to develop before serving.

Zesty Lemon Dressing

¼ cup freshly squeezed lemon juice	*Zest of ¼ lemon*
¼ cup extra virgin olive oil	

Mix the lemon juice and olive oil. Stir in the lemon zest.

Per serving: *Calories 596 (From Fat 362); Fat 40g (Saturated 5g); Cholesterol 0mg; Sodium 419mg; Carbohydrate 54g; Dietary Fiber 8g; Protein 13g.*

Seitan Peanut Saté

Seitan, also known as "wheat meat," is a tasty source of protein and replaces traditional chicken in this dish. It's also low in fat and makes a quick, delicious lunch. Although it's great served with the Asian Noodle Salad with Tamari-Lime Dressing (see the recipe elsewhere in this chapter), it can also work well in a pita garnished with fresh salad greens.

Preparation time: *5 minutes*

Cooking time: *10 minutes*

Yield: *4 servings*

One 8-ounce packet seitan, drained	1 teaspoon mustard
1 teaspoon toasted sesame oil	2 cups mustard greens or bok choy
½ cup water	3 tablespoon roasted organic peanuts
2 teaspoons tamari	1 cup bean sprouts (optional)

1 Cut the seitan into ¼-inch slices.

2 Add the oil to a large skillet. Sauté the seitan slices in the oil over medium heat for about 4 minutes.

3 Dissolve the tamari and mustard in the water and pour the mixture over the seitan.

4 Add the greens and peanuts, cover, and simmer over medium heat for 5 minutes.

5 Turn off the heat and mix in the sprouts, if desired. The heat from the other ingredients will cook the sprouts.

6 Serve with noodles or in a pita.

Per serving: Calories 134 (From Fat 48); Fat 5g (Saturated 1g); Cholesterol 0mg; Sodium 360mg; Carbohydrate 7g; Dietary Fiber 1g; Protein 16g.

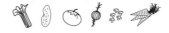

Asian Noodle Salad with Tamari-Lime Dressing

Noodles are the perfect complement to any saté dish, like the Seitan Peanut Saté (see the recipe elsewhere in this chapter). This Asian noodle salad is full of fresh crisp vegetables and lots of aromatic herbs.

Preparation time: *20 minutes*

Cooking time: *10 minutes*

Yield: *4 servings*

¼ cup carrots prepared julienne	*4 slices ginger cut into matchsticks*
1½ cups snow peas	*One 12-ounce package buckwheat noodles*
¼ of a red pepper prepared julienne	*¼ cup fresh cilantro*
3 spring onions cut into thin slices	*¼ cup fresh parsley*

1 In a shallow, medium saucepan, bring ½ inch of water to boil.

2 Cook the carrots, snow peas, and red pepper over high heat so they're crunchy yet tender (1 to 3 minutes). Remove each kind of vegetable before cooking the next.

3 Drain well and transfer to a large mixing bowl. Add the onions and ginger.

4 Prepare the noodles according to the package instructions. Rinse with cold water and drain.

5 Add the noodles, cilantro, and parsley to the vegetables. Mix the ingredients together.

6 Drizzle the dressing over the salad and toss gently so the noodles are covered.

7 Divide into 4 portions and serve.

Tamari-Lime Dressing

1 tablespoon tamari	*1 tablespoon water*
1 tablespoon fresh lime juice	

Mix the tamari, lime juice, and water to make the dressing.

Per serving: *Calories 333 (From Fat 14); Fat 2g (Saturated 0g); Cholesterol 0mg; Sodium 238mg; Carbohydrate 68g; Dietary Fiber 2g; Protein 11g.*

Indian Summer Coconut and Butternut Squash Soup

This warming soup, infused with just a hint of summer flavors, is perfect for welcoming the cooler days of fall.

Preparation time: *20 minutes*

Cooking time: *1 hour, 15 minutes*

Yield: *4 servings*

⅔ cup raw pumpkin seeds	1 cup coconut milk
1 medium butternut squash	1 teaspoon sunflower oil
2 onions, chopped	5 to 6 cups water
1 chili, seeded and chopped	⅓ to ½ teaspoon sea-salt
3 cloves garlic, crushed	4 to 8 slices of crusty sourdough bread

1 Preheat the oven to 350 degrees Fahrenheit.

2 Toast the pumpkin seeds in a heavy skillet over medium heat for a few minutes, stirring constantly until they are puffed, popping, and fragrant.

3 Set aside half the seeds for garnish and blend the remaining half in a blender until finely ground.

4 Poke several holes in the squash with a fork and set it on a baking sheet. Bake at 350 degrees Fahrenheit for 30 to 40 minutes until it's tender.

5 Remove the squash from the oven, scoop out the seeds and fibers after the squash is cool enough to handle, and cut the flesh into cubes.

6 In a skillet on medium-low heat, sauté the onion, chili, and garlic in the oil for 6 to 8 minutes. (If you're using the ginger [see the VaryIt!], add it to the skillet and sauté it with the other ingredients.)

7 Bring the water to a boil, and then add the squash and sautéed vegetables. Cover, reduce the heat to low, and simmer for 15 minutes, or until the vegetables are tender.

8 Add the ground pumpkin seeds and sea salt. Simmer for another 10 to 15 minutes until the soup thickens.

9 Stir in the coconut milk until you get the desired consistency and cook for an additional 5 minutes.

10 Pour the soup into a tureen and sprinkle with the remaining pumpkin seeds. Serve with sourdough bread.

Per serving: Calories 502 (From Fat 234); Fat 26g (Saturated 13g); Cholesterol 0mg; Sodium 698mg; Carbohydrate 58g; Dietary Fiber 8g; Protein 15g.

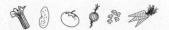

Crunchy Boiled Salad with Pumpkin Seed Dressing

Boiled salad is a super-delicious alternative to a lettuce-based salad. You can use whatever is in your fridge and as little or as many vegetables as you like. The idea is to lightly cook the vegetables in the same water, starting with the lightest flavored vegetables and working up to the stronger flavors.

Tools: *Steamer basket*

Preparation time: *10 minutes*

Cooking time: *10 minutes*

Yield: *4 servings*

¼ cup carrots, cut into diagonals	*1 cup broccoli florets*
1 cup snow peas	*1 tablespoon fresh parsley*
¼ cup red radish, cut into quarters	

1 Place 1½ to 2 inches of water in a medium saucepan and bring to a boil.

2 Place the carrots in a steamer basket and steam in the boiling water for 2 to 3 minutes. Remove and place in mixing bowl.

3 Repeat Step 2 with the snow peas. Repeat again with the radishes and again with the broccoli.

4 Add the parsley to the vegetables.

5 Drizzle the Pumpkin Seed Dressing over the vegetables, toss lightly, and serve.

Pumpkin Seed Dressing

1 tablespoon pumpkin seeds	*1 tablespoon grated fresh ginger*
1 tablespoon shoyu (or tamari)	*1 tablespoon freshly squeezed lemon juice*
1 tablespoon water	

1 Toast the pumpkin seeds in a small skillet over medium heat until brown.

2 Combine the shoyu and water in a small saucepan and simmer over low heat for 3 minutes.

3 Remove the pan from the heat. Add the ginger, lemon juice, and pumpkin seeds, and stir well.

Per serving: Calories 43 (From Fat 11); Fat 1g (Saturated 0g); Cholesterol 0mg; Sodium 242mg; Carbohydrate 6g; Dietary Fiber 2g; Protein 3g.

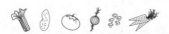

Brown Rice Sesame Sushi with Ginger-Tamari Dipping Sauce

Vegetarian sushi is a wonderful, nutritious lunch that can be made with leftover rice in just a few minutes! Play around with the filling — you can experiment with crisp fresh vegetables, fish, or even fruit. Almost any leftover can be used. Think about color and presentation. Sushi makes for wonderful appetizers, lunch, or main course.

Tools: *Sushi mat, rice paddle*

Preparation time: *10 minutes*

Cooking time: *15 minutes*

Yield: *4 servings*

½ cup short-grain brown rice	*¼ cucumber cut into strips the length of a nori sheet*
½ cup sweet brown rice	*½ avocado*
1 tablespoons brown rice vinegar	*Handful of watercress*
½ tablespoon mirin	*1 to 2 pieces pickled daikon, cut into thin strips*
4 sheets nori, toasted	*1 tablespoon black-and/or-white toasted sesame seeds*
1 small carrot cut into strips (and/or red bell pepper)	*1 to 2 teaspoons umeboshi paste*

1 Cook the rice and allow it to cool to room temperature, or use leftover rice.

2 Place the rice in a large bowl and drizzle it with the brown rice vinegar and mirin. Gently toss the rice.

3 Lay a nori sheet shiny side down on the sushi mat. Spread ¼ cup of rice over the nori using the rice paddle or your hands dipped in water, leaving ¼ inch bare on top edge. Sprinkle ¼ of the sesame seeds over the rice.

4 Make a canal with the rice paddle across the middle of the rice-covered nori sheet.

5 Place ¼ of the carrot, cucumber, avocado, watercress, and pickled daikon in neat lines across canal. Add a thin line of umeboshi paste across the vegetables.

6 Starting with the end nearest to you, roll the sushi, making sure the filling is contained in the middle of the roll.

7 Unroll the mat, moisten the top edge of the sheet, and roll until the nori is sealed.

8 Cut the sushi into halves, and then quarters, using a slant or straight cut. Dip your knife into a bowl of water after each cut for easier cutting.

9 Repeat Steps 3 through 8 with the remaining nori sheets.

10 Serve with Ginger-Tamari Dipping Sauce.

Vary It!: *Try these other filling combinations: carrots and green onion; shitake and wasabi; shitake and sprouts or green onion; tofu, miso, grated carrots, and green onion; dill pickle; mustard sprouts.*

Ginger-Tamari Dipping Sauce

2 tablespoons tamari

2 tablespoons water

¼ teaspoon grated fresh ginger

Mix all the ingredients together in a small bowl.

Per serving: *Calories 420 (From Fat 59); Fat 7g (Saturated 1g); Cholesterol 0mg; Sodium 1,052mg; Carbohydrate 82g; Dietary Fiber 7g; Protein 10g.*

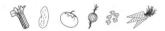

Sour Plum Corn on the Cob

Who doesn't love fresh corn on the cob? This delicious recipe comes with a twist — instead of flavoring with butter, just rub each ear of corn with umeboshi plum for a new and exciting taste experience. Sweet, salty, and a touch of lively sour! Try it.

Tools: *Steamer tray*

Preparation time: *5 minutes*

Cooking time: *8 minutes*

Yield: *4 servings*

4 ears of corn with husks and silk removed

2 small umeboshi plums (Japanese sour plums)

1 Place about 1½ inches of water in a large pot and bring to a boil.

2 Place the corn in a steamer tray, place the tray in the pot, and cover.

3 Reduce the heat to medium and steam the corn for 5 minutes or until tender.

4 Remove the corn and rub each piece with a small amount of umeboshi plum flesh before serving.

Per serving: *Calories 86 (From Fat 9); Fat 1g (Saturated 0g); Cholesterol 0mg; Sodium 597mg; Carbohydrate 20g; Dietary Fiber 2g; Protein 3g.*

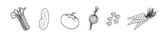

Summer Salad Wrap with Garden Greens and Balsamic Vinaigrette

Wraps are a unique and quick way to create a satisfying lunch. Although this recipe uses salad ingredients, you can also make wraps with leftovers, rice and beans, tofu and veggies — the list is endless! Feel free to add other ingredients to the salad.

Preparation time: *10 minutes*

Cooking time: *3 minutes*

Yield: *1 serving*

½ avocado	¼ cup cucumber cut into julienne pieces
1 small carrot	1 tablespoon chopped, fresh cilantro
Juice of ¼ lemon	1 tablespoon chopped, fresh mint
1 organic tortilla wrap	Sea salt
1 tablespoon hummus	Handful garden greens

1 Cut the avocado into thin slices.

2 Grate the carrot into a bowl and squeeze the lemon juice over the carrot.

3 Warm the tortilla in the broiler or toaster oven for 2 to 3 minutes, being careful not to overcook it or it will be too crispy to wrap.

4 Spread a thin layer of hummus over whole wrap. Place the avocado, cucumber, grated carrot, cilantro, and mint in the middle of the tortilla. Sprinkle a pinch of sea salt and a little of the salad dressing over the filling.

5 Fold in the bottom and top of the wrap until they overlap. Fold in one side to overlap, and then the remaining side. This should seal the wrap. Place on serving plate.

6 Pour the dressing over the garden greens and toss lightly. Serve with the wrap.

Balsamic Vinaigrette

A few drops of balsamic vinegar	Sprinkle of pressed garlic
1 tablespoon extra virgin olive oil	Sprinkle of finely chopped fresh basil
Pinch of sea salt	

In a small bowl, mix the dressing ingredients until they're well-blended.

Per serving: Calories 828 (From Fat 633); Fat 70g (Saturated 10g); Cholesterol 0mg; Sodium 399mg; Carbohydrate 50g; Dietary Fiber 14g; Protein 9g.

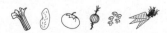

Chunky Carrot and Split Pea Soup with Crunchy Croutons

Split peas are members of the legume family that cook fairly quickly, are loaded with nutrients, and make delicious and hearty soups. It also remains delicious the next day, so it makes happy leftovers!

Preparation time: *10 minutes*

Cooking time: *30 minutes*

Yield: *4 servings*

1-inch piece kombu	*Pepper*
1 large carrot, cut into chunks	*1 to 2 tablespoons shoyu*
1 onion, diced	*1 cup watercress, finely sliced*
6 cups water	*½ teaspoon minced garlic (optional)*
1 cup green split peas	*1 teaspoon rice wine vinegar*
Sea salt	

1 Place kombu, carrots, and onion in a large pot and cover with 2 cups of water. Bring to a boil over medium heat and simmer for 2 minutes.

2 Add the split peas and the remaining water. Cover and bring to boil over medium heat for 2 to 3 minutes.

3 Reduce the flame to low and cook for about 20 minutes.

4 Remove saucepan from the heat. Season with a pinch of salt and pepper, the rice vinegar, and shoyu.

5 Turn the flame very low, add the watercress and garlic, and cook for 3 minutes.

6 Serve garnished with croutons.

Croutons

1 to 2 slices of bread	*1 teaspoon shoyu*	*1 to 2 teaspoons of water*
1 tablespoon sesame oil	*Dried basil or oregano*	

1 Heat the oven to 350 degrees Fahrenheit.

2 Cut the bread into small cubes and place them on a baking sheet.

3 Mix the sesame oil, shoyu, herbs, and water. Pour the mixture over the bread cubes, making sure each one gets covered.

5 Bake the bread cubes in the oven at 350 degrees Fahrenheit for 15 minutes until they're crispy and golden.

Per serving: Calories 251 (From Fat 35); Fat 4g (Saturated 1g); Cholesterol 0mg; Sodium 410mg; Carbohydrate 41g; Dietary Fiber 1g; Protein 15g.

Vegetable and Chickpea Couscous Salad

Couscous is made from ground semolina and is super-quick and easy to turn into delicious meals and side dishes. This yummy salad will appeal to all of your taste buds!

Preparation time: *10 minutes*

Cooking time: *30 minutes*

Yield: *4 servings*

2 cups water (divided)1 medium carrot, diced

1 stalk celery, diced

1 small onion, diced

¼ cup fresh or frozen peas

Few pieces roasted red pepper, diced

1 cup cucumber, diced

2 tablespoons parsley, minced

1 cup cooked chickpeas (can use organic canned chickpeas)

Sea salt

1 cup couscous

Mint sprigs and lemon slices for garnish

1 In a shallow saucepan, bring ³/₄ cup of water to boil and blanch the carrots, celery, onion, and peas for 2 to 3 minutes. Cool.

2 Place the cooled vegetables, red pepper, cucumber, parsley, and chickpeas in a large serving bowl and mix.

3 Add 1¹/₄ cups of water and a pinch of sea salt in a medium saucepan and bring it to a boil over medium heat.

4 Add the couscous, stir, and turn off the flame. Cover the couscous and let it sit for 5 minutes.

5 Fluff the couscous and add it to the vegetables. Mix the ingredients together.

6 Pour the dressing over the couscous and mix gently.

7 Serve garnished with mint and lemon slices.

Dressing

1 teaspoon sea salt

1 tablespoon tahini

1 tablespoon extra virgin olive oil

Juice of 2 small lemons

¼ cup water

1 Place the salt, tahini, olive oil, and lemon juice in a small bowl and blend the ingredients together.

2 Mix in enough water to create a smooth, creamy dressing.

Per serving: *Calories 310 (From Fat 61); Fat 7g (Saturated 1g); Cholesterol 0mg; Sodium 230mg; Carbohydrate 52g; Dietary Fiber 7g; Protein 11g.*

Chapter 15

Appealing Appetizers to Divine Dinner Recipes

In This Chapter

▶ Whetting your appetite with appetizers

▶ Dishes to mix and match for dinner

This chapter offers some quick and easy macrobiotic appetizer recipes you can whip up in no time. Many of them originate from different cultures, but all have the same plant-based deliciousness that makes them healthy, economical, and savory.

In the second part of this chapter, I explain the importance of dinner from a nutritional perspective and then roll out all sorts of divine dinner recipes guaranteed to expand your recipe repertoire and tasty enough to impress family and friends.

Cooking Up Anytime Appetizers

The appetizers below are savory recipes that can be prepared for social events, dinners, or just as light snacks.

Hearty Hummus with Pita Triangles

Hummus is a staple food in many Middle Eastern counties and always a surefire winner at any party. This recipe creates a hearty hummus that beats anything you can buy in a store. For chunkier hummus, don't blend the ingredients very long. Stop when the ingredients are blended but not smooth.

Preparation time: *10 minutes*

Cooking time: *8 minutes*

Yield: *4 servings*

2 cups canned chickpeas

2 to 3 large cloves garlic, chopped

1/3 cup tahini

2 tablespoons extra virgin olive oil

1/3 cup water

2/3 cup fresh lemon juice

2 tablespoons chopped green onions

1/2 teaspoon ground cumin

1/2 teaspoon sea salt

4–6 pitas

A few sprigs fresh parsley or fresh olives for garnish (optional)

1 Preheat the oven to 350 degrees.

2 Put all the ingredients but the pitas and parsley into a food processor or blender and blend until creamy.

3 Cut the pitas into triangles, drizzle with olive oil, sprinkle with a pinch of sea salt, and bake at 350degrees for 5 to 8 minutes.

4 Place the hummus in a serving bowl and the pita triangles on a plate to serve. Garnish with the parsley or olive slices, if desired.

Per serving: Calories 388 (From Fat 177); Fat 20g (Saturated 3g); Cholesterol 0mg; Sodium 559mg; Carbohydrate 44g; Dietary Fiber 9g; Protein 13g.

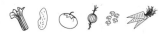

Tasty Tempeh Sticks with Mustard Dip

Eaten throughout Asia, particularly in Indonesia, tempeh is an excellent source of protein and a great way to offer your guests a crunchy, nutritious snack.

Preparation time: *5 minutes*

Cooking time: *15 minutes*

Yield: *4 servings*

1-pound block tempeh	*Few slices fresh ginger*
1-inch strip kombu	*2 tablespoons tamari*
1 cup water	*Safflower oil for deep-frying*
Few slices garlic	*Mild black olives*

1 Cut the tempeh in to ¹/₂-inch wide sticks (about 1¹/₂ inches long). Place the tempeh, kombu, water, garlic, ginger, and tamari into a medium saucepan. Cover and bring to a boil.

2 Reduce the heat to medium-low and simmer for about 10 minutes.

3 In a deep frying pan, heat the oil on low. Turn the temperature to high when the tempeh is ready to be fried.

4 Deep-fry the tempeh for about 3 minutes, or until crispy and golden brown. Remove the tempeh from the oil and drain on paper towels.

5 Serve the tempeh and olives with the mustard dip.

Mustard Dip

1 tablespoon mustard	*1 teaspoon tahini*
2 teaspoons brown rice vinegar	*¹/₄ cup water*
1 to 2 teaspoons shoyu	

1 Place the mustard, vinegar, shoyu, and tahini into a small bowl.

2 Mix until blended. Add enough water to make a smooth dip.

Per serving: Calories 338 (From Fat 210); Fat 23g (Saturated 3g); Cholesterol 0mg; Sodium 952mg; Carbohydrate 15g; Dietary Fiber 6g; Protein 23g.

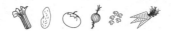

Summer Soba Salad

This cool, tangy salad is a light and delicious appetizer, or you can serve it a la carte for a refreshing summer lunch.

Preparation time: *10 minutes*

Cooking time: *30 minutes*

Yield: *4 servings*

1 medium cucumber	12-ounce package soba noodles
6 radishes	5 kale leaves, lightly blanched
2 scallions	1/2 cup water
1/2 cup dry wakame	1 tablespoon crushed toasted black sesame seeds
1/2 teaspoon sea salt	

1 Finely slice the cucumbers, radishes, scallions, and wakame.

2 Place the sliced vegetables in a medium bowl, add the salt, and let sit for about 15 minutes.

3 Cook the noodles according to the directions on the package, rinse under cool water, and drain.

4 Pour the excess liquid off the vegetables and add the noodles.

5 Pour the orange and sesame dressing over the salad and mix gently. Let sit for 15 minutes.

6 Wash the kale. Cut off the stalk and roughly chop.

7 Boil the boil in a shallow pan. Add the kale and cook over a high heat for 1-2 minutes to blanch the leaves.

8 Serve on a bed of blanched kale garnished with the sesame seeds.

Orange and Sesame Dressing

3 tablespoons shoyu	Juice of half an orange
2 tablespoons mirin	6 tablespoons brown rice vinegar

Place the shoyu, mirin, orange juice, and vinegar in a small bowl and mix together.

Per serving: *Calories 293 (From Fat 15); Fat 2g (Saturated 0g); Cholesterol 0mg; Sodium 1,135mg; Carbohydrate 58g; Dietary Fiber 5g; Protein 15g.*

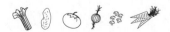

Chickpea Fritters with Spicy Avocado Dressing

These bite-size fitters will be the hit of any social gathering. The crisp coating unfolds to a delicious chickpea interior, and a smattering of yummy avocado dressing completes the taste sensation.

Preparation time: *10 minutes*

Refrigeration time: *30 minutes*

Cooking time: *20 minutes*

Yield: *20 pieces*

1 cup organic cooked chickpeas

3 scallions, finely chopped

1 clove garlic, finely chopped

1 teaspoon ground cumin

¹/₄ cup coriander (cliantro), chopped

Sesame or vegetable oil for deep frying

Sprig of coriander or cilantro for garnish (optional)

1 Blend the chickpeas in a food processor with the scallions, garlic, cumin, and coriander until it makes a smooth paste.

2 Press the mixture into patties (roughly the size of a tablespoon) and place them on a baking sheet. Refrigerate the patties for 30 minutes.

3 Heat the oil in a deep fryer or a large skillet, and deep-fry the patties in batches until they're golden brown and crisp. Place on paper towels to remove the excess oil.

4 Serve the fritters warm with a small spoonful of spicy avocado dressing on top of each one. Garnish with a sprig of coriander or cilantro, if desired.

Spicy Avocado Dressing

1 avocado

2 teaspoons lime juice

1 tablespoon dried chili flakes

Peel the avocado and remove the pit. Mash the flesh until smooth and mix it with the lime juice and chili flakes.

Per serving: Calories 278 (From Fat 113); Fat 13g (Saturated 2g); Cholesterol 0mg; Sodium 10mg; Carbohydrate 34g; Dietary Fiber 12g; Protein 11g.

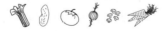

Basil and Plum Cucumbers

This dish combines the fresh taste of cucumber with the tart flavors of umeboshi vinegar and lemon juice. It can be served as an appetizer or as a salad side dish.

Preparation time: *15 minutes*

Cooking time: *None*

Yield: *4 servings*

1 English seedless cucumber	*1 teaspoon umeboshi vinegar*
½ teaspoon sea salt	*1 tablespoon fresh lemon juice*
¼ block tofu, diced	*1 tablespoon fresh basil, finely sliced*

1 Peel the cucumber and chop on an angle.

2 Place the cucumbers and sea salt in a medium bowl. Mix gently and let sit for at least 10 minutes.

3 Place the tofu and vinegar into a small bowl and let sit for about 10 minutes.

4 Combine the tofu and cucumbers. Add the lemon juice and basil, mix gently, and serve.

Per serving: *Calories 23 (From Fat 8); Fat 1g (Saturated 0g); Cholesterol 0mg; Sodium 292mg; Carbohydrate 2g; Dietary Fiber 1g; Protein 2g.*

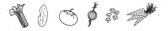

Easy Edamame Ecstasy

Commonly served in Japanese restaurants, this delicious soybean appetizer can be addictive! It's a "down-and-dirty" food that you eat with your hands, squeezing the beans from the pod into your mouth.

Preparation time: *0 minutes*

Cooking time: *8 minutes*

Yield: *4 servings*

1 16-ounce package of frozen edamame	*Sea salt to taste*

1 In a medium saucepan, cook the edamame according to the package directions.

2 Drain and place the edamame in a serving bowl.

3 Sprinkle a couple of teaspoons of sea salt over the edamame, making sure that all the pods get a few granules, and serve.

Per serving: Calories 605 (From Fat 163); Fat 18g (Saturated 0g); Cholesterol 0mg; Sodium 763mg; Carbohydrate 54g; Dietary Fiber 24g; Protein 48g.

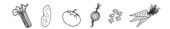

Stuffed Orange and Walnut Celery Sticks

This is a super-quick and delicious appetizer that will delight your taste buds with the combination of orange, walnut, and celery. Simplicity with amazing taste!

Preparation time: *10 minutes*

Cooking time: *8 minutes*

Yield: *10 servings*

3 tablespoons walnuts	*1 teaspoon brown rice miso*
1 tablespoon orange juice	*5 celery stalks*
½ teaspoon orange rind	

1 Roast the walnuts in a dry skillet until toasted, about 5 to 8 minutes. Remove the nuts from the skillet and finely chop them.

2 Place the orange juice, orange rind, and miso into a small bowl and mix well.

3 Add the walnuts and mix together.

4 Place a small amount of the walnut mixture along the center of the celery. Cut into bite-size pieces and serve.

Per serving: Calories 54 (From Fat 34); Fat 4g (Saturated 0g); Cholesterol 0mg; Sodium 124mg; Carbohydrate 5g; Dietary Fiber 2g; Protein 2g.

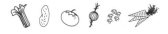

Rich Red Lentil Pate

This is an easy recipe to make that is satisfying and sustaining. It can go with tortillas, pitas, crackers, rice cakes, and bread.

Preparation time: *5 minutes*

Cooking time: *40 minutes*

Refrigeration time: *Overnight*

Yield: *4 servings*

2 cups dried red lentils	2 to 3 garlic cloves, minced
1 piece wakame, soaked and diced	½ teaspoon dried basil
4 cups water	1½ cups walnut pieces, lightly pan roasted
Shoyu, to taste	¼ cup fresh parsley, minced
Sea salt, to taste	Umeboshi vinegar to taste
1 teaspoon olive oil	Balsamic vinegar to taste
3 shallots, diced	

1 Sort out small stones and other inedible pieces from the lentils, and then rinse the lentils well.

2 Place the lentils, wakame, and water in a heavy pot over medium heat. Bring the contents to a boil and continue to boil uncovered for 10 minutes.

3 Reduce the heat to low, cover, and simmer for 20 minutes, or until the lentils are creamy.

4 Season lightly with shoyu and a pinch of sea salt. Simmer another 5 minutes.

5 Heat the olive oil in a large skillet over medium heat. Cook the shallots, garlic, and basil 3 to 4 minutes or until softened, stirring constantly.

6 Add the lentils and stir well.

7 Place the lentils, walnuts, parsley, and a dash of shoyu in a blender or food processor and puree until the mixture is smooth.

8 Pour into a serving bowl and lightly sprinkle the pate with the vinegars. Mix well.

9 Refrigerate the mixture overnight.

10 Serve on crackers, toasted whole wheat bread, or pitas.

Per serving: Calories 575 (From Fat 231); Fat 26g (Saturated 3g); Cholesterol 0mg; Sodium 194mg; Carbohydrate 63g; Dietary Fiber 17g; Protein 29g.

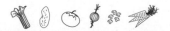

Traditional Rice Ball Treats

Rice balls are an ideal travel food. The pickled plum and the nori wrapped around the outside preserve the rice for several days — longer in winter, shorter in summer. These are good to have on hand when you need some fiber and an energy supply in a convenient snack.

Preparation time: *10 minutes*

Cooking time: *None*

Yield: *4 rice balls (4 servings)*

2 cups cooked short-grain brown rice

2 pickled umeboshi plums with pits removed, or umeboshi paste

3 sheets nori

1 With moistened hands, form firm balls of cooked brown rice (about the size of a golf ball). Keep a bowl of water nearby to wet hands.

2 Poke a hole in the center of the rice ball and insert ¹/₂ plum or 1 teaspoon of umeboshi paste. Reseal the hole. Repeat Steps 1 and 2 until no more rice remains.

3 Toast the nori by waving it over a hot burner.

4 Fold the nori into pieces that are large enough to cover the rice ball and tear it along the folds. Cover the rice ball by pressing the nori around it with slightly moist hands. Repeat this step until all the rice balls are covered.

Per serving: Calories 124 (From Fat 2); Fat 0g (Saturated 0g); Cholesterol 0mg; Sodium 575mg; Carbohydrate 28g; Dietary Fiber 1g; Protein 2g.

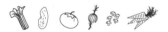

Guacamole with Crunchy Triangle Bread

Originating hundreds of years ago from Aztec culture in Mexico, guacamole is still a delicious creamy snack suitable for any occasion. Simply serve up this easy-to-make dish and watch it disappear instantly. Guaranteed!

Preparation time: *10 minutes*

Cooking time: *0 minutes*

Yield: *4 servings*

2 avocados	½ tomato, seeded and roughly chopped
1 tablespoon extra virgin olive oil	½ red onion, finely chopped
1 tablespoon fresh lemon juice	2 tablespoons fresh cilantro, finely chopped
1 teaspoon chopped garlic	Sea salt (optional)
½ teaspoon umeboshi paste	4 slices whole wheat bread

1 Peel and pit the avocados. Mash the flesh in a medium mixing bowl. Fold in the olive oil, lemon juice, garlic, umeboshi paste, tomato, onion, and cilantro, and season with a pinch of sea salt, if desired.

2 Scoop onto a serving platter.

3 Remove the crust from the bread, cut it into triangles, and toast.

4 Place the toast on the platter with the guacamole and serve.

Per serving: Calories 182 (From Fat 144); Fat 16g (Saturated 3g); Cholesterol 0mg; Sodium 44mg; Carbohydrate 11g; Dietary Fiber 8g; Protein 3g.

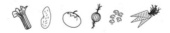

Dining Well at the End of the Day

Dinner is actually an English word that originated from a word that meant "to eat," or more specifically, "to dine." Dinner is usually considered the main meal of the day and eaten sometime in the late afternoon to early evening.

Supper is an English word that is derived from an old German word that meant "to sup." However, supper is usually referred to as the evening meal or last meal of the day, while dinner can be an earlier meal (in the UK, dinner is still considered lunch). Often, the last meal frequently marked a social or festive occasion.

The most important thing we need to think about when it comes to dinner, at least in terms of our overall health, is that it should be the *lightest* meal of the day.

Somehow in the 21st century, we've got it all backwards — we make the last meal of the day the mother of all meals, stuff ourselves royally, and then even have a snack before bed! This ensures that we'll have a disruptive sleep with excessive dreaming and awaken the next morning feeling groggy, dull, and more than likely, full of gas. Sleep is a time for regeneration, not digestion.

If you want to have a good, healing sleep, be sure not to overeat at dinner, get to bed early, and make sure you don't eat for at least three hours before you retire for the night.

Sometimes, a light, after-dinner walk can help activate more efficient digestion.

What follows are several divine dinner recipes of unique cultural variety — and even some familiar favorites. You can mix and match these recipes to create well-balanced meals. Here are my suggestions:

- Millet Mashed Potatoes + Mustard-Tamari Tempeh with Sautéed Carrots and Onions
- Baked Sole with Kalamata Olives and Capers + Water-Fried Kale, Swiss Chard, and Broccoli with Sour Plum and Lemon Dressing
- Winter Warming Carrot and Corn Kasha Varnishkas + Lemon Broccoli + Dulse Onion Soup
- Shiitake Wild Rice with Tahini-Bechamel Topping + Stir-Fried Tofu with Basil and Tamari + Collard Greens with Citrus Dressing
- Cuban Rice and Corn with Spicy Black Beans + Watercress with Parsley
- Millet, Butternut Squash, and Corn Cakes + Mustard Green Salad with Tangy Citrus Dressing
- Basil Walnut Pesto with Linguine + Fennel Mesclun Salad with Lemon Poppy Seed Dressing

Millet Mashed "Potatoes"

Millet makes an excellent substitute to traditional mashed potatoes. It's a satisfying accompaniment to any meal!

Preparation time: *5 minutes*

Cooking time: *40 minutes*

Yield: *4 servings*

1 cup millet	1/4 teaspoon salt
3 cups water	1 teaspoon tamari
1 cup cauliflower florets	Sprig of parsley for garnish (optional)

1 Lightly roast the millet in a medium skillet by stirring over medium-low heat until it smells toasty (about 5–8 minutes).

2 Bring the water to a boil in a large saucepan over high heat, and add the millet, cauliflower, and salt.

3 Cover the pan, reduce the heat to low, and simmer for 25 minutes.

4 Add the tamari and cook for an additional 5 minutes.

5 Mash the millet and cauliflower using a potato masher or a hand blender, adding water if necessary.

6 Place in a serving bowl and garnish with the parsley, if desired.

Per serving: Calories 454 (From Fat 35); Fat 4g (Saturated 1g); Cholesterol 0mg; Sodium 233mg; Carbohydrate 90g; Dietary Fiber 6g; Protein 14g.

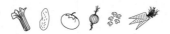

Mustard-Tamari Tempeh with Sautéed Carrots and Onions

Tempeh is a great bean product that can be cooked in many different ways. You can mix tempeh with a variety of different vegetables to create a nutritious bean/vegetable dish.

Preparation time: *15 minutes*

Cooking time: *10 minutes*

Yield: *4 servings*

½ tablespoon toasted sesame oil	*2 tablespoons tamari*
½ pound tempeh, cut into 1-inch cubes	*1 teaspoon natural mustard*
1 tablespoon wakame	*1 garlic clove*
1 large onion, chopped	*4 tablespoons water*
2 carrots, cut into thin strips	*1 cup of fresh parsley, finely chopped*

1 In a cast iron skillet or steel pan, heat the oil over medium heat. Add the tempeh cubes and sauté them, turning to brown each side, until they're golden brown.

2 In a small bowl, soak the dried wakame in water for 5 minutes until it's fully hydrated. Drain the wakame and squeeze out the water. Finely chop the wakame and set it aside.

3 In a medium saucepan, heat the remaining oil and lightly fry the onions, garlic and carrots until soft. Add the vegetables to the skillet with the tempeh and stir the ingredients together. Place back on a medium heat for 2-3 minutes.

4 Mix the tamari and mustard in a small bowl. Dilute the mixture with 4 tablespoons of water. Add this mixture and the wakame to the tempeh and vegetables in the final minutes of cooking, stirring to make sure all the ingredients are covered. Continue to cook for a further 2-3 minutes.

5 Sprinkle the fresh parsley over the tempeh and vegetables, and serve.

Per serving: Calories 171 (From Fat 73); Fat 8g (Saturated 2g); Cholesterol 0mg; Sodium 532mg; Carbohydrate 14g; Dietary Fiber 5g; Protein 13g.

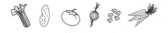

Baked Sole with Kalamata Olives and Capers

Sole is a delightful, light white fish that is complemented by the tart flavors of olives and capers.

Preparation time: *10 to 15 minutes*

Cooking time: *30 minutes*

Yield: *4 servings*

Four 4- to 5-ounce sole fillets	*1 tablespoon toasted sesame oil*
1 to 2 teaspoons tamari	*2 tablespoons capers, drained*
1 cup water	*1¹/₂ cups kalamata olives, pitted and chopped*
Juice of one lemon	*Splash of rice wine vinegar*
2 leek stalks, thin-cut lengthways	*Fresh parsley or basil, chopped, for garnish (optional)*
Pinch of sea salt	
1 medium onion, chopped	

1 Preheat the oven to 400 degrees.

2 Rinse the sole fillets and place them in a glass or ceramic baking dish.

3 In a small bowl, dilute the tamari with the water and lemon juice. Drizzle the liquid over the fillets until they're covered.

4 Add the leeks and sea salt and bake at 400 degrees for 20 to 30 minutes, or until the center of the flesh is thoroughly cooked.

5 In a medium skillet, heat the oil and fry the onions over medium heat until they're golden brown.

6 Add the capers, olives, and vinegar, and sauté for 1 minute.

7 Remove the fish from the oven and place onto serving plates. Spoon the olive and caper topping over the fish. Garnish with the parsley or basil, if desired.

Vary It!: *For a vegetarian version of this dish, replace the sole with extra-firm tofu. Slice 1 pound of tofu into thick slices. In a large, preheated skillet, fry the tofu slices and leeks with 1 tablespoon of toasted sesame oil over medium-high heat until the tofu is golden brown on both sides. Place the tofu on a serving dish and spoon the olive and caper topping over it. Garnish with chopped parsley or basil, if desired.*

Per serving: Calories 237 (From Fat 108); Fat 12g (Saturated 2g); Cholesterol 53mg; Sodium 702mg; Carbohydrate 12g; Dietary Fiber 1g; Protein 20g.

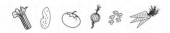

Water-Fried Kale, Swiss Chard, and Broccoli with Sour Plum and Lemon Dressing

This is a quick, easy, and nutritious dish that adds delicious greens to any meal.

Preparation time: *15 minutes*

Cooking time: *10 minutes*

Yield: *4 servings*

1 tablespoon Sesame seeds	*1 bunch Swiss chard*
1 bunch kale	*1 bunch broccoli*

1 Toast the sesame seeds for approximately 10 minutes in a small, dry skillet over medium heat. Stir frequently to avoid burning.

2 Wash the greens thoroughly in a colander. Chop them into uniform small pieces and cut the broccoli into florets.

3 Bring 1 to 1$^1/_2$ cups water to a boil in a medium saucepan and add the greens and broccoli.

4 Partially cover the pan and simmer over medium heat for 4 to 6 minutes.

5 Drain the greens and broccoli, and place them in serving dish. Drizzle with the Sour Plum and Lemon Dressing, and garnish with the sesame seeds.

Sour Plum and Lemon Dressing

2 teaspoons umeboshi plum paste	*Water*
Juice of $^1/_2$ a lemon	

Mix the umeboshi plum paste with the lemon juice and thin with water.

Vary It!: *You can mix most combination of greens for this dish. This recipe also works well with bok choy, chard, and cabbage.*

Per serving: *Calories 81 (From Fat 11); Fat 1g (Saturated 0g); Cholesterol 0mg; Sodium 385mg; Carbohydrate 15g; Dietary Fiber 7g; Protein 8g.*

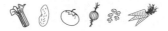

Winter Warming Carrot and Corn Kasha Varnishkas

Kasha Varnishkas is a traditional Jewish dish that my mother used to make that combines pasta (traditionally bow tie noodles) with buckwheat. This is a very warming and hearty winter dish.

Preparation time: *15 minutes*

Cooking time: *35 to 40 minutes*

Yield: *4 servings*

8 ounces of farfalle pasta	*1 cup toasted kasha*
2 teaspoons sesame oil	*2 cups water*
1 large onion, chopped	*Pinch Sea salt*
1 large carrot, finely chopped	*2 tablespoons shoyu or tamari*
1 cup corn	*1 tablespoon fresh parsley*

1 Cook the pasta according to the instructions on the package. Drain the pasta, rinse under cold water, and set it aside.

2 Heat the oil in a large skillet and sauté the onion over medium heat for 3 minutes.

3 Add the carrots and corn to the onion and continue cooking for another 3 to 5 minutes or until the onion is golden brown.

4 In a large saucepan, bring the water to a boil over high heat, add the kasha and salt, reduce the heat to low, cover, and simmer for 10 minutes.

5 Pour boiling water over the pasta to reheat and shake to remove any excess water.

6 Add the pasta, vegetables, and shoyu to the kasha and mix gently.

7 Transfer to a serving dish and garnish with parsley.

Per serving: *Calories 431 (From Fat 42); Fat 5g (Saturated 1g); Cholesterol 0mg; Sodium 485mg; Carbohydrate 86g; Dietary Fiber 8g; Protein 16g.*

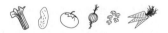

Lemon Broccoli

Broccoli is full of disease-fighting goodness and makes a great side dish for any meal. Add some punch with the easy lemon dressing, and you'll never look at broccoli the same way again!

Preparation time: *5 minutes*

Cooking time: *5 minutes*

Yield: *4 servings*

3 heads broccoli	*¹/₂ cup water*
1 to 2 tablespoons olive oil	*Juice of 1 lemon*
¹/₂ to 1 teaspoon sea salt	

1 Rinse the broccoli and cut the head into small florets and the stem into small pieces.

2 Warm a large skillet over medium heat, add the olive oil, and turn the flame to high.

3 Add the broccoli and sea salt and sauté 1 to 2 minutes until the broccoli is coated in oil.

4 Add the water and cover. Steam for 2 minutes.

5 Mix the lemon juice with a little water and a pinch of salt.

6 Place the broccoli in a serving bowl and season with the lemon dressing.

Per serving: *Calories 96 (From Fat 38); Fat 4g (Saturated 1g); Cholesterol 0mg; Sodium 350mg; Carbohydrate 13g; Dietary Fiber 7g; Protein 7g.*

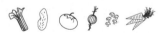

Dulse Onion Soup

Dulse is a super sea vegetable that offers an abundance of vitamins and minerals in one simple and delicious soup! This thick and hearty soup will keep you warm on a cold winter day.

Preparation time: *5 minutes*

Cooking time: *25 minutes*

Yield: *4 servings*

1 medium onion, diced	½ cup rolled oats
1 teaspoon sesame oil	2 tablespoons white miso
½ cup dried dulse	1 tablespoon parsley, finely chopped
4 cups water	

1 Heat a large saucepan over medium heat, add the oil, and cook the onion for 2 to 3 minutes.

2 Rinse the dulse under cold water and cut it into small pieces.

3 Add the water, oats, and dulse to the saucepan and bring everything to a boil. Reduce the heat to low, cover, and simmer for 15 minutes.

4 Dilute the miso using a small amount of the soup broth.

5 Stir the miso into the broth and cook for 3 to 4 more minutes.

6 Serve with a garnish of parsley or other favorite herb.

Per serving: *Calories 82 (From Fat 18); Fat 2g (Saturated 0g); Cholesterol 0mg; Sodium 239mg; Carbohydrate 14g; Dietary Fiber 2g; Protein 3g.*

Shiitake Wild Rice with Tahini-Bechamel Sauce

Although wild rice may not be a true whole grain (it's a seed), it blends nicely with brown rice to create a delicious partnership.

Tools: *Pressure cooker*

Preparation time: *10 minutes*

Cooking time: *1 hour to 1 hour and 10 minutes*

Yield: *4 servings*

³/₄ cup brown rice

14 cup wild rice

Pinch Sea salt

1 chopped onion

3 cups chopped shiitake mushrooms

1 tablespoon toasted sesame oil

2 to 3 teaspoons tamari

1 cup chopped almonds

1 cup fresh parsley

1 Rinse rice and wild rice together by placing in a pot with enough water to cover. Swirl your hands around the grain to loosed dust and drain. Do this two to three times, as the grain is often quite dusty or even dirty.

2 Soak the grain in enough fresh water to cover for at least two and up to an ideal four hours. This soaking helps with assimilation, making the grain easier to digest.

3 Drain water from soaking grain and place into pressure cooker with 1¹/₂ cups of water. Bring to a boil with the lid loosely covered; then add sea salt.

4 Seal the lid and bring to full pressure. Most pressure cookers have a jiggling part that the steam moves back and forth to make a noise as well as a colored (usually red) metal prong that the pressure rises so you know the pressure is reached. When the pressure comes up, immediately turn down stove to low heat.

5 Allow to cook for 30 minutes. Then turn off the heat and allow the pressure cooker to remain undisturbed for 25 minutes so that the rice continues to cook in its own heat. Then remove the pot from the stove, open the release valve to make sure all steam is vented, and gently stir. Transfer the rice to a serving bowl.

6 In a medium skillet over medium heat, sauté the onions and shiitake mushrooms in sesame oil until the onions are soft and the mushrooms are almost cooked. Add the tamari and simmer on low heat for 3 to 4 minutes.

7 Combine the mushrooms and onion with the rice. Add the chopped almonds and parsley. Pour the Tahini-Bechamel Sauce over the dish, mix, and serve.

Tahini-Bechamel Sauce

2 tablespoons tahini

5 tablespoons water

4 teaspoons tamari

Pinch of sea salt

1 Mix the tahini and water in a small bowl.

2 Add the tamari and salt and mix.

Per serving: *Calories 566 (From Fat 208); Fat 23g (Saturated 3g); Cholesterol 0mg; Sodium 369mg; Carbohydrate 79g; Dietary Fiber 11g; Protein 18g.*

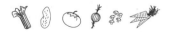

Stir-Fried Tofu with Basil and Tamari

Tofu adds a smooth texture to a quinoa salad. It can be served as a side dish, mixed into a salad, or served with rice or noodles. Basil adds its own unique flavor of Italy!

Preparation time: *5 minutes*

Cooking time: *15 minutes*

Yield: *4 servings*

1 pound firm tofu	*2 to 3 tablespoons water*
1¼ teaspoon toasted sesame oil, divided	*Squeeze of fresh lemon juice*
1 tablespoon tamari	*½ bunch basil, chopped*

1 Cut the tofu into 1-inch cubes.

2 Add the oil to a large skillet and heat over medium-high heat, making sure the oil doesn't smoke. Sauté the tofu for 2-3 minutes.

3 Cover the skillet and let the tofu puff up, cook for about 3 minutes.

4 In a small bowl, mix the tamari, water, a dash of oil, and a squeeze of lemon. Pour the mixture over the tofu.

5 Add the basil, cover, and cook about 8 minutes, or until the tofu reaches the desired consistency.

Vary It!: *You can use any herb for this dish, but if you substitute sage for the basil, be sure to chop it very fine and use a small amount because sage is very bitter.*

Per serving: *Calories 178 (From Fat 100); Fat 11g (Saturated 2g); Cholesterol 0mg; Sodium 246mg; Carbohydrate 5g; Dietary Fiber 3g; Protein 19g.*

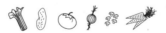

Collard Greens with Citrus Dressing

Collard greens, a staple of the American South, are full of vitamins and nutrients. They're delicious when served as a simple side dish.

Preparation time: *5 minutes*

Cooking time: *3 to 4 minutes*

Yield: *4 servings*

8-10 large collard green leaves

Juice from ½ orange

1 teaspoon umeboshi paste

1 Wash the collard leaves well and drain. Cut the middle stem from each of the leaves and chop the stem finely.

2 Fold the leaves in half lengthwise and roll them up like a jelly roll. Starting at one end of the roll, slice the greens into thin strands.

3 Bring ½ inch of water to boil in a shallow saucepan. Place the greens and stems in the water and cook for 2 to 3 minutes.

4 In a small bowl, mix the orange juice and umeboshi paste with about 1 tablespoon of water to make the citrus dressing.

5 When the greens are tender, remove them from the pan and drain. Place the greens in a serving bowl and drizzle with the dressing. Lightly toss and serve.

Per serving: *Calories 38 (From Fat 4); Fat 0g (Saturated 0g); Cholesterol 0mg; Sodium 124mg; Carbohydrate 8g; Dietary Fiber 2g; Protein 3g.*

Cuban Rice and Corn with Spicy Black Beans

Rice and black beans is a staple dish of many South American countries. Black beans are one of the most nutritious beans; they're full of fiber and magnesium. Try this quick and easy Cuban specialty for an especially big "yum" dinner.

Tools: Steamer

Preparation time: 5 minutes

Cooking time: 20 minutes

Yield: 4 servings

4 cups cooked long-grain brown rice or basmati rice

1 tablespoon sesame oil

1 onion, diced

2 cloves garlic, crushed

2 cups organic black beans

1/4 teaspoon chili powder or 1/2 teaspoon chipotle powder + 1 teaspoon cumin

Pinch sea salt

1 tablespoon of finely chopped parsley

2 ears of corn

1 Cook the rice according to the package directions.

2 Heat the oil in a large saucepan and fry the onions and garlic over medium heat for 5 minutes or until the onion is tender.

3 Add the black beans, chili powder, and salt, and cook 3 to 4 minutes.

4 Stir in the parsley and cook 1 minute.

5 Transfer the beans to a serving dish and garnish with a parsley sprig.

6 Bring 1/2 inch of water to boil in a small saucepan.

7 Cut the kernels from the ears of corn and place them in a steamer over the boiling water. Cook over medium heat for 3 to 4 minutes.

8 Mix the corn with the rice and place in a serving bowl.

9 Serve the beans over rice.

Per serving: Calories 342 (From Fat 61); Fat 7g (Saturated 1g); Cholesterol 0mg; Sodium 51mg; Carbohydrate 56g; Dietary Fiber 10g; Protein 15g.

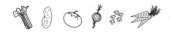

Watercress with Parsley

Watercress is packed full of vitamins and nutrients and is the perfect bitter side dish to the Cuban Rice and Corn with Spicy Black Beans (you can find this recipe elsewhere in this chapter).

Preparation time: *5 minutes*

Cooking time: *5 minutes*

Yield: *4 servings*

3 bunches watercress, chopped

¼ cup parsley, finely chopped

¼ teaspoon tamari (optional)

1 In a shallow saucepan, bring ½ inch of water to a boil.

2 Add the watercress and cook for 3 minutes.

3 Add parsley and tamari, if desired. Cook the greens for 2 minutes. Drain and serve.

Per serving: *Calories 4 (From Fat 1); Fat 0g (Saturated 0g); Cholesterol 0mg; Sodium 32mg; Carbohydrate 1g; Dietary Fiber 0g; Protein 1g.*

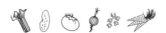

Millet, Butternut Squash, and Corn Cakes

Millet is a very versatile grain with a sweet, nutty flavor that goes exceptionally well with squash. Traditional Chinese medicine recommends millet for problems of blood sugar and the pancreas. You can make fresh millet for this recipe or use leftover millet by simply steaming it and allowing it to cool.

Preparation time: *10 minutes*

Cooking time: *35 to 40 minutes*

Yield: *4 servings*

1 cup millet	*$\frac{1}{2}$ cup cooked corn*
1 teaspoon mustard seeds	*$2\frac{1}{2}$ cups water*
1 teaspoon curry powder	*$\frac{1}{2}$ teaspoon sea salt*
2 cups peeled and diced butternut squash	*1 clove garlic, crushed*
1 teaspoon freshly grated ginger	*$\frac{1}{2}$ cup fresh chopped cilantro*

1 After washing and rinsing the millet, dry roast the millet in a large skillet over medium heat for about 4 minutes. Stir constantly until the millet starts to pop.

2 Remove the millet from the skillet, and set aside.

3 Toast the mustard seeds and curry powder in the skillet over medium heat for 1 to 2 minutes until they're aromatic.

4 Mix the millet, mustard seeds, squash, ginger, corn, water, and sea salt in a large saucepan. Bring to a boil over high heat.

5 Reduce the heat to low, cover, and simmer for 25 minutes or until the millet has absorbed all the water.

6 Remove the pan from the heat. When the mixture is cool, add the cilantro.

7 Wet your hands and blend the mixture to a uniform consistency. Form the mixture into 12 cakes and grill for approximately 3 minutes on each side, or until golden. Alternatively, dust the cakes with a coating of flour, heat a tablespoon of oil into a skillet and lightly fry for 3-4 minutes each side.

8 Serve hot.

Per serving: *Calories 501 (From Fat 40); Fat 4g (Saturated 1g); Cholesterol 0mg; Sodium 306mg; Carbohydrate 102g; Dietary Fiber 8g; Protein 15g.*

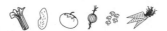

Mustard Green Salad with Tangy Citrus Dressing

Mustard greens provide a nice tartness to the sweet millet cakes (you can find the recipe for these elsewhere in the chapter). The greens are full of nutrients and add a robust flavor to the meal.

Preparation time: *5 minutes*

Cooking time: *None*

Yield: *4 servings*

1 cup extra virgin olive oil	*Squeeze of fresh lemon juice*
2 tablespoons finely chopped fresh parsley	*Pinch of sea salt*
½ teaspoon minced fresh or dried basil	*4 cups mustard greens*
½ teaspoon minced fresh or dried oregano	

1 Mix the oil, parsley, basil, oregano, lemon juice, and salt together in a medium bowl and beat with a fork until mixed thoroughly.

2 Drizzle the dressing over the greens. Gently toss until the greens are covered. Serve.

*****Per serving:*** *Calories 494 (From Fat 487); Fat 54g (Saturated 7g); Cholesterol 0mg; Sodium 160mg; Carbohydrate 3g; Dietary Fiber 2g; Protein 2g.*

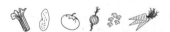

Basil Walnut Pesto with Linguine

When you're hungry for pasta, nothing is more satisfying than a delicious bowl of pasta with pesto. This is a quick and simple way to create a satisfying lunch or dinner, and this dish keeps well for second-day leftovers. Pesto can be kept refrigerated for two to three days.

Preparation time: *10 minutes*

Cooking time: *15 minutes*

Yield: *4 servings*

¹/₂ cup pine nuts	*2 tablespoons olive oil*
2 cups fresh basil, chopped	*1 teaspoon salt or 2 tablespoons tamari*
2 to 3 cloves garlic, pressed	*10 to 12 ounces of dry or fresh linguine*
¹/₂ cup finely chopped walnuts	

1 Heat a heavy skillet over a medium heat. Place the pine nuts into the skillet and dry roast the pine nuts until they are golden brown (approximately 5 minutes).

2 Puree the pine nuts, basil, garlic, walnuts, olive oil, and salt or tamari to a food processor or blender until the ingredients are smooth and creamy. Add a little water if necessary to create a thick, smooth consistency.

3 Prepare the linguine according to the directions on the package. Drain the pasta.

4 Stir the pesto into the hot pasta. Garnish with fresh basil and serve.

Per serving: *Calories 456 (From Fat 182); Fat 20g (Saturated 3g); Cholesterol 0mg; Sodium 587mg; Carbohydrate 58g; Dietary Fiber 5g; Protein 16g.*

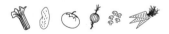

Fennel Mesclun Salad with Lemon Poppy Seed Dressing

Mesclun is the perfect light accompaniment to the richness of pesto sauce, so consider serving this salad with Basil Walnut Pesto with Linguine (you can find the recipe for this dish elsewhere in this chapter). Choose organic greens, and wash and drain them well before serving.

Preparation time: *5 minutes*

Cooking time: *None*

Yield: *4 servings*

4 cups mesclun greens	*1 bulb fennel, finely sliced*
½ cup fresh herbs (parsley, dill, or cilantro)	*Sea salt, to taste*
10 to 12 cherry tomatoes	

1 Place the greens, herbs, tomatoes, and fennel in a large serving bowl.

2 Sprinkle with a little sea salt and drizzle the salad dressing over the salad.

3 Gently toss the salad and serve immediately.

Lemon Poppy Seed Dressing

2 tablespoons light miso	*¼ cup water*
2 tablespoons lemon juice	*¼ teaspoon poppy seeds*

Whisk the miso, lemon juice, water, and poppy seeds together until blended.

Per serving: Calories 54 (From Fat 9); Fat 1g (Saturated 0g); Cholesterol 0mg; Sodium 364mg; Carbohydrate 10g; Dietary Fiber 4g; Protein 3g.

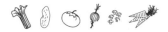

Down-Home American Spaghetti Marinara and Meatless Meatballs

Here's a variation of a familiar dish that has become an American institution. The use of *seitan* (also known as *wheat meat*) simulates meatballs. By using prepared tomato sauce and packed seitan, this dish is one of those convenient "no time for dinner" dishes. It's best served with salad greens and vinaigrette dressing. For the dressing, I recommend natural food labels such as Annie's, Westbrea, or Eden.

Preparation time: *10 minutes*

Cooking time: *20 minutes*

Yield: *4 servings*

2 teaspoons olive oil

2 medium brown onions, finely chopped

10 medium shiitake mushrooms, chopped, stems discarded

1 package seitan

Jarred tomato sauce, to taste

10 to 12 ounces dry or fresh spaghetti

½ teaspoon salt

Dash of tamari

1 tablespoon dried parsley

1 Heat a large skillet over medium heat, add the olive oil, and sauté the onions for about 5 minutes or until they're soft and translucent.

2 Add the mushrooms and sauté for 5 minutes.

3 Carve the seitan into balls or cut it into squares, and add it to the skillet.

4 Add the tomato sauce and stir gently. Cook everything in the skillet for 5 minutes.

5 Cook the pasta according to the directions on the package.

6 Drain the pasta and return it to the empty pot.

7 Stir the seitan, onions, mushrooms, and tomato sauce into the pasta. Add the dried parsley and serve.

Per serving: *Calories 527 (From Fat 88); Fat 10g (Saturated 2g); Cholesterol 0mg; Sodium 1,387mg; Carbohydrate 85g; Dietary Fiber 9g; Protein 26g.*

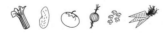

Spanish-Style Tempeh Paella

Paella has long been a favorite dish in Spain. This version with tempeh adds a nice twist to a traditional recipe and can be a real family dinner treat. I suggest serving this dish with your favorite green salad and vinaigrette.

Tools: *Pressure cooker*

Preparation time: *10 minutes to 2 hours*

Cooking time: *1 hour*

Yield: *4 servings*

1 to 2 strips kombu	½ cup cubed burdock
1½ cups uncooked brown rice	8 ounces tempeh cut into 1/4" cubes
1 tablespoon Dark sesame oil	1–1½ tablespoons Tamari
1 cup cubed celery	2 cups of water
1 cup cubed onion	Fresh ginger juice, to taste
1 cup cubed carrots	

1 Soak the kombu for two hours or use a strip leftover from another dish. Soak the rice for 1–2 hours and drain.

2 Brown the rice with a little oil in a large skillet over medium heat for 5 minutes or until it's lightly brown and fragrant. Set aside.

3 Pan-fry the vegetables individually in a little oil over high heat until they are soft. Cook the celery first, remove it from the skillet, and then repeat with the onion, the carrot, and finally the burdock.

4 Cut the kombu into small squares.

5 In a medium skillet, pan-fry the tempeh with the tamari over medium heat until dry.

6 Layer the vegetables in a pressure cooker (or large pot) in the same order you cooked them, followed by the kombu, tempeh, and rice. Gently add the water. Add a few drops of tamari and a pinch of sea salt to taste.

7 If using a pressure cooker, bring to full pressure, then reduce heat to low and cook for 40 minutes. Remove from heat and allow the pressure to subside before opening. (If you're boiling the ingredients in a large pot, use 2½ cups of water.)

8 Mix all the ingredients together in a large serving bowl and season with fresh ginger juice.

Per serving: Calories 517 (From Fat 92); Fat 10g (Saturated 2g); Cholesterol 0mg; Sodium 314mg; Carbohydrate 88g; Dietary Fiber 11g; Protein 21g.

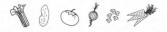

Brown Rice, Vegetable, and Tofu Stir-Fry with Sliced Almonds

Creating a stir-fry dish is a great way to use leftover rice and any vegetables you have on hand. You can replace any of the vegetables in this dish with what's in your fridge. You can't go wrong — it's quick, easy, and delicious!

Preparation time: *10 minutes*

Cooking time: *15 minutes*

Yield: *4 servings*

1 tablespoon extra virgin olive oil

4 medium carrots, cut julienne

1 cup chopped fresh shitake mushrooms

2 stalks celery, cut into slices

Pinch of sea salt

2 small zucchini, cut julienne

4 green onions, cut on the diagonal

1/2 red onion, cut on the diagonal

1 cup finely chopped leafy greens, such as kale or bok choy

1 pound firm tofu, cut into 1/2-inch cubes

Almond slices

2 cloves fresh garlic, thinly sliced

1 teaspoon minced fresh ginger

3 tablespoons tamari

1/3 cup water

2 cups cooked brown rice

1 In a large wok or skillet, heat the olive oil until it's very hot but not smoking.

2 Add the carrots, mushrooms, celery, ginger, garlic and a pinch of salt and stir-fry over medium-high heat for 3 minutes.

3 Add the zucchini, onions, and tofu, and cook for 2 minutes.

4 Add the greens and stir-fry until they are just wilted (add a little water if necessary).

5 Stir the almonds into mixture.

6 Mix the tamari with 1/3 cup water and pour over the stir-fried vegetables. Cook for another 2 to 3 minutes.

7 Transfer the vegetables to a serving dish and serve with cooked brown rice.

Per serving: *Calories 435 (From Fat 157); Fat 18g (Saturated 2g); Cholesterol 0mg; Sodium 789mg; Carbohydrate 49g; Dietary Fiber 10g; Protein 27g.*

Chapter 16

Delectable Desserts and Beverages

Although the concept of desserts is a more Westernized one, we do love our desserts. For many people, the main meal often is just a formality to get to that mouth-watering dessert. However, the degree of longing you experience for dessert may have some physiological basis. A low blood sugar condition, easily produced in some individuals by waiting long periods between meals, can inspire sweet cravings (or increase the desire to overeat). Knowing how to regulate your blood sugar with specific foods and eating more frequently can make a big difference.

Beyond dessert recipes, I also include a variety of hot teas and beverages to conclude this chapter.

Ending Your Meal with Healthy and Tasty Desserts

The word *dessert* was first recorded around 1600 and was derived from a French word that meant "to clear the table." Usually, a sweet food was served as the final course of a meal, or sometimes a strongly flavored one, such as slices of cheese.

Dessert is best thought of as a treat, not as an integral part of the daily meal. If you're healing and are restricted to simple sugars — despite the fact that simple sugars come from natural food origins (barley malt, rice syrup, maple syrup, and so on) — you should still limit the number and amount of desserts you eat.

Hurricane Key Lime Pie

This Florida key lime pie is delicious and has the same sweet-and-sour punch as any conventional pie. It was created by a friend when she was confined at home in Florida during a hurricane. It's perfect for a dinner party or afternoon tea treat!

Preparation time: *40 minutes*

Cooking time: *20 minutes*

Refrigeration time: *4 hours*

Yield: *6 servings*

1 pressed sweet crust	*⅓ cup key lime juice*
3 teaspoons arrowroot	*1 teaspoon agar agar flakes (yes, that's the actual name)*
1 cup apple juice, divided	
1 cup soy milk	*¼ teaspoon salt*
¾ cup sweetener (half brown rice syrup and half maple syrup)	*½ teaspoon vanilla extract*
	Tofu topping

1 Prepare the pressed sweet crust (recipe follows).

2 Mix the arrowroot with ¼ cup of apple juice in a small bowl.

3 Place the remaining apple juice, soy milk, key lime juice, agar flakes, salt, and vanilla extract in a medium saucepan and bring the mixture to a gentle roll over medium heat.

4 Add arrowroot mixture and simmer over medium-low heat for 2 to 3 minutes.

5 Remove the pie filling from the heat and let it cool for 15 minutes.

6 Pour the filling into the crust and chill until firm (at least 4 hours).

7 Top the chilled pie with the tofu topping and garnish with thin slices of key lime.

Pressed Sweet Crust

1 cup toasted pecans	*Pinch of nutmeg*
1 cup of whole wheat pastry flour (or half whole wheat and half white)	*Pinch of salt*
	⅛ cup walnut oil or evoo (extra virgin olive oil)
1 teaspoon cinnamon	*¼ cup brown rice syrup or maple syrup*

1 Preheat the oven to 350 degrees.

2 Grind the pecans and flour in a food processor until they're the consistency of bread crumbs.

3 Add the cinnamon, nutmeg, and salt. Mix.

4 Add the oil and syrup and blend. The mixture should hold together without being sticky.

5 Press the mixture into a 9-inch, greased pie dish and bake at 350 degrees for 20 minutes or until golden.

Tofu Topping

1 pound silken tofu

1/2 cup maple syrup

1/8 teaspoon salt

1/2 teaspoon vanilla extract

Mix all the ingredients together in a food processor and chill.

Per serving: *Calories 979 (From Fat 402); Fat 45g (Saturated 5g); Cholesterol 0mg; Sodium 505mg; Carbohydrate 134g; Dietary Fiber 8g; Protein 21g.*

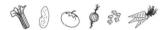

Dreamy Rice Pudding

This recipe is a perfect way to use leftover rice to create a delicious and traditional dessert.

Preparation time: *5 minutes*

Cooking time: *30 minutes*

Yield: *4 to 6 servings*

1 cup amasake (or rice milk)

1/2 cup apple juice

2 cups brown rice

3 tablespoons raisins

3 tablespoons sunflower seeds

1 teaspoon cinnamon

1 teaspoon vanilla (optional)

1 Combine all the ingredients except the vanilla in a large saucepan.

2 Simmer over medium-low heat for 20 to 30 minutes, stirring often to prevent sticking, until thick and creamy.

3 Stir in the vanilla and serve warm or chilled.

Per serving: *Calories 218 (From Fat 40); Fat 5g (Saturated 1g); Cholesterol 0mg; Sodium 29mg; Carbohydrate 41g; Dietary Fiber 4g; Protein 5g.*

Yum-Yum Oatmeal and Raisin Cookies

Who doesn't like cookies? These delicious treats are winners and great with an afternoon cup of tea or grain coffee.

Preparation time: *15 minutes*

Baking time: *15 to 18 minutes*

Yield: *8 to 10 servings*

⅓ cup maple syrup	¾ cup whole wheat pastry flour
⅓ cup rice syrup	1 teaspoon ground cinnamon
3 tablespoons water	½ teaspoon sea salt
½ cup canola oil	½ cup roasted almonds
1 tablespoon almond butter	1½ cups rolled oats
1¼ teaspoons vanilla extract	½ cup raisins
¾ cup unbleached white flour	

1 Preheat the oven to 375 degrees. Grease two baking sheets, or line them with parchment paper.

2 In a large mixing bowl, combine the maple and rice syrups, water, oil, almond butter, and vanilla with an electric mixer on medium speed until the ingredients are well blended.

3 In a large bowl, stir together the flours, cinnamon, and salt.

4 Add the wet mixture to the dry ingredients, folding in gently with a wooden spoon or rubber spatula.

5 Chop the almonds. Add the almonds, oats, and raisins to the mixture and stir well.

6 Place a teaspoonful of the cookie dough onto the cookie sheet. Flatten the dough slightly with the back of a damp fork. Repeat with the remaining dough.

7 Bake the cookies at 375 degrees for 15 to 18 minutes or until the edges of the cookies are slightly browned.

8 Remove the baking sheets from the oven and allow the cookies to cool slightly before removing them from the baking sheet.

9 Place the cookies on a large plate and serve or store in an airtight container.

Per serving: *Calories 456 (From Fat 190); Fat 21g (Saturated 2g); Cholesterol 0mg; Sodium 181mg; Carbohydrate 63g; Dietary Fiber 5g; Protein 8g.*

Refreshing Seasonal Fruit Kanten

Light and refreshing, this dessert is the nearest thing to a natural version of Jell-O. Agar agar is a tasteless, dried sea vegetable commonly used as a texturizing agent, emulsifier, stabilizer, and thickener in ice cream, sherbets, jellies, soups, sauces, canned soups, and even canned meat and fish. Agar agar is a vegetable gelatin that appeals to vegetarians because true gelatin is generally made from calf's feet.

Agar agar acquires the flavor of whatever fruit you prepare it with. Change this dessert as the seasons change and you'll always delight your dinner guests and kids.

Note: Soft fruits such as cherries, berries, peaches, or melons don't need to be cooked with agar agar. However, firmer fruits such as apples or pears need to be peeled, chopped, and cooked in the agar agar and juice mixture to soften them.

Preparation time: *30 minutes*

Cooking time: *15 to 20 minutes*

Yield: *4 to 6 servings*

2½ cups apple juice or other fruit juice

3 tablespoons agar agar flakes

1½ to 2 cups of bite-size fresh fruit (use seasonal fruits)

Pinch of salt

1 Combine the juice, salt, and agar agar in a medium saucepan. Bring to a slow boil over a low heat. (Boiling too quickly will make the agar agar sink to the bottom of the pot before it can dissolve.)

2 Simmer 10 to 15 minutes, stirring frequently until the agar is dissolved.

3 Place the fruit pieces into a glass serving dish and slowly pour the agar agar mixture over the fruit.

4 Allow the mixture to stand for 30 minutes.

5 Garnish with a mint leaf, and refrigerate until you're ready to serve it.

Great fruit combinations include blackberries, blueberries, and pomegranate; melon, papaya, strawberries, and mint; apples and blackberries; strawberries and oranges.

Per serving: *Calories 102 (From Fat 2); Fat 0g (Saturated 0g); Cholesterol 0mg; Sodium 5mg; Carbohydrate 26g; Dietary Fiber 2g; Protein 1g.*

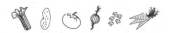

Scrumptious Boca Brownies

Here I present super-scrumptious brownies with a difference — they're sugar free and dairy free — and just as delicious as the real thing. Surprise your family and friends with a healthy and devilishly delicious dessert!

Preparation time: *15 minutes*

Baking time: *45 minutes*

Yield: *9 brownies*

³/₄ cup unsweetened applesauce

2 tablespoons water

2 teaspoons vanilla extract

1¹/₃ cups maple syrup granules

1 cup whole wheat pastry flour

¹/₃ cup semolina flour

³/₄ cup unsweetened cocoa powder

¹/₂ teaspoon baking powder

Pinch of sea salt

Vanilla soy milk

³/₄ cup hazel or macadamia nuts, coarsely chopped

1 cup nondairy, grain-sweetened chocolate chips

1 Preheat the oven to 350. Lightly grease an 8-inch square baking pan.

2 In a large bowl, mix the applesauce, water, vanilla, and maple syrup granules.

3 Stir the flours, cocoa powder, baking powder, and sea salt together in a medium bowl. Fold them into the wet ingredients gently so the mixture is just combined.

4 Stir in the soy milk to create a smooth batter.

5 Gently fold in the nuts and chocolate chips until well mixed.

6 Pour the mixture into the prepared baking pan and bake at 350 degrees for 40 to 45 minutes, until the center is firm when touched lightly.

7 Remove the brownies from the oven. After they have cooled, cut them into squares. Serve or store in an airtight container.

Per serving: *Calories 566 (From Fat 215); Fat 24g (Saturated 7g); Cholesterol 0mg; Sodium 62mg; Carbohydrate 91g; Dietary Fiber 11g; Protein 14g.*

Old-Fashioned Baked Apples with Tahini Raisin Filling

This is a super-easy desert that can be used with virtually any type of apple for a sweeter or sharper flavor. It works perfectly with a generous scoop of Rice Dream ice cream.

Preparation time: *15 minutes*

Baking time: *15 minutes*

Yield: *4 servings*

4 ripe apples	*$^1/_3$ cup chopped pecans*
$^3/_4$ cup tahini (sesame seed paste)	*$^1/_4$ teaspoon cinnamon*
1 cup apple juice, divided	*Dash of nutmeg*
3 tablespoons raisins	*Dash of vanilla*
$^3/_4$ cup of boiling water	

1 Preheat the oven to 375 degrees. Lightly oil a 9x13" baking dish

2 With a paring knife, remove the apple core to $^1/_2$ inch of the bottom of each apple (ideally, best to have an apple corer). Make the holes about $^3/_4$ to an inch wide. Use a spoon to dig out the seeds. Set the apples in a shallow baking dish, top side up.

3 In a small bowl, vigorously mix the tahini and $^1/_2$ cup of the apple juice. Add the raisins, walnuts, cinnamon, and nutmeg, and mix the ingredients together.

4 Fill each cored apple with this filling.

5 Add boiling water to the baking pan.

6 Pour a bit of the remaining apple juice over each apple before baking.

7 Bake the apples at 375 degrees for 30 to 40 minutes until tender but not mushy.

8 Remove the apples from the oven and baste the apples several times with the remaining juices and serve warm.

Tip: As a traditional dessert, this recipe especially nice to serve with a scoop of vanilla natural soy ice cream (non dairy) or rice dream.

Per serving: *Calories 386 (From Fat 220); Fat 24g (Saturated 3g); Cholesterol 0mg; Sodium 19mg; Carbohydrate 41g; Dietary Fiber 7g; Protein 8g.*

Melt-in-Your-Mouth Banana Coconut Bread

This is a delicious summer dessert that you can make in a short time, but it's long on taste.

Preparation time: *10 minutes*

Baking time: *40 to 50 minutes*

Yield6-8 *servings*

⅔ *cup walnuts*	*1 teaspoon baking powder*
2¾ *cups sliced bananas*	*1 teaspoon baking soda*
½ *cup canola oil*	*1 teaspoon coconut*
½ *cup brown rice syrup*	½ *teaspoon sea salt*
1 cup whole wheat pastry flour	½ *teaspoon ground allspice*
1 cup unbleached white flour	*Pinch ground cardamom*

1 Preheat the oven to 375 degrees. Grease a 9-by-5-inch glass loaf pan.

2 Chop the walnuts and place them on a baking sheet. Roast the walnuts at 375 degrees for 5 to 8 minutes.

3 Blend the banana and oil together in a food processor until just combined.

4 In a large mixing bowl, stir the banana mixture and the rice syrup.

5 Mix the flours, baking powder, baking soda, coconut, sea salt, allspice, and cardamom together in a medium bowl.

6 Add the dry ingredients and walnuts to the wet ingredients and mix the wet and dry ingredients together until they're well blended.

7 Pour the mixture into the prepared loaf pan and bake at 375 degrees for 40 to 50 minutes.

8 Using a skewer or thin knife, test the middle to check that the center of the bread is cooked. It should come out clean.

9 Remove the bread from the oven and gently insert a knife around the sides of the pan to loosen the bread and remove it from the pan. Place on a wire rack to cool.

10 Serve or store in an airtight container.

Per serving: *Calories 839 (From Fat 383); Fat 43g (Saturated 4g); Cholesterol 0mg; Sodium 793mg; Carbohydrate 109g; Dietary Fiber 7g; Protein 11g.*

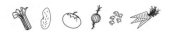

Almond Date Delights

If you love dates and coconut, you're gonna love these tasty treats. One is just not enough!

Preparation time: *5 minutes*

Cooking time: *20 minutes*

Yield: *4 to 6 servings (10–14 balls)*

2 cups almonds

11 cup shredded coconut

1 cup chopped pitted dates

1¹/₂ cup raisins

1 Preheat the oven to 375 degrees. Place the almonds on a baking sheet and roast them for about 5 minutes until brown.

2 After the almonds are cooled, chop them in a food processor.

3 Preheat the oven to 325 degrees. Place the coconut on a baking sheet and toast for about 10 minutes until golden brown.

4 Remove the coconut from the oven and set aside to cool.

5 In a food processor, blend half of the dates and raisins until the ingredients start to combine. Add a small amount of water if necessary.

6 Gradually add the remaining dates and raisins and continue to blend into a paste.

7 Add the almonds and continue to blend until the mixture forms a ball.

8 Roll out the date mixture into 1-inch balls and cover them with the coconut.

Per serving: *Calories 765 (From Fat 365); Fat 41g (Saturated 6g); Cholesterol 0mg; Sodium 31mg; Carbohydrate 98g; Dietary Fiber 14g; Protein 19g.*

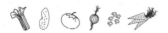

Fresh Fruit Slices

This is the quickest and simplest dessert you can imagine. Just take a few of your favorite locally grown seasonal fruits, slice them, and attractively arrange them on a plate. Voîla! That's it; just sweet, refreshing, and simple. They're a lovely after-dinner treat or a midmorning or afternoon snack.

Preparation time: *10 minutes*

Cooking time: *None*

Yield: *4 servings*

Delicious Berry Mix	**Tasty Tropical Fruits**
1 cup raspberries	*3 ripe kiwi fruits*
1 cup blueberries	*¼ of a watermelon*
1 cup strawberries	*½ of a papaya*

Apple Coconut Island Medley	**Citrus Delight**
2 large apples, cored	*1 large orange*
1 cup raisins	*2 tangerines*
¼ of fresh coconut	*1 large grapefruit*

1 Slice any fruit that needs slicing into bite-size pieces.

2 Arrange the fruit on plates or in bowls. Be creative!

Per serving: *Calories 66 (From Fat 2); Fat 0g (Saturated 0g); Cholesterol 0mg; Sodium 1mg; Carbohydrate 17g; Dietary Fiber 3g; Protein 1g.*

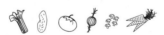

Marvelous Maple-Walnut and Chocolate Chip Cookies

Chocolate chip cookies are irresistible. This is a dairy- and sugar-free recipe that doesn't lose any of the scrumptiousness of regular chocolate chip cookies. Bake, chew well, and enjoy!

Preparation time: *10 minutes*

Cooking time: *30 minutes*

Yield: *8 to 10 servings (approximately 3 dozen cookies)*

1 cup walnuts

½ cup coconut oil

¼ cup tahini

1 cup maple syrup

1 teaspoon vanilla extract

3 cups pastry or spelt flour

½ teaspoon sea salt

2 teaspoons baking powder

1 cup (rice syrup or barley malt sweetened) chocolate chips

1 Preheat the oven to 350 degrees.

2 Finely chop the walnuts, place them on a baking sheet, and lightly roast at 350 degrees for 10 minutes.

3 Place the coconut oil, tahini, maple syrup, and vanilla extract into a blender and blend well.

4 Place the flour, salt, and baking powder into a large mixing bowl and whisk lightly with a hand whisk. Stir in the chocolate chips.

5 Add the wet ingredients to the dry ingredients and gently mix with a spatula to form a dough. Let the dough sit for at least 15 minutes.

6 Cover 2 cookie sheets with parchment paper. Place a teaspoonful of the cookie dough onto the cookie sheet. Slightly flatten the dough with the back of a damp fork. Repeat with the rest of the cookie mixture.

7 Bake the cookie dough at 350 degrees for 20 minutes, or until the edges of the cookies brown slightly.

8 Allow the cookies to cool slightly before removing them from the cookie sheet.

9 Place the cookies on a large plate and serve, or store in an airtight container.

Per serving: *Calories 603 (From Fat 288); Fat 32g (Saturated 15g); Cholesterol 0mg; Sodium 247mg; Carbohydrate 80g; Dietary Fiber 8g; Protein 9g.*

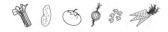

"Snacks" should mean "healthy snacks!"

Not eating for a long period can increase your hunger, which can result in sweet cravings (like dessert) and the desire to overeat. And one thing you don't want to overindulge in is dessert.

A snack combats hunger for a larger meal. However, snacks have gotten a bad rap — for many people, snack means "food treat." Ideally, a snack should be a small nourishing and simple meal that reduces appetite and slightly elevates blood sugar.

Wholesome snacks can increase energy, take the edge off of hearty appetites, and provide healthful nutrition. Try including fruits, nuts, seeds, and some raw vegetables such as carrots or celery (especially nice with a bean dip). When traveling, soup from a wide-mouth thermos can be very satisfying with a hearty piece of bread and a bean or hummus spread. Simple leftovers can do wonders when your appetite hits a low. Real whole food regains its taste after several chews. Rarely do you have to warm it up to "taste" it.

Drink to Your Health! Herbal, Grain, and Specialty Beverages

Liquid is the lightest part of your meal and a healthy and satisfying way to end a formal meal. If you watch most people while they're eating, they tend to drink *with* the meal. Actually, they're not drinking with the meal; they're *washing down* the meal. This reflects not only our poor chewing habits, but the fact that most refined food after several chews doesn't taste good any longer. Most meats lose their initial flavor and are frequently swallowed in large chunks.

If a meal is chewed thoroughly, you'll rarely crave fluid as you eat. In fact, Gandhi's suggestion was to "Drink your meal and chew your fluid." In other words, chew well enough that the food is reduced to a fluid mass in the mouth, and liquids should be combined with saliva and gradually swallowed. If you eat as Gandhi suggests, you'll discover that you don't need to "wash" anything down.

After you complete a meal, make some tea and sip it gradually. Mild heat has a medicinal effect, while extreme heat isn't recommended. In fact, research suggests that cold fluid just before a meal suppresses gastric secretions.

Traditional Chinese medicine favors hot tea over cold after a meal. Cold drinks, according to ancient texts, damage your ability to process food and fluids. The belief is that cold decreases activity (think of ice) and warmth increases activity (think of boiling water). The act of digestion is a warm process, as is life itself (think of the saying "stone cold dead"). Therefore, cold fluids were thought to *decrease* the digestive fire (cold negates heat).

Kukicha Twig Tea

A Japanese compound word meaning "stalk" *(kuki)* and "tea" *(cha)*, *kukicha* is a popular tea served in many macrobiotic restaurants. You can use twigs in a loose form or in a teabag version. Loose twigs can be reused — just add $\frac{1}{2}$ teaspoon of fresh twigs to each new brew. Discard the used twigs after three or four uses.

Preparation time: *5 minutes*

Cooking time: *0 minutes*

Yield: *1 serving*

1 kukicha twig teabag or 1 cup of loose twigs	*1 cup boiling water*

Steep the teabag in the water for 3 to 5 minutes and serve, or bring the twigs and water to a boil and simmer for 3 to 5 minutes. Serve.

If the tea is allowed to simmer, the color deepens, but then you risk the tea becoming slightly bitter. A boiled kukicha that is allowed to infuse away from the heat will be light in color, subtly sweet, and slightly astringent.

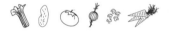

Tea trivia

All true teas actually stem from the plant *camellia Sinensis*. This bush is an attractive perennial shrub about 5 feet tall with gentle rounded leaves and thin tender twigs. Teas are green, black, or other varieties depending on the time of harvest, as well as the way they are cured and handled.

Made from the twigs and stems of the same plant that black and green teas come from, kukicha (also known as twig tea) is aged after harvest and then roasted. It has a soothing, unique flavor and is very low in caffeine. Where one cup of brewed coffee can contain as much as 150–180 milligrams of caffeine, black tea 65–100 milligrams, and green tea 10–60 milligrams, kukicha can range from 1 to 9 milligrams.

Kukicha is a healthy choice for grain-, vegetable-, and bean-based diets due to its alkaline qualities and extremely low caffeine level. Its natural tannins aid in digestion of grains and give it the unique ability to neutralize acid and alkaline elements in foods we eat.

Bancha Tea

Often confused with kukicha, bancha tea contains twigs *and* leaves. Its caffeine content averages from 9 to 15 milligrams, depending on the tea quality and brewing.

Preparation time: *3 to 5 minutes*

Cooking time: *None*

Yield: *1 serving*

Bancha twig teabag   1 cup boiling water

Steep the teabag in the water for 3 to 5 minutes and serve.

Mint Tea

Mint tea can be a delicious option after a meal and, according to some herbal writings, helps aid digestion, helps with gas, and stimulates bile flow. However, I should warn you about using peppermint: It's also known to have muscle relaxant properties and may relax the lower esophageal sphincter, allowing stomach contents to move upward into the esophagus (food pipe). For this reason, people with gastroesophageal reflux disease (GERD) should want avoid mint or mint-based teas.

Preparation time: *3 to 5 minutes*

Cooking time: *None*

Yield: *1 serving*

1 mint teabag   1 cup boiling water

Steep the teabag in the water for 3 to 5 minutes and serve.

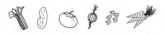

Dandelion Root Tea

This hearty tea is considered a tonic for the liver and helps reduce the desire to continue eating after a meal. It's popular with Italian culture. Some herbal writings suggest that dandelion strengthens the walls of the heart.

Preparation time: *3 to 5 minutes*

Cooking time: *None*

Yield: *1 serving*

1 dandelion root teabag	*Roasted chicory (optional)*
1 cup boiling water	*Lemon juice (optional)*

1 Steep the teabag in the water for 1 to 3 minutes. (This tea gets strong pretty quickly!)

2 Add a pinch of roasted chicory, if desired.

3 Add a squeeze of lemon juice, if desired.

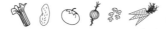

Roasted Barley Tea

This rich, full-bodied, and soothing after-meal tea is known in Japan as *mugi-cha*. In Japanese, *mugi* means barley. This tea can be purchased in commercial Japanese markets as well as large natural-food markets.

Preparation time: *3 to 5 minutes*

Cooking time: *None*

Yield: *1 serving*

1 roasted barley teabag	*1 cup boiling water*

Steep the teabag in the water for 3 to 5 minutes and serve.

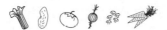

Red Bush Tea (Rooibos Tea)

Popular in South Africa for generations and now consumed in many countries, Rooibos (pronounced *roy-boss*), sometimes called African Red Bush Tea, contains a high level of antioxidants and no caffeine. It has low tannin levels compared to fully oxidized black tea or unoxidized green tea leaves and has a subtle sweet natural taste with a hint of nut flavoring.

Preparation time: *3 to 5 minutes*

Cooking time: *None*

Yield: *1 serving*

1 rooibos teabag   *1 cup boiling water*

Steep the teabag in the water for 3 to 5 minutes and serve.

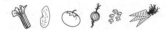

Grain Café Latte

Grain coffee is a nice way to complete breakfast. Made from grains (usually rye and barley), it contains zero caffeine and is a hearty finish to a meal. Several brands are available in natural food stores: Roma, Cafix, Pero, Barley Brew, Dandelion Blend, and Instant Yannoh to name a few. You can make a grain latte with boiling water and a splash of soy or rice milk.

Preparation time: *2 minutes*

Cooking time: *3 to 4 minutes*

Yield: *1 serving*

½ cup soy or rice milk   *Vanilla, nutmeg, or cinnamon for garnish (optional)*
½ cup water
1 heaping teaspoon of grain coffee

1 Bring the milk and water to a gentle boil.

2 Add the grain coffee. Stir well and serve the beverage in a tall glass or cup.

3 Mix in a dash of vanilla with a sprinkle of nutmeg or cinnamon for an added treat.

Hot Lemon Water

Cunningly simple and practically an American herbal tradition, this is simply squeezing $\frac{1}{2}$ of fresh lemon into a cup of boiled water. Lemon neutralizes excessive salt in the body, enhances the skin, acts as a mild diuretic, and according to traditional Chinese medicine, its sour taste is beneficial to the liver.

Preparation time: *3 minutes*

Cooking time: *None*

Yield: *1 serving*

Several wedges of lemon (approximately $\frac{1}{8}$ of a small lemon)   *1 cup boiling water*

Add the fresh lemon juice to the water and serve.

Unless you're sure of the organic quality of the lemon, don't allow the rind to steep in the cup.

Umeboshi Tea

Umeboshi tea is excellent for digestive problems. For overeating, gas, cramps, sea sickness, hangovers, etc. Its alkalizing properties are legendary and should be in every home first aid kit — I rarely travel without them.

Preparation time: *3 to 5 minutes*

Cooking time: *None*

Yield: *1 serving*

Kukicha twig tea (optional)   *$\frac{3}{4}$ teaspoon umeboshi paste*

$\frac{3}{4}$ cup boiling water   *$\frac{3}{4}$ teaspoon shoyu*

1 If desired, steep the teabag in the water for 3 to 5 minutes, or simmer the twigs and water for 3 to 5 minutes.

2 Pour the liquid into a cup, add the umeboshi paste and shoyu, and stir until blended.

Dried White Radish Tea

White radish (also known as *daikon*) is a good relaxant and aids healing. It is sometimes useful for bringing down mild fevers and also acts as a diuretic. This delicious tea can be refrigerated and reheated before drinking. This tea can also be made with red or black radish if white radish isn't available. Many natural food markets also carry a dried version.

Preparation time: *2 minutes*

Cooking time: *10 minutes*

Yield: *1 serving*

1 teaspoon dried daikon   *1 cup water*

1 Add the dried daikon to the water in a small saucepan, cover and bring to a boil.

2 Reduce the heat to low and simmer for 10 minutes.

3 Strain and serve.

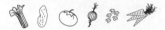

Fresh White Radish Tea

Fresh daikon tea is also effective for reducing mild fevers and helping to discharge excessive fluid (diuretic). Sometimes, the fresh version is used to support weight loss and the elimination of animal protein.

Preparation time: *5 minutes*

Cooking time: *None*

Yield: *1 serving*

1 tablespoon finely grated daikon   *Sea salt*
Several drops of fresh ginger juice   *1 cup boiling water*

1 Place the daikon gratings and ginger juice in a mug. Add a pinch of sea salt.

2 Add the water and steep for 3 minutes.

3 Drink the gratings.

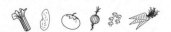

Chapter 17

Making Healthy Restaurant Choices

*T*his chapter offers guidance about making healthy choices when eating out in the real world. Sometimes you're going to have to explain your dietary needs to a server who may know nothing about macrobiotics. I give you a few tips for getting through those situations.

Basic Strategies for Eating Out

When you first start changing your diet to a more plant-based, whole-foods approach, the prospect of eating out can seem overwhelming. Although macrobiotic restaurants aren't on every corner, you'll be surprised at just how many restaurants you can enjoy a healthy "macro-ish" meal. You may also feel unsure of how to handle invitations to dinner parties and weddings or how to order a meal on a flight.

Following a macrobiotic diet doesn't have to be complicated for you or for anyone around you. Here are some easy-to-follow strategies that remove the stress from dining out.

✔ **Choose food from the vegetarian selections on the menu.** Most people now understand the term *vegetarian,* and it's socially acceptable in most foreign countries to not eat meat. Most restaurants have at least a couple of vegetarian options, although they may not all be dairy free.

> ✔ **Plan ahead to eat smaller portions.** The portion size in American restaurants is typically larger than that served in other countries. If you don't want to overeat or are watching your weight, share an entrée with a friend or take home your leftovers and enjoy them later.

Enquiring about Ingredients

Waiters can be intimidating people. They're always in a rush, usually have more tables than they can handle, and despite whatever they say, they're usually looking to get you in and out so the next party can fill the table. That said, don't be afraid to ask the waiter exactly what's in a dish. I always ask the waiter about the ingredients so I'm not surprised when it arrives at the table.

Because of the increasing number of dietary requirements people have, most servers are used to customers customizing their orders. Here are some typical concerns to ask the waiter about:

> ✔ Ask if certain dishes are steamed or fried. Is lard or vegetable oil used?

> ✔ Ask about sauces. Does it contain meat broth, pork bits, sugar, or MSG? Is the soup from a package mix? If there's anything you don't like, don't order it.

> ✔ Clarify with your server if your additions (like extra vegetables) will be charged as extra or as a side dish. That way, the bill won't make your eyes cross on first look.

Don't be afraid. You're paying the bill! Have a conversation because it's the only way you'll get what you want. Just remember to smile and be friendly and courteous. The server has a lot to do, and he's not the person who's actually cooking your food. He's really just a messenger. It's up to you to communicate your needs clearly so the message gets conveyed to the kitchen.

Ordering the Lesser of Menu Evils

I have a bunch of favorite restaurants, and I know just what to order in each of them. Equally, I've gotten to know which local restaurants don't offer much of an appetizing selection for me, so I avoid them.

Ethnic restaurants tend to offer healthier vegetarian choices and are less likely to use dairy products in their dishes.

As for ordering beverages in a restaurant, water is the best option. You can order hot tea as well. I like to bring my own teabags with me so I can enjoy a warm drink after dinner. Most restaurants will give or sell you a cup of hot water for your tea. It doesn't matter what others think if you bring teabags or condiments. You're taking a positive step to better control your health. This is a good thing. Be proud.

When I travel or dine out, I try to search ahead of time on the Internet for whole-foods, macrobiotic, vegetarian, vegan, or raw-foods restaurants or natural/whole food stores. If none of these are available, I use simple time-tested strategies, which I explain in the following sections, to choose a restaurant and order from the menu.

Breakfast

Many restaurants serve breakfast menus of eggs, bacon, sausage, and pancakes — foods that don't really fit a macrobiotic diet. However, don't give up on enjoying breakfast out. Many restaurants and cafes serve great oatmeal; whole-wheat or buckwheat pancakes; sugar-free or low-sugar muffins; English muffins; or whole-wheat or rye toast. You may even find scrambled tofu or soup on some menus!

If you order scrambled eggs, ask to have vegetables cooked into the eggs or served on the side. You can try spinach or broccoli or even cut cabbage and chopped tomato, which helps break down fat. Always make your ratio of animal protein to vegetables as small as possible.

Italian restaurants

Dining in an Italian restaurant is easy. Simply look for pasta dishes that aren't laden with cheese, cream, meat, or fish, and you'll usually find a handful of great options. Linguine *pomodoro* is a favorite of mine. It's a simple pasta with a tomato-and-basil sauce (sometimes called marinara sauce). Typically I ask for broccoli and mushrooms to be included in the sauce, and if these aren't available, I order whatever the vegetables of the day are.

Unless they're part of a chain, Italian restaurants are usually very accommodating. You may be able to customize your dish by adding or subtracting one or more ingredients. You can usually order side dishes of vegetables; just watch out for hidden oils or butters added to vegetables during cooking. Also be aware of items made with animal proteins, even if the menu description reads as though it's vegetarian. *Risotto,* a traditional Italian rice dish, is often made with chicken stock and topped off with butter and cheese. Be sure to check with your server before ordering.

Pizzas are typically served with a layer of cheese. Order a cheese-free pizza with lots of vegetables for a tasty meal. Some restaurants now offer a whole-wheat crust. Ask them.

Indian restaurants

For all you pungent food lovers, Indian restaurants offer lots of choices of rice, bean, chickpea, and vegetable dishes. Although some Indian dishes are made with ghee (clarified butter), you'll find plenty without it. Ask the waiter if the Indian breads contain yeast or if they serve whole-wheat chapatti.

My favorites are vegetable rice biryani (rice and vegetables), channa masala (chickpeas), daal (lentils), and aloo gobi (cauliflower with potatoes).

Mexican restaurants

These are the king of rice-and-bean restaurants. Typically, Mexican and other Latin American restaurants use a lot of meat in their dishes, particularly pork. However, rice and black or pinto beans are staples to any meat dish and are readily available to vegetarians.

Check that no animal products are used in the cooking of beans (many restaurants use lard or chicken stock in their cooking). Order dishes such as enchiladas, fajitas, or burritos without cheese or sour cream. (Mexicans love to put cheese over everything!) A side order of vegetables will complete your meal.

Japanese restaurants

Japanese food is delicious. Choose vegetable-filled nori rolls made with brown rice or summer rolls. However, beware of the hidden sugars in nori rolls. Sticky rice is generally sweetened using rice wine vinegar or mirin; many restaurants now use regular sugar instead, so you may find the sushi too sweet. If possible, bring your own tamari or shoyu. Most restaurants use low-quality, high-sodium soy sauce.

Finding healthy snacks: Sometimes you have to provide your own

Healthy snacks can sometimes be more challenging to find, especially when you're out and about. So rather than turn to muffins, donuts, or candy bars, try to keep snacks such as nuts, dried fruit, carrot sticks, celery stalks with a bit of nut butter spread in them, and tea bags on hand. Keep these items at home and take them with you when you travel or go to work. This strategy may prevent you from being tempted by accessible junk food.

Most Japanese soups are full of vegetables and noodles in a delicious broth. Check that miso soup is made fresh and not from a packet. If it's from a packet, chances are that it contains a good amount of MSG. Tempura vegetables, while tasty, are high in oil because they're deep-fried. They are best eaten infrequently and with some daikon radish to balance the oil.

American restaurants

You may find a simple pasta dish, vegetable burgers, and a selection of salads or baked potatoes on most American menus. If you eat animal protein, select the minimum. Choose the healthiest of salad dressings (oil and vinegar) and avoid creamy dressings such as ranch or Caesar because they may contain eggs or dairy. Most restaurants give you the option to order a salad instead of French fries.

Middle Eastern restaurants

Many menu items from Middle Eastern restaurants fit well into a macrobiotic diet: hummus, tabouli, couscous, falafels (chickpea patties), lentil soup, vegetable stews, and salads. Middle Eastern restaurants are usually an excellent choice — just go easy on the delicious breads and order humus without extra olive oil!

Thai restaurants

The flavors of Thai herbs and spices are just too good not to have in your diet. Choose Thai dishes carefully because coconut milk is a key ingredient in many dishes, and it's high in saturated fat and often sugar. Pad Thai is a simple and delicious noodle dish with nuts and vegetables. Ask the waiter to have it made without sugar or the sweet sauce on the side.

You can try many other great noodle dishes and soups, such as tom yum gai — a delicious spicy vegetable soup (check to see whether the stock is vegetarian).

Chinese restaurants

Although Chinese restaurants have an abundance of rice, noodle, and vegetable dishes on their menus, you need to check if they use MSG (monosodium glutamate) in their cooking. *MSG* is a controversial flavor enhancer that has been known to cause reactions such as headaches, sweating, chest pain, shortness of breath, and nausea, among other symptoms. Although none of these symptoms necessarily require medical treatment, why put yourself through eating MSG when you don't have to? Look for restaurants displaying signs stating they don't use MSG. Also watch out for the use of chicken stock, sugar, and eggs in dishes.

Airline food

Most airlines (those that still offer meals) generally have a reasonable selection of vegetarian options. Although macrobiotic foods may not be one of the choices, the closest you can get is the Asian vegetarian. You can also choose from vegan, lactose free, kosher, or standard Western (maybe). Choose dairy-free or Asian options when possible, because cheese seems to be a featured ingredient in most airline food.

Food at airports, train or bus terminals, or service stops on the highway is rarely vegetarian friendly. I usually bring my own lunch or a thermos of hot soup with some bread or crackers to keep me going until I get to my destination.

Special events, conferences, and birthday and dinner parties

It's quite acceptable and expected these days that at least one person attending a special event will favor vegetarian meals. Give plenty of notice to the organizers so they can plan ahead for your meal. You don't have to give a full list of foods that you can and can't eat, but do make it known that you'd prefer to have a dairy-free meal.

Part V
The Part of Tens

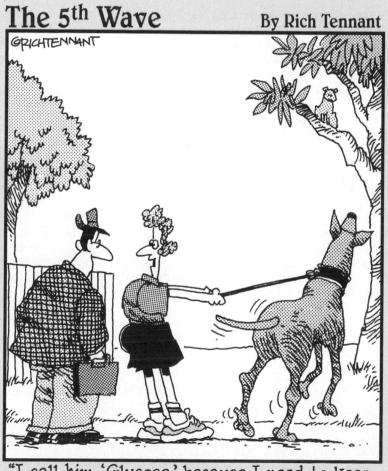

The 5th Wave   By Rich Tennant

"I call him 'Glucose,' because I need to keep him under control every day."

In this part . . .

This part presents helpful information in lists of ten items each. You can read about the ten sure-fire ways to handle sweet cravings, as well as the ten tips for prompt and permanent weight-loss, and tailoring your macrobiotic journey more to your personal needs.

Chapter 18

Ten Sure-Fire Ways to Handle Your Sweet Tooth

Annually, Americans spend more than $23 billion on candy and gum alone. In 1915, the national average of annual sugar consumption was approximately 15 to 20 pounds per person. Today, the average person consumes his own weight in sugar, plus more than 20 pounds of corn syrup! Devoid of nutrients, refined sugar depletes the body of vitamins, minerals, and enzymes, makes cell fluids acidic, and fosters inflammation and immune dysfunction. It takes as little as 100 grams of sugar (this could even be from a fruit juice source) to paralyze immune cells for up to five hours. If you're healthy, this effect may not be relevant, but if your health is compromised by disease or weakness, you can't afford for the immune cells to leave their post.

I don't mean to imply that you should never eat sweet foods, but if one type of food tends to make people lose control, it usually contains sugar.

The idea is not to *fuel* those cravings so that they grow to the point where you feel out of control and suddenly "gotta have something sweet." You crave sweet foods for physiological as well as psychological reasons. Sometimes sweet foods can even be medicinal, such as for an excess alkaline condition.

However, if you find yourself obsessing about sugar, or just want to take a sugar holiday, the following ten strategies, compiled from years of client feedback, personal experience, and study, can help you reduce your need for sugar. Then, when you do decide to have something sweet, you can enjoy a quality sweet without the compulsion to eat as much as you can get your hands on. You may find one or two of the strategies beneficial, and applying several of them may help you conquer your sweet tooth.

Tame Your Animal Appetite

The more animal protein you eat, the more you find yourself craving sugar. It may be because of the complement that sugar has with meat: Meat has no carbohydrates, and sugar has no protein. Therefore, they complement each other in a rather extreme way. The salt in the meat may also trigger a sugar craving. (See the next section for more about the love-hate relationship between salt and sugar.) When you eat a lot of meat, your appetite for sugar can easily become compulsive.

So what can you do to combat your cravings? First, try cutting your animal protein consumption in half. If this fails, experiment with eating a macrobiotic vegetarian diet for two weeks and note your positive changes.

Go Easy on the Salt

Salt and sugar have a dynamic relationship. The more salt you eat, the more you crave sugar. On average, you require $\frac{3}{4}$ to 1 teaspoon of sodium daily. North Americans consume an average of 2 to 3 teaspoons of salt a day. You crave this taste only when your body has an excess of internal acid (typically from sugar, alcohol, or overeating).

Cut your salt intake dramatically and change to sea salt. Only add salt toward the end of your cooking time. Food should not taste salty; although some dishes may have a salty accent for medicinal purposes, in general, salt should only *enhance* a food's natural flavor. If you've eaten too much salt, one of the quickest ways to counteract excess sodium is by drinking hot water and lemon.

Eat More Meals

Eating more frequently reduces your craving for volume and sugar. Poor blood sugar management is one of the most common reasons for sugar cravings. Waiting too long between meals makes your blood sugar hit bottom. When that happens, the craving for something sweet becomes overwhelming. Typically, most people experience a drop in blood sugar when they eat a light early lunch and then fast throughout the afternoon. They arrive home with a voracious dinner appetite. If this profile fits you, try to eat at least every four hours to maintain even blood sugar.

Eat Less

Miss Piggy once said, "Never eat more than you can lift." That's good advice when it comes to curbing sugar cravings. When you overeat, you may feel mentally dull and physically tired. Then you find yourself craving a stimulant, such as sugar, caffeine, or salt, to restore your energy. So as strange as it may sound, if you avoid overeating, you'll cut back on your cravings.

Steer Clear of Sugar (Duh)

Of course, this sounds obvious, but the frequency with which you eat sugar determines how extensive your cravings are. Simply put, the more you eat it, the more you crave it.

When you crave something sweet, see if you can replace that craving with a less concentrated, milder sweet, such as fruit. Eating the skin of fruits like apples, peaches, and grapes helps stabilize your blood sugar because the skin is fibrous.

Pretend You're Being Followed (Get Moving!)

Start walking — fast — on a daily basis. Consistent exercise increases circulation, which in turn increases your well-being, will, self-discipline, and energy. Exercise also makes you more sensitive to the fatiguing effects of sugar and inspires you to make healthier choices.

Stop EBB!

EBB is a pervasive practice that leads to poor sleep, fatigue, and sugar cravings. I'm talking about *eating before bed*. Give your hard-working stomach three hours to digest dinner before hitting the sack. You'll have a deeper sleep and feel more refreshed when you wake up. Otherwise, you get out of bed feeling somewhat numb from digesting all night and having a disturbed, dream-filled sleep. Then you wander into the kitchen craving something sweet to act as a stimulant, like the popular combo of coffee and a Danish.

Support the Broccoli Lobby

Increase your consumption of whole grains, vegetables, and beans. Diets devoid of these foods create intense cravings for an immediate sugar source. Or, put another way, if you have logs (complex carbohydrates) burning in the fireplace, you don't need to throw in newspaper (simple sugars).

Beware of Food Associations

This is not a corporate warning — and they're not following you! What I mean is that you need to be aware of certain experiences that trigger food cravings.

Many of us have specific psychological and emotional associations with food rituals, such as eating ice cream when you're sad, snacking on certain treats when you go to the movies, or regressing into bad food habits you formed in your childhood. Many times these comfort foods are sugar-laden treats. Often these habits provide emotional comfort, but when they endanger your health, it's time to find healthier substitutes. So have a piece of fresh fruit instead of ice cream, or maybe drink a mug of green tea instead of hot chocolate.

Express Yourself

It's harmful to your body and spirit to suppress your feelings. When you don't express your emotions, especially negative ones, you often end up frustrated and then try to numb those feelings by eating. Unfortunately, this is an ineffective and short-lived solution. Instead of eating when you're upset, try the following:

- ✔ Make a list of all the things that you're upset about and list two possible solutions for each problem.

- ✔ Get some exercise and then see how you feel about your problems. Exercise often opens up new perspectives, as well as strengthens your coping ability.

- ✔ Give your emotional stress levels a break by focusing on a creative activity. Compose a song, write a poem, work with clay, draw, journal, do some challenging yoga, or participate in some other fun activity that appeals to you. Activities that put you in the moment also refresh your perspective and strengthen your coping skills.

- ✔ Reflect on what is upsetting you and determine whom you have to express those feelings to. If you're not sure, write down your points for more clarity so you can articulate your concerns to the appropriate person.

Chapter 19

Ten Tips for Prompt and Permanent Weight Loss

You can probably recite at least a half-dozen perils of weight gain, and American bestseller lists feature more diet books than you can shake a carrot stick at. Despite all the knowledge and resources Americans have about maintaining a healthy weight, we're still one of the most obese nations on the planet. Something is clearly not working.

Although many people experience immediate weight loss as a result of a high-protein diet, the loss is usually not the result of consuming more protein but simply stems from cutting calories. In the long run, a high-protein diet can lead to obesity, gout, colon cancer, and many other conditions.

In addition to our physical design, maintaining a healthy and slender body is also based on lifestyle habits. The solutions to weight loss that I present in this chapter can help you love and honor the body you live in.

Here are ten sure-fire solutions to keeping weight off, halting the aging clock, and increasing your vitality — or ten ways to keep yourself from feeling confined to a black wardrobe or sucking in your gut every time you pass a mirror.

Get Active!

Regular exercise increases your willpower and physical sensitivity, so you end up appreciating how fit and trim your body is, while reducing the likelihood of indulging. In terms of exercise, shopping, cleaning, or running after your children doesn't qualify. Two kinds of exercise are recommended:

- ✔ Get a daily minimum of 30 minutes of aerobic exercise, such as biking, brisk walking, hiking, or swimming.

- ✔ Try strength training with weights two to three times a week. Strength training not only helps you burn calories faster, but it also gives your metabolism a significant boost. In her book *Strong Women Stay Slim*, Miriam Nelson, a Tufts University researcher, showed that a group of women following a weight-loss diet *and* doing strength-training exercises lost 44 percent more fat than those who only followed the diet.

Mind Your Blood Sugar

When you're going through your daily routine, your body uses the sugar in your blood and muscles to fuel its activities. If you don't eat and replenish the body's supply of fuel, your blood sugar falls to a low extreme. When this happens, your need for sugar is severe, and you're likely to throw caution to the wind and succumb to sugar-laden foods that can threaten your weight. Forget willpower. At this point, if your hunger is extreme enough, you'll do anything to score a sweet treat. These slip-ups can be avoided — and your self-respect can remain intact — if you simply eat more frequently. Low blood sugar is one reason people overeat. Eat a small meal every four hours to avoid these blood sugar lows.

Avoid Late-Night Eating

If you like any of the following, then by all means, eat right before bed:

- ✔ Getting the most unsatisfying, dream-filled, and restless sleep imaginable
- ✔ Waking up feeling like you were run over
- ✔ Awaking puffy-faced and irritable

If none of these outcomes sounds appealing, it may serve you better to avoid eating for three hours before going to bed.

The old adage of eating like royalty for breakfast, comfortable citizens for lunch, and paupers for dinner makes the most sense. The less digestion you do when sleeping means the deeper, shorter, and more immune enhancing your sleep will be.

Reduce Dietary Fat and Sugar

In the basic American diet (BAD!), nearly 40 percent of total calories come from fat. A goal of 15 to 20 percent would be far healthier. But avoiding fat altogether isn't a good idea, because doing so can increase fat cravings; so although you may be avoiding fats, you may compensate by overeating. So having *some* dietary fat is the right solution.

You can reduce the amount of fat you eat and still make food amazingly tasty. It's best to consume 1 to 3 teaspoons of fat (the daily maximum) in sautéed dishes or salad dressings or through nuts sprinkled into food as a garnish. Reducing fat is easier when you're eating whole foods with macrobiotic principles and avoiding refined foods (sugar, white flour, and so on).

An excess of simple sugars frequently ends up around your waist, buttocks, abdomen, or thighs. That's the nature of excess sugar; it becomes a fat. Sugar also makes you feel bloated and less connected to your body. In this condition of reduced sensitivity, you're not as likely to care about what you eat or attempt to discipline yourself.

Select Beverages Wisely

Alcohol is high in calories. Liquors, sweet wines, and mixed drinks contain anywhere from 150 to 450 calories per glass. By contrast, water, sparkling water, and light fruit spritzers are calorie free or at least lower in calories. If you choose to drink alcohol, limit yourself to one drink and select light wine or beer.

Include More Quality Complex Carbohydrates

Complex carbohydrates are fruits, vegetables, and whole grains. Add 1 to 1½ cups of whole grain to your daily diet. This does not mean bread, breadsticks, pasta, or rice cakes! It means *whole* grain! Try brown rice, oats (rolled oats are permissible here), quinoa (great in salads), barley (great in soups or cooked with lentils), and so on. Whole grains will bond to toxins in your gut and help keep your blood clean, as well as ensure bowel regularity.

Eating more vegetables and preparing them in different ways (see Chapter 13) can create an appealing sense of variety. This is essential for a meal plan that will nourish and satisfy. Beans, in the form of tofu or tempeh, or even canned beans, also create a more satisfying meal so that your cravings for foods that produce weight gain are minimized. You can use beans in soups, as a dip or spread, as a side dish, or tossed into a salad.

Eat a Light Snack Before Going to Social Events

It's a bad idea to arrive at a party famished. It's like going grocery shopping when you're starving. You set yourself up for a big test, which you'll probably fail. Not only are you more likely to overeat, but you're also *less* likely to resist the temptation of eating the higher-fat and higher-calorie foods. Try eating a small amount of healthy food before leaving the house to reduce the urge to overindulge.

"Portionize" to Avoid Overeating

Your stomach is slightly larger than your fist. Think about this the next time you pile food on your plate. Serve food straight onto smaller plates instead of placing serving bowls on the table. You'll eat less and will be less likely to have seconds. You can always eat again later. If you're in a restaurant and are unsure of the portion sizes, order an appetizer or share an entrée with a friend.

Plan Your Meals

When you think about what you're going to eat ahead of mealtime, you stay focused on your eating plan and aren't tempted by other influences. Fewer trips to the market lessen the temptation to make impulse purchases. Make sure you have some healthy snacks, such as nuts or raw vegetables, or interesting leftovers available for possible snack attacks.

Watch Emotional Triggers

Don't ignore the stresses that push your buttons and make you seek comfort in food. Work problems, relationships, and home life can bring up unresolved conflicts that make you just want to get naughtily numb with more food than your body needs.

After you recognize and accept these triggers, find non-food ways to soothe your unsettled feelings. Exercise, deep breathing, and relaxation techniques such as massage and yoga work wonders for effectively releasing stress. You can also make a note of what you're feeling and promise yourself to sort out the situation at another time when you're not so upset.

Part VI
Appendixes

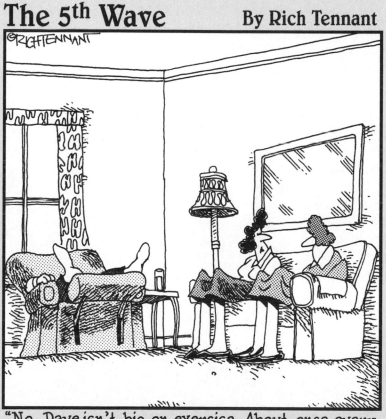

The 5th Wave   By Rich Tennant

"No, Dave isn't big on exercise. About once every
three years we take him to the doctor's and
have his pores surgically opened."

In this part . . .

Appendix A provides you a sample menu for an entire week of cooking. Appendix B gives you an idea of where macrobiotics came from by briefly describing the lives of the pioneers of the movement.

Appendix A

Sample Menu for One Week

· ·

*T*he key to menu planning is organization and variety. Selecting different ingredients, tastes, and textures is pleasing to your palate and good for an overall balanced diet.

Each day, your food intake should include some whole grain (from short grain brown rice or other whole grains), protein (from bean products or minimal amounts of optional animal protein, such as fish), sea vegetables, fermented foods (like pickles), and lots of fresh vegetables, especially dark leafy greens such as kale and collard greens. Balance is always key.

When all your meals are balanced with flavors, textures, and nutrients, you'll feel it! It's a great feeling.

Day 1

Breakfast	Lunch	Dinner
Hearty Miso Rice Porridge with Nut Sprinkle; Toast; Herbal Tea	Vegetable and Chickpea Couscous Salad; Water-Fried Kale, Swiss Chard, and Broccoli with Sour Plum and Lemon Dressing	Baked Sole with Kalamanta Olives and Capers; Summer Soba Salad

Desserts (Optional)	Snacks (Optional)
Refreshing Seasonal Fruit Kanten	Tasty Tempeh Sticks with Mustard Dip

Day 2

Breakfast	Lunch	Dinner
Boston Baked Beans; Sour Dough Toast; Twig Tea	Sour Plum Corn on the Cob; Crunchy Boiled Salad with Pumpkin Seed Dressing	Millet Mash; Mustard-Tamari Tempeh with Sautéed Carrots and Onions

Desserts (Optional)	Snacks (Optional)
Old-Fashioned Baked Apples with Tahini-Raisin Filling	Easy Edamame Ecstasy

Day 3

Breakfast	Lunch	Dinner
Mouth Watering Breakfast Muffins; Grain Café Latte	Summer Salad Wrap with Garden Greens and Balsamic Vinaigrette	Shiitake Wild Rice with Tahini-Bechamel Sauce; Stir-Fried Tofu with Basil and Tamari

Desserts (Optional)	Snacks (Optional)
Yum Yum Oatmeal Raisin Cookies	Hearty Hummus and Pita Triangles

Day 4

Breakfast	Lunch	Dinner
Spiced Mexican Tofu Scramble with Tortilla Chips; Bancha Tea	Brown Rice Sesame Sushi with Ginger-Tamari Dipping Sauce	Millet, Butternut Squash, and Corn Cakes; Mustard Green Salad with Tangy Citrus Dressing

Desserts (Optional)	Snacks (Optional)
Melt-in-Your-Mouth Banana Coconut Bread	Guacamole with Crunchy Triangle Bread

Day 5

Breakfast	Lunch	Dinner
Winter Warming Oatmeal with Roasted Almonds, Raisins, and Cinnamon; Roiboos Tea	Veggie Nut Bulgur Salad; Seitan Peanut Saté	Cuban Rice and Corn with Spicy Black Beans; Watercress with Parsley

Desserts (Optional)	Snacks (Optional)
Fresh Fruit Slices	Traditional Rice Balls

Day 6

Breakfast	Lunch	Dinner
Whole Wheat Toast; Tamari/Tahini Topping; Kukicha Tea	Vegetable Miso Soup with Spelt Noodles; Tasty Tempeh Sticks with Mustard Dip	Down-Home American Spaghetti Marinara and Meatless Meatballs; Garden Green Salad

Desserts (Optional)	Snacks (Optional)
Almond Date Delights	Basil and Plum Cucumbers

Day 7

Breakfast	Lunch	Dinner
Banana Pecan Pancakes; Tempeh Bacon Roibos Tea	Chunky Carrot and Split Pea Soup with Crunchy Croutons	Brown Rice, Vegetable, and Tofu Stir-Fry with Sliced Almonds

Desserts (Optional)	Snacks (Optional)
Hurricane Key Lime Pie	Chickpea Fritters with Spicy Avocado Dressing

Macrobiotic Pioneers

. . . .

*I*n attempting to assemble a history of macrobiotics, it's difficult to actually mark where the starting point begins; the prime movers and shakers of macrobiotics had multiple, often unaccredited historical influences, so establishing an exact origin quickly becomes an illusive and arbitrary task.

George Ohsawa (1893-1966) is often regarded as the "founder" of macrobiotics. But while he did synthesize a blueprint of adopted principles and healing strategies from different sources under the banner of *macrobiotics* — a name he no doubt borrowed from German physician Christopher Hufeland's 1797 book — Ohsawa was not, in fact, the originator by any means. In his writings, he credits the Japanese medical doctor, Sagen Iskizuzka, as his first mentor and teacher. Ishizuka formed much of his theory from traditional Chinese Medicine, which was developed over several thousand years.

Christopher William Hufeland (1762–1836)

If anyone deserved the title of "Great Grandfather of Macrobiotics," Hufeland would probably win it hands down. He was one of the most eminent German physicians of his time. Hufeland vigorously championed the idea of preventive medicine. During a time when the medical science of the day focused on symptomatic disease treatment, he claimed that the ultimate goal of human medicine was not to treat illness but to maximize life. Of his many writings, his most popular book, *Makrobiotik, or The Art of Prolonging Human Life,* was published in 1796, became a best seller and was translated into many languages.

Hufeland embraced the Hippocratic principle of a natural healing force that existed. He insisted on treating the whole person, stressing the value of a sensible lifestyle, intellectual stimulation, humor and joy and a vegetarian diet with regular exercise.

His packaging of the "Makrobiotik" dietary program fueled the healthy eating movement of the past 200 years, shaping the teachings of health leaders such as Sylvester Graham, W.H. Kellogg, Bernard McFadden, Paul Bragg, George Ohsawa, Bernard Jensen, Michio Kushi, and Herman Aihara — all of whom positively influenced the health and lives of millions with their dedication, insight and tenacity.

Ekken Kaibara (1630–1714)

Ekken Kaibara (1630–1714), sometimes referred to as the "Great-Grandfather of Macrobiotics," was a Japanese Neo-Confucian scholar born on the island of Kyushu, in southern Japan. After his father taught him nutrition and medicine, his hunger to learn embraced many fields of study related to health and spiritual teachings.

He advised eating grain as a staple food with plentiful amounts of seasonal vegetables; recommended consuming foods that were peacefully prepared and balanced according to the five tastes of sweet, sour, salty, bitter, and pungent; suggested the avoidance of fatty meats and recommended animal protein to be eaten in minimum amounts; was not fond of greasy, raw, or overcooked fare or foods that were unripe; warned of overeating and suggested leaving 10 to 20 percent of one's capacity empty; recommended giving thanks to all the elements that conspired to bring food to one's table; suggested refraining from eating when upset or prior to bed; and endorsed brief walks after eating to promote circulation. His recommendations are surely a template for what was to evolve as a macrobiotic directive.

Sagen Ishizuka (1850–1910)

Sagen Ishizuka righteously deserves the title of "Grandfather of Macrobiotics." Born to Samurai parents in 1850, Ishizuka was drawn to medicine at an early age and eventually became a physician in the Japanese army. Suffering throughout his life from a chronic kidney condition, he was unable to find relief from the allopathic medicine that he had practiced as a physician.

Researching Oriental medicine, Ishizuka was inspired to pursue studies and experiment with his daily nourishment. Influenced by classical texts as well as the teaching of Kaibara, he gave up the modern Japanese western influences of milk, animal meats, and refined rice for a more traditional diet of grain, vegetable, beans, seaweeds, and fermented foods. Soon, his illness reversed and Ishizuka was motivated to experiment with his patients.

Ishizuka saw health imbalance in terms of two universal extremes: conditions from inflammation (characterized by an excess of potassium-based factors) or conditions of constriction (based on an excess of sodium). Often, many sicknesses were composed of both extremes. According to Ishizuka, the destiny of our health is controlled by our choice and preparation of food that influences our sodium-potassium chemical balance.

George Ohsawa (1893–1966)

George Ohsawa, born as Yukikazu Sakurazawa, was a gifted original thinker, entrepreneur, tireless writer, lecturer, social activist, student, and philosopher who collectively synthesized the teachings of his predecessors into a cohesive format of diet, philosophy, spiritual teaching, and behavioral principle. It was a package he later, in the last decade of his life, introduced as *macrobiotics*.

Ohsawa developed a severe case of intestinal and pulmonary tuberculosis at the age of 18, ironically the same disease he witnessed consume his mother's life when he was 12. Refusing to undergo the same westernized "medical treatments" that failed to save her, Ohsawa chose his own path, encouraged by discovering Ishizuka's first book, *A Chemical Nutritional Theory of Long Life*. The book detailed Ishizuka's dietary suggestions, concentrating on balancing the ratio of sodium and potassium in the blood through a combination of whole traditional foods that includes sea vegetables and fermented foods.

Diligently following Ishizuka's program from the book, Ohsawa's symptoms soon disappeared. The realization of food's innate power to change the course of sickness proved a turning point in the life of young Ohsawa.

He wrote hundreds of books, pamphlets, and articles about all aspects of folk medicine, nutrition, philosophy, chemistry, martial arts, language, cultural arts, and principles of well-being. With his ever-present wife Lima, a consummate teacher of cooking arts and fierce dedication to his work, they traveled throughout the world, making new friends wherever their journeys took them.

Ohsawa's presentation of macrobiotics, his views on healing, sickness and health seemed quite radical to many. He articulated his ideas in archaic terms borrowed from Taoist Yin-Yang philosophy layering his expression in complexity and alien to many. He championed Japanese foods that had, according to him, necessary medicinal value and frequently suggested, in lieu of fasting, an exclusive diet of brown rice, which he claimed could cure most diseases.

George Ohsawa lived as he had taught others to live: adventurously with a spirit of play, a strong social concern for human welfare, and a deep commitment to leave the world healthier and better then he had found it. According to the testimony of others, Ohsawa helped countless people regain their health and personified joy and gratitude in much of what he did.

Herman Aihara (1920–1998)

Herman (Nobuo) Aihara began his initial studies with George Ohsawa in 1940. Attracted by the philosophy and world peace goals that Ohsawa was then teaching, Aihara studied with Ohsawa on and off while he experimented with a change of diet. He arrived in New York in 1952 and eventually, with fellow student, Michio Kushi, became President of the Ohsawa Foundation in New York. In the early 1960s, he ventured with his wife, Cornelia, to Chico, California where a small community of macrobiotic people had settled.

On the west coast, the unassuming and intelligent Aihara began to teach and write, eventually establishing one of the first United States macrobiotic magazines and often traveling throughout the U.S. by car with Cornelia and children in tow offering public lectures and cooking classes.

Later, the Aihara's began another organization, The George Ohsawa Macrobiotic Foundation (GOMF) that sponsored his talks and acted as a publishing arm for his writings. Eventually, he started another institute of macrobiotic studies for students and teachers called The Vega Institute.

The Aihara's annual summer camp in the High Sierras meets every July (to this day) for 10 days of camping that includes outdoor lectures beneath tall pines and redwoods, meals prepared in fire pits of extraordinary simplicity and taste, and a number of other classes from acupuncture massage to cooking and martial arts.

Michio Kushi (1926–)

Michio Kushi was born into a family of educators. After meeting and studying with Ohsawa, Michio decided to come to the United States to continue Ohsawa's work under the banner of macrobiotics.

Kushi and his wife Aveline lectured throughout the United States, settling in Boston and beginning one of many foundations and various business ventures (East West Journal, Erewhon, Redwing books, Sanae and The Seventh

Inn Restaurants, Kushi Foods,) as well as a seven-day yearly congress known as the Kushi Conference, usually occurring on east coast college campuses.

Along with Aveline, Kushi has authored dozens of books, including *The Book of Macrobiotics* (Japan Publications) and *The Cancer-Prevention Diet* (St. Martin's Press, 1983).

The Kushi Institute continues in rural Beckett, Massachusetts, offering three levels of accreditation and various graduate programs for students and those who want to teach Kushi's interpretation of macrobiotics.

Index